MW01285066

THE
PINEAL
GLAND

CURRENT ENDOCRINOLOGY: BASIC AND CLINICAL ASPECTS
Louis V. Avioli, *Series Editor-in-Chief*

THE
PINEAL
GLAND

Edited by
Richard Relkin, M.D.

Director of Medicine
Chief, Endocrinology and Metabolism
Easton Hospital, Easton, Pennsylvania
Professor of Medicine
Hahnemann Medical College and Hospital
Philadelphia, Pennsylvania

ELSEVIER BIOMEDICAL
New York · Amsterdam · Oxford

Elsevier Science Publishing Co., Inc.
52 Vanderbilt Avenue, New York, New York 10017

Distributors outside the United States and Canada:
Elsevier Science Publishers B.V.
P.O. Box 211, 1000 AE Amsterdam, The Netherlands

Library of Congress Cataloging in Publication Data

Main entry under title:

The Pineal gland.
    (Current endocrinology)
    Includes bibliographies and index.
    1. Pineal body. 2. Melatonin—Physiological effect. I. Relkin, Richard.
    II. Series. [DNLM: 1. Pineal body. WK 350 P649021]
QP188.P55P554   599.01'42   82-7371
ISBN 0-444-00714-8   AACR2

Manufactured in the United States of America

CONTENTS

FOREWORD

Although endocrinology textbooks satisfy a fundamental educational need and are routinely used as reference standards, an information gap often exists between the current state of the art and the published contents. Refinements in laboratory methods and assay techniques, the ever increasing awareness of metabolic and endocrine correlates that were once unapparent, and the dramatic discoveries in molecular biology and genetics make it extremely difficult to present an up-to-date volume at time of publication. The endocrinology textbook may effectively serve the academic community only for 3–5 years.

Despite the constant change in the state of the art, new discoveries defining relationships between endocrinology and molecular biology, physiology, genetics, biochemistry, biophysics, and immunology do not proceed at comparable rates. In fact, certain areas of endocrinology have been dormant for years.

In an attempt to offer timely reviews, a number of well-established authorities were offered the challenge of editing small editions that characterize the state-of-the-art in *specific* areas of endocrinology. This format relieves the editor (or editors) from the nearly impossible task of producing a "current textbook" of endocrinology and facilitates the process of rapid and timely revision. Moreover, a specific endocrine discipline review can be revised if and when necessary without revising an entire textbook.

Endocrine Control of Growth, edited by W. Daughaday, was the first review in this series, *Current Endocrinology: Basic and Clinical Aspects*. This has been followed by individual texts on *Glucagon, Prostaglandins, Prolactin, Clinical Reproductive Neuroendocrinology*, and *Endocrine Aspects of Aging*. The series presents those current aspects of endocrinology of interest to the basic scientist, clinician, house officer, trainee, and medical student alike. These initial volumes will be followed by others on *Thyroid, Posterior Pituitary, Biochemical Action of Steroid Hormones, The Adrenal*, and *Gastrointestinal Hormones*. We are confident that this complete series and its revised editions, when appropriate, will serve the academic community well.

Louis V. Avioli, M.D.

PREFACE

It is only in the past decades that burgeoning research into the functions of the mammalian pineal has given us a body of knowledge about this neuroendocrine gland which has brought it out of the dark ages into the realm of modern science. An organ that at various times in the past has been considered to have a spiritual function or to be vestigial, is now thought of primarily as a neuroendocrine transducer, its hormonal secretion being prominently influenced by stimuli from environmental lighting.

It is difficult at this time to predict what place the pineal will eventually occupy in terms of its relative importance in the mammalian—and especially the human—endocrine system. From present indications, however, it would appear that this gland could one day assume a paramount position in mammalian endocrinology.

Richard Relkin, M.D.

CONTRIBUTORS

DAVID E. BLASK, M.D., Ph.D.
Associate Professor of Anatomy, Department of Anatomy, University of Arizona School of Medicine, Tucson, Arizona

THOMAS S. KING, Ph.D.
Postdoctoral Fellow, Department of Anatomy, The University of Texas Health Science Center at San Antonio, 7703 Floyd Curl Drive, San Antonio, Texas

ALFRED J. LEWY, M.D., Ph.D.
Director, Sleep and Mood Disorders Laboratory, Department of Psychiatry; Assistant Professor, Departments of Psychiatry and Pharmacology, Oregon Health Sciences University, Portland, Oregon

HARRY J. LYNCH, Ph.D.
Laboratory of Neuroendocrine Regulation, Lecturer, Department of Nutrition and Food Science, Massachusetts Institute of Technology, Cambridge, Massachusetts

PAUL PÉVET, Ph.D.
Netherlands Institute for Brain Research, IJdijk 28, Amsterdam, The Netherlands; Department of Anatomy and Embryology, University of Amsterdam, Amsterdam, The Netherlands

RUSSEL J. REITER, Ph.D.
Professor, Department of Anatomy, The University of Texas Health Science Center at San Antonio, 7703 Floyd Curl Drive, San Antonio, Texas

RICHARD RELKIN, M.D.
Director of Medicine, Chief, Endocrinology and Metabolism, Easton Hospital, Easton, Pennsylvania; Professor of Medicine, Hahnemann Medical College and Hospital, Philadelphia, Pennsylvania

BRUCE A. RICHARDSON, Ph.D.
Postdoctoral Fellow, Department of Anatomy, The University of Texas Health Science Center at San Antonio, 7703 Floyd Curl Drive, San Antonio, Texas

MARY K. VAUGHAN, Ph.D.
Assistant Professor, Department of Anatomy, The University of Texas Health Science Center at San Antonio, 7703 Floyd Curl Drive, San Antonio, Texas

PAUL PÉVET, Ph.D.

ANATOMY OF THE PINEAL GLAND OF MAMMALS

From a phylogenetic point of view, few organs have undergone as much change in form and cytological differentiation as has the pineal gland. Among the primitive nonmammalian vertebrates, the pineal organ is a sense organ containing photoreceptors and nerve cells; in mammals, it is a typical glandular organ. In reptiles and birds and even in some lower forms, a structural change to an endocrine gland is apparent (see details in refs. 1–6).

This review will deal exclusively with the anatomy of the mammalian pineal gland. It is very clear, however, that the way in which the mammalian pineal functions has very old phylogenetic roots and that such evolution should not be forgotten, especially when correlations between morphological and physiological observations are made.

GROSS MORPHOLOGY

Ontogenetically originating from that part of the diencephalic roof that is situated between the habenular commissure rostrally and the posterior commissure caudally, the pineal is an epithalamic structure. In mammals, it is a solid parenchymatous median dorsal intracranial organ.

From the Netherlands Institute for Brain Research, IJdijk 28, Amsterdam, and the Department of Anatomy and Embryology, University of Amsterdam, The Netherlands.

1

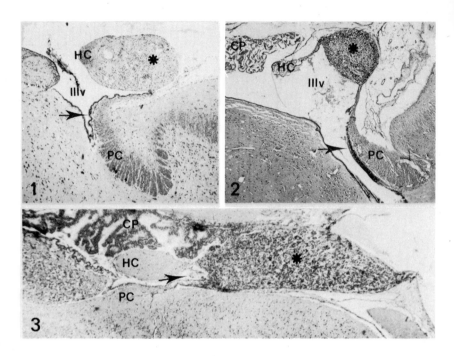

FIGURES 1 and 2. Sagittal sections through the pineals (*) of the tenrec *(Centetes ecaudatus)* (Figure 1) and of the fruit bat *(Eidolon helvum)* (Figure 2). Note the more or less large amount of pineal tissue in close contact with the cerebrospinal fluid present in the third ventricle (IIIv). Following the classification proposed by Vollrath (8), these pineals are of type A. **Arrows** = pineal recess; **HC** = habenular commissure; **PC** = posterior commissure; **arrow** = subcommissural organ; **CP** = choroid plexus. (Hematoxylin-eosin × 80, × 75.) *From Pévet and Racey and Pévet and N'Diaye Alassane, unpublished data.*

FIGURE 3. The length of the pineal (*) of the mole-rat *(Spalax ehrenbergi)* reaches twice (or more) the greatest width of the organ and is thus classified type AB (Vollrath, 8). **Arrow** = pineal recess; **CP** = choroid plexus; **HC** = habenular commissure; **PC** = posterior commissure. (Hematoxylin-eosin × 120.) *From Pévet (81).*

However, its morphological aspects, its anatomical position, as well as its size, vary according to species.

In most of the mammalian species—in exactly 42 of the 57 species examined [combination of the observations reported (7–9) and our own unpublished ones]—the pineal is of the proximal type (Figures 1–3) [types A and AB of Vollrath (8), to whom we refer for a useful classification system]. This means that a fairly large amount of pineal tissue may come into close contact with the third ventricle and, notably, with nerve fibers of central origin. In some other species, such as the rabbit and the guinea pig, the pineal is a long and more-or-less rodlike organ reaching the cerebellum and lying closely related to the skull (Figure 4) (type ABC; 8). In the rat and hamster, as in some other rodents, most

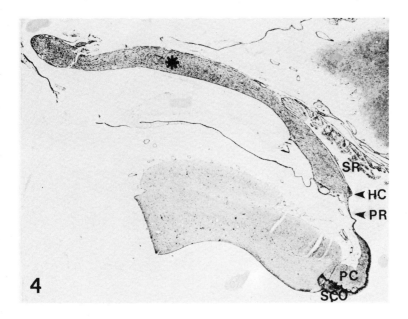

FIGURE 4. Long, more or less rodlike pineal organs reaching the cerebellum and lying closely related to the skull—as exemplified here in the rabbit—belong to type ABC (Vollrath, 8). **PR** = pineal recess; **HC** = habenular commissure; * = pineal; **PC** = posterior commissure; **SR** = suprapineal recess; **SCO** = subcommissural organ. (Bodian × 25.) *From Romijn (51), by courtesy.*

of the pineal cells leave their original position between the two commissures to move, during ontogenesis and postnatal development (Figure 5), in a dorsocaudal direction, forming the so-called superficial pineal—the pineal, for most authors. The few pineal cells left between the commissures form the so-called deep pineal. The deep pineal—which represents, in the hamster, 3–12% (10) and, in the rat, 0.5–2.5% (9) of the total volume of the pineal—and the superficial one are connected by a pineal stalk that is primarily composed of myelinated and unmyelinated nerve fibers, connective tissue, and blood vessels (11,12), but in which parenchymal cells can also be observed, at least in the rat (11,13).

Such variation and complexity in the morphology of the pineal in the different mammalian species immediately raise the question of the validity of pinealectomy, a widely used technique to study pineal function. Pinealectomy—which is an operation practically impossible to realize without lesioning the brain in most of the mammalian species in which the pineal is of type A or AB—can be, and is easily, accomplished in the rodents commonly used in the laboratory, e.g., the rat and the hamster, in which the pineal lies superficially. Such pinealectomy, however, corresponds only to a superficial-pineal pinealectomy, the deep pineal not being touched during the operation. However, although not

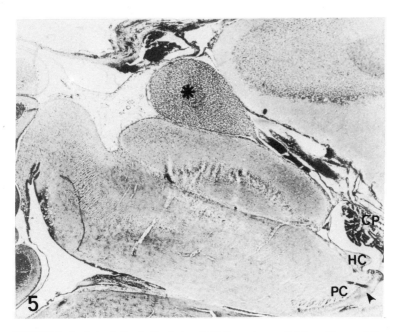

FIGURE 5. In the rat, the bulk of pineal (*) tissue has a distal position and the organ is classified as type C or αC when a deep pineal is present. HC = habenular commissure; PC = posterior commissure; **arrowhead** = subcommissural organ; CP = choroid plexus. (Bouin × 120.) *From Ariëns Kappers, unpublished data; by courtesy.*

complete, pinealectomy is a very effective operation, at least in the hamster, in which it abolishes dark-induced gonadal atrophy. This means that under this condition the deep pineal is either too small to be effective or that superficial pinealectomy could act, via an interruption of the sympathetic innervation, at the level of the deep pineal (see under Innervation). This effect of superficial pinealectomy could also be due to the fact that the deep pineal is not concerned with this phenomenon. Thus, it seems important to determine whether these two parts of the pineal, present in only a few rodents, are similar or dissimilar in structure and function.

The deep pineal is very small and lies so concealed that it is virtually inaccessible to routine biochemical studies and is often neglected by morphologists. Histologically, however, the deep and superficial pineal appear very much alike, the only notable difference being the greater number of glial cells in the deep pineal (14). However, in the hamster and the rat, different circadian nuclear size changes of pinealocytes were observed in the superficial and deep pineal (9). Dissimilarities in function also become apparent in the rat after osmotic stress; only the superficial pineal is affected (9). It has also been demonstrated in the rat that the deep pineal (more exactly, the area containing the deep pineal) does not exhibit the day/night changes in serotonin-N-acetyltransferase and hydroxyindole-O-methyltransferase (HIOMT) activities characteristic of the superficial pineal (15). Moreover, no HIOMT activity has been detected in the deep pineal of the hamster (16).

All these results suggest that in the rat and hamster, if there is no apparent structural difference, the superficial and deep parts of the pineal are functionally not identical. This finding immediately raises the question of whether differences in function also exist in the apparently uniformly structured pineals present in most species. Such a question could also be related with the physiological significance of the existence of a cortex and a medulla in the pineal of some mammals (see ref. 9). Although some results, especially electrophysiological ones, seem to support this idea, it is at present impossible to answer this question.

As just explained, in most mammalian species the pineal is closely related to the third ventricle, and in rodents, where it is superficially located, a deep pineal is present. The question of the often-postulated (17) release of pineal hormone either in the region of the pineal recess or via the suprapineal recess into the third ventricle has to be examined.

In mammals, the pineal is a solid, compact organ. The release of substances produced by cells that are not closely related to the pineal or the suprapineal recesses is, thus, difficult to conceive. The pineal recess, which indicates the opening of the lumen of the original saccular pineal "anlage" into the third ventricle, is lined by ependymal cells. There is thus no direct contact of pinealocytes with the cerebrospinal fluid (CSF). In numerous species, part of the dorsal surface of the gland is covered by the suprapineal recess of the third ventricle. Between the ependymal wall of this recess and the pineal parenchyma at the dorsal surface of the organ, there is the pial covering of both this recess and the pineal, as well as a variable amount of loose pia-arachnoid tissue, forming part of the so-called velum interpositum. In these conditions, it is difficult to conceive that the products synthesized by the pineal parenchyma are released directly into the internal cerebrospinal fluid containing the suprapineal or pineal recess (18). It is not possible, however, to exclude completely the possibility that part of the compounds synthesized by pinealocytes are released directly into the third ventricle. Hewing (19,20), indeed, has observed that in the hamster, vole, guinea pig, and rhesus monkey the ependymal lining of the pineal recess is discontinuous and that some pinealocytes are in direct contact with the CSF. The number of such pinealocytes, however, is very small. Thus, if part of the substance produced by the pinealocytes can be released directly into the third ventricle, it is a very small part and we do not think that this release, if present, is an important functional principle. This does not mean, however, that the interactions between pineal and CSF are not of physiological importance. Fleischhauer (21), for example, has shown that a fluorescent dye injected into the lateral ventricle completely penetrated the pineal parenchyma in the cat. It seems, thus, that the hormonal principles secreted by the pineal cells—excluding the ependymal cells, which, as suggested by Pavel (22,23), can release their secretory products, if existing, directly into the third ventricle (see following)—are released, like those of all other endocrine glands, into the general circulation, but that the substances present in the CSF could be taken up by the pineal via the ependymal cells.

Pineal volume, which has been studied in a great number of species with the aim of relating it to body weight or brain weight (24–26), shows great interspecific variations, as indicated by the absolute volume as well as by the relative volume (to body or brain weight) or by the epiphysial index (definition and details, refs. 25,27). It is known that the state of activity of the pineal is correlated with pineal volume, and variations in adult pineal volume have been studied in detail in at least three species of rodents (28–30). However, it appears that interspecific differences in adult pineal volume are far greater than variations stemming from daily or seasonal cycles, or from other factors. Interspecific differences in adult pineal volume have, thus, a primary genetic basis. Larger size does not automatically indicate greater "importance" in a functional sense. However, it is probably sound to assume that very large pineals play a larger physiological role than do extremely small ones and, in the extreme case, in species lacking a pineal body, certainly the latter must be considered as somehow functionally different from those in which the pineals are large and apparently vigorously active.

It seems increasingly evident that the pineal is principally involved in the integration of information about environmental conditions, especially daylength in temperate zones, as already demonstrated in some rodents (31–33), as well as other information such as temperature, rainfall, food, separately or in association, depending on the ecological situation in which the species concerned lives (34–38). It seems, thus, necessary to examine the variation in pineal size in the context of the adaptations that organisms have made to geographical, climatological, and meteorological conditions.

It appears that animals having a very large pineal, such as the sea lion, seal, walrus (39), northern fur seal (40), Weddell seal (41), elephant seal (Figures 6 and 7), and some cervidae (42), are all Arctic or Holarctic species, ranging to very high latitudes as well as high altitudes, whereas animals such as the anteater, sloth, armadillo (Figure 8) and pangolin (1,42–43), which have no pineal, or such as the rhinoceros, elephant dugong (1,42,44), and red kangaroo (Figure 9), which have a small pineal, are all mammals limited to tropical/equatorial zones. A latitudinal trend in relative pineal size, clearly demonstrated in some rodents (Figure 10), is, thus, very apparent in mammals.

Some other correlations that are not necessarily related to geography have also been observed. In general, smaller pineals tend also to be correlated with nocturnality and larger pineals with diurnality (42). More interestingly, there would also seem to be a fairly good correlation between pineal size and degree of homeothermia in mammals. Many of the heterothermic endotherms have a small pineal. This has to be correlated with the capacity of the species concerned for adaptation to the thermal environment. For example, endothermic mammals (and nonmammals, ref. 42) that live in the more harsh thermal environments—for example in Arctic zones—that maintain a constant, warm body tem-

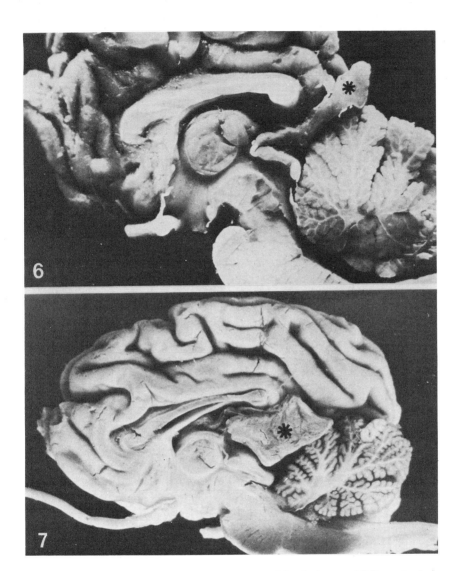

FIGURES 6 and 7. Sagittal sections through the brain of the elephant seal *(Mirouga leonina)*. Note in the adult (Figure 6) as in the neonatal (Figure 7) brains of this animal living in the polar zone the very large size of the pineal (*). *From Griffiths, unpublished data; by courtesy.*

perature, and that, by necessity, have a seasonally limited and synchronized reproductive pattern tend to have a well-developed pineal organ (details in ref. 42).

The essence of seasonal reproductive cycles is that animals are prohibited from breeding, and more especially from delivery of young, during seasons that would not allow for optimal survival of the offspring

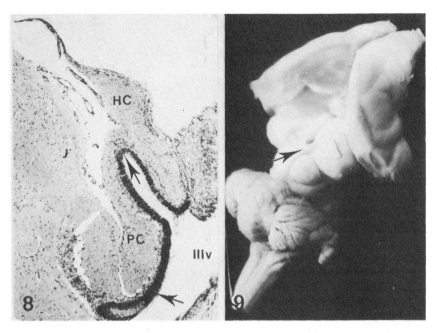

FIGURE 8. Sagittal section of the roof of the nine-banded armadillo *(Dasypus novemcinetus)* diencephalon. Note the absence of pineal tissue. **HC** = habenular commissure; **PC** = posterior commissure; **arrow** = subcommissural organ; **IIIv** = third ventricle. (× 50.) *From Phillips, unpublished data, by courtesy.*

FIGURE 9. Macrophotography of a kangaroo brain *(Macropus robustus)* exposed in the Netherlands Brain Research Institute's Museum. Note the small pineal **(arrow)** of this subtropical animal. *From Pévet, unpublished data.*

and thus of the species. The great variation in pineal size observed in the different mammalian species should, in our opinion, be associated with the adaptive importance of the pineal in this process. The more the environmental conditions of life for the animal are difficult, the more synchronization of the diverse activities of the animals, and especially reproductive activity, with the environment is indispensable; the more so would the function of the pineal be important. For example, in the equatorial/tropical zones, the major climatic regions of the world, which are essentially characterized by the fact that the monthly mean temperatures do not show much seasonal fluctuation (45), the pressure of the environment is not very strong when compared to that of temperate and, especially, Arctic zones. This is particularly true in the equatorial wet regions, where not only mean temperatures but also rainfall, and consequently the availability of food, remain high and constant throughout the year. Most mammalian and also nonmammalian species characterized by absence of the pineal live in tropical/equatorial zones. Moreover, when the pineal is present, it tends to be smaller. Except in the equatorial wet forests, most of the tropical zones are characterized by a

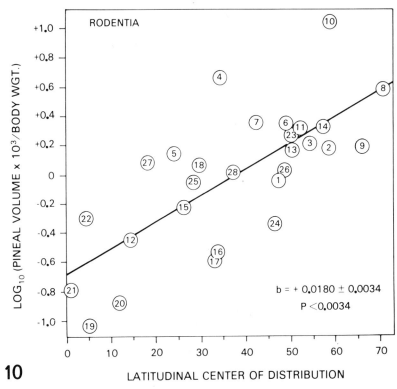

FIGURE 10. Relationship between relative pineal volume in rodent species and their latitudinal centers of north-south geographic distribution. Each circle represents a particular species:

SCIURIDAE
  1. *Citellus citellus*
  2. *Marmota marmota*
  3. *Sciurus vulgarus*

CRICETIDAE
  Tribe: Hesperomyini
  4. *Peromyscus leucopus*
  5. *Sigmodon hispidus*
  Tribe: Cricetini
  6. *Cricetus cricetus*
  7. *Mesocricetus auratus*

SUBFAMILY: MICROTINAE
  8. *Dicrostonyx*
     groenlandicus
  9. *Lemmus lemmus*
  10. *Microtus orcadensis*
  11. *Microtus*
      pennsylvanicus
  12. *"Microtus*
      senegalensis"
  13. *Phenacomys*
      intermedius
  14. *Synaptomys borealis*

SUBFAMILY: GERBILLINAE
  15. *Meriones crassus*
  16. *Meriones libycus*
  17. *Meriones persicus*
  18. *Meriones shawi*

MURIDAE
  19. *Cricetomys*
      gambianus
  20. *Dasymys incomtus*
  21. *Lemniscomys striatus*
  22. *Praomys (Rattus)*
      morio

GLIRIDAE
  23. *Eliomys quercinus*
  24. *Glis glis*
  25. *Graphiurus*
      graphiurus
  26. *Muscardinus*
      avellanarius

CAVIIDAE
  27. *Cavia aperea*

CAPROMYIDAE
  28. *Myocastor coypus*

seasonal rhythm in the annual rainfall and most animal species present an annual sexual cycle, more-or-less well-synchronized with the rainfall (45). In desert zones, the conditions of life are difficult for animal species. This could perhaps explain why in some tropical/equatorial species the pineal has been reported to be large and very active (see under Histology).

Under higher-latitude temperate and Arctic-zone variations in climatological conditions, especially, the annual variations of temperature and food availability are large. The animals have to adapt to these variations of the environment, whose magnitude depends on the altitude as well as on the latitude. In particular, they must—to ensure the survival of the species—synchronize their reproductive activity with the period of the year (i.e., 6–7 months in southern temperate zones, to 2–3 weeks in northern territories of the Northern Hemisphere) in which the conditions of life are optimal for the offspring. Under such conditions, in which physiological processes of adaptation, especially the maintenance of a warm and constant body temperature and synchronization of seasonal reproductive patterns are very important, the animals tend to have well-developed pineal organs.

In such a concept, the increase in pineal size at high latitude should be related to the increase in the critical value of neuroendocrine transduction for timing and exact phase tuning of biological rhythms. The validity of this suggestion has to be tested by comparative and quantitative physiological studies using many species and geographical sites. In our opinion, it would be necessary to look especially at the correlations between pineal size, not with latitude, but with latitude-related biotopes such as equatorial wet forest, savanna, desert zones, and temperate, Holarctic, and Arctic zones, combined with the zonation in altitude (details in ref. 45); i.e., all biotopes in which the pressure of the environment is not the same.

INNERVATION

The pineal contains principally four groups of nerve fibers, namely sympathetic, parasympathetic, commissural, and peptidergic fibers. Among these fibers, however, only the sympathetic ones, of which the physiological function in pineal activity has been amply studied, appear to be largely distributed within the gland. The commissural and peptidergic fibers, the role of which has still to be elucidated, appear to be only locally distributed, whereas the parasympathetic ones have been described in only two species.

Morphological Structure and Distribution of the Sympathetic Nerve Fibers

The central nervous system (CNS) pathway from the retina to the pineal is described in detail in another chapter of this book. We will therefore concentrate our study on the internal aspect of the pineal sympathetic innervation.

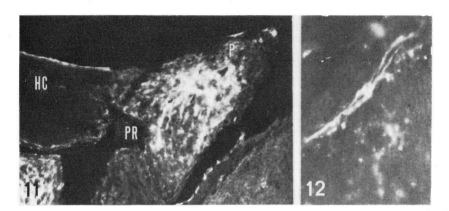

FIGURE 11. Noradrenergic innervation of the pineal gland (**P**) of the hedgehog visualized by the Falck and Hillarp technique. **HC** = habenular commissure; **PR** = pineal recess. (× 80.) *From Pévet (81).*

FIGURE 12. Higher magnification of a noradrenergic fiber. (× 350.) *From Pévet (81).*

The presence of sympathetic nerve fibers within the pineal, which has long been suspected (see references in ref. 11), was clearly established by Ariëns Kappers (11), who showed that in the rat, after superior cervical ganglionectomy, intrapineal nerve fibers were almost completely lacking after 2 months. These findings were later amply confirmed in the rat and other species by means of different techniques, such as surgical and chemical sympathectomy, electron microscopy, and, especially, fluorescence histochemistry (Figures 11 and 12). This last-mentioned technique has also permitted the demonstration that not only the green fluorescence, due to the presence of noradrenaline, but also a yellow fluorescence characteristic of serotonin was detectable in these nerve fibers. The presence of serotonin is explained by the fact that in numerous species such as rat, mouse, guinea pig, and dog (46–48), the sympathetic fibers take up and retain the serotonin released from pinealocytes (48), amounting to about 30% of the total pineal serotonin content, at least in the rat (49). Autoradiographic work has also demonstrated that the nerve endings can take up not only serotonin but also many other amines such as dopamine, adrenaline, and 5-hydroxytryptophan (50).

Most of the sympathetic nerve fibers observed in the pineal originate from the paired superior cervical ganglia of the sympathetic trunk. They reach the pineal in two somewhat different ways. In some species, such as calf, cat, dog, hedgehog, macaque, and rabbit, many fibers, which are mostly unmyelinated, enter the gland via the perivascular space of arterioles, venules, and capillaries vascularizing the organ. In the rabbit, this type of sympathetic innervation can even be observed along the entire surface of the pineal, especially along the great cerebral vein (51).

Postganglionic sympathetic fibers reach the gland also by the way of two bilateral symmetrical nervi conarii (Figures 13 and 14), which in

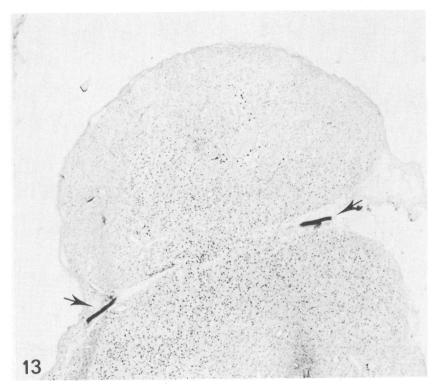

FIGURE 13. Branches of the right and left nervus conarii **(arrows)** penetrating the pineal organ of the rabbit at its lateral sides, somewhat rostral to the tip. (× 90.) *From Romijn (66), by courtesy, with permission of the publisher.*

some species such as cat, bat, and man may fuse before entering the pineal, generally at its caudal pole (see details in 9). It seems, however, that in most of the species, like the rat (11), the majority of sympathetic fibers reach the organ by way of the nervi conarii.

As demonstrated by means of Falk and Hillarp fluorescence and electron-microscopical techniques, either together or not combined with pharmacological studies, the intrapineal distribution of sympathetic fibers and their varicosities varies from species to species. In the guinea pig (48) and the Mongolian gerbil (52), they are found almost exclusively around vessels, whereas in chinchilla (53) and sheep (9) these nerve fibers are mainly confined to the parenchyma. In the cat, ground squirrel, hamster, rat, and rabbit, the intrapineal adrenergic nerves are distributed around vessels as well as in the parenchyma (references in 9,54). This seems to be the case also in cattle and pigs, species in which, singularly, only very few isolated adrenergic nerves were found (55). In species such as the hamster, Mongolian gerbil, and rat, in which the pineal consists of a complex of different parts (see earlier), the sympathetic nerve fibers are not restricted to the superficial pineal (termed "the

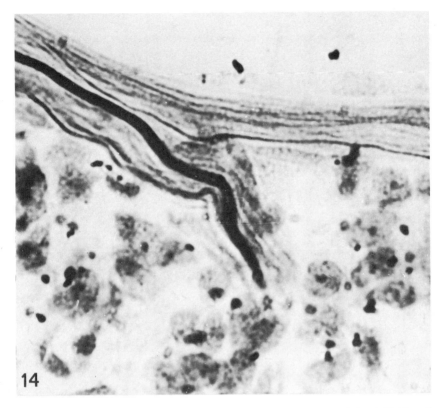

14

FIGURE 14. Branch of the left nervus conarii entering the rabbit pineal gland. Thick and thin fiber bundles as well as single fibers can be distinguished. (× 1500.) *From Romijn (66), by courtesy, with permission of the publisher.*

pineal" by most authors including myself); they are, indeed, also observed in the deep pineal. In the rat, sympathetic fibers leaving the superficial pineal can be followed through the pineal stalk to the deep pineal. Following superior cervical ganglionectomy in the rat (56), or pinealectomy in the hamster (57) (which, in this species, corresponds only to an elimination of the superficial pineal), the fibers present in the deep pineal disappeared. This demonstrated that the sympathetic fibers present in the deep pineal originate from the superior cervical ganglia and reach the deep pineal via the superficial one.

At the ultrastructural level, the noradrenergic postganglionic nerve fiber terminals have been intensively studied. These endings are essentially characterized by the presence of dense-core vesicles of about 100 nm in diameter and electron-lucent vesicles of 45–60 nm in diameter (Figure 15). For some authors (58), two populations of electron-lucent (or clear) vesicles, round and flat ones, can be distinguished. In intact rats and mice, 30–60% of the vesicles examined contain a dense core (58–60), the proportion being 75–90% in rabbits (61). Moreover, in rats

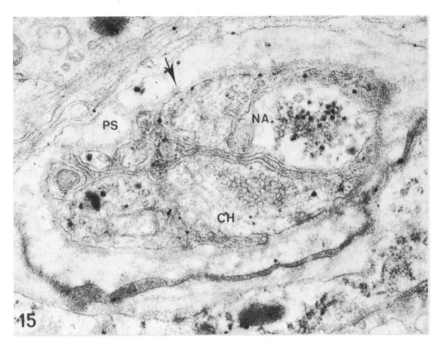

FIGURE 15. Nerve bundle running in the perivascular space **(PS)**. Noradrenergic **(NA)** and cholinergic **(CH)** nerve endings can be observed. **Arrow** = basal lamina. (× 40,000.) *From Romijn (66), by courtesy, with permission of the publisher.*

and ground squirrels about 2–5%, and in chinchilla about 10%, of the total number of vesicles are large dense-core vesicles (53). As demonstrated by Machado (62), all these results are, however, greatly dependant on the fixative solution used. Moreover, they also depend on the time of the day, since it appears, at least in the mouse (58), that the number of small dense vesicles present a circadian evolution, showing a marked decrease after the onset of darkness. This decrease may be correlated with the release of noradrenaline from the nerve fibers. The electron-lucent or clear vesicles, at least the flat ones, also present a circadian evolution exactly opposite to that of the small dense-core vesicles, a result that is in accordance with the idea that the flat clear vesicles represent depleted dense-core vesicles (for more details and references, see ref. 9).

At the ultrastructural level, the effect of various drugs on the dense-core vesicles has been studied in detail, and cytochemical methods have been frequently applied to analyze the content of both the dense-core and clear vesicles (see ref. 9). From both these pharmacological and cytochemical studies, it is clear that the small dense-core vesicles, as well as the electron-lucent vesicles, are largely implicated in the storage and release of noradrenaline and serotonin, or their precursors. Whether

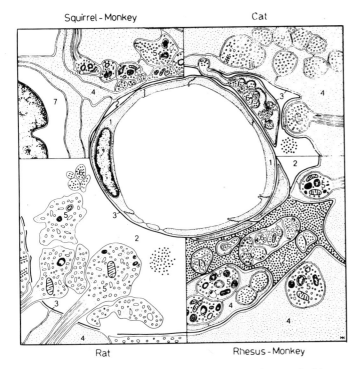

FIGURE 16. Topography of perivascular spaces in the pineal of four mammalian species: **(1)** endothelium; **(2)** perivascular space; **(3)** basal lamina; **(4)** glial cell cytoplasm; **(5)** pinealocyte processes; **(6)** sympathetic nerve processes. *From Wartenberg (132), by courtesy, with permission of the publisher.*

or not all the clear vesicles are functionally identical is difficult to determine (ref. 9). The large dense-core vesicles remained unaffected by all the drugs used, suggesting that they do not contain amines. Some cytochemical observations, on the contrary, suggest that they contain noradrenaline and serotonin associated with another substance that is reserpine (or other drugs) -resistant (63). This could explain the negative results observed by other authors. These large dense-core vesicles could, thus, be functionally basically similar to the small ones (see details in 9).

Sympathetic nerve fibers and their transmitter substance, noradrenaline, are of the utmost importance for the regulation of pinealocyte function. The ultrastructural relationships between these fibers and the pinealocytes are, thus, important to consider. The terminals of noradrenergic postganglionic fibers do not form true synaptic contacts with the pinealocytes, these fibers ending freely either in the parenchyma or, in most cases, in the pericapillary spaces. Thus, it appears that the neurotransmitter reaches the pinealocytes by way of diffusion. The neurotransmitter released from nerve fiber endings or varicosities diffuses through the perivascular space, at least in the majority of species, and reaches the target cells more or less directly, depending on whether or not the ending of the pinealocyte process is covered by the basal lamina and on the presence or absence of a glial barrier (more details, ref. 64) (see also Figure 16).

Parasympathetic Innervation and Intramural Neurons

A parasympathetic innervation of the pineal of the macaque monkey was briefly described by Kenny (65). In the rabbit, this innervation has been studied in great detail by means of light and electron microscopy, by enzyme histochemistry, and experimentally (51,61,66,67). This parasympathetic innervation in the rabbit appears to be very complicated because it consists of both intra- and extrapineal nerve cells. Consequently, pre- and postganglionic parasympathetic fibers are present in the gland. As depicted schematically in Figure 17, preganglionic acetylcholinergic fibers originating in the superior salivary nuclei leave the brain stem with the facial nerves to run with the greater superior petrosal nerves. Some of these fibers synapse with postganglionic parasympathetic nerve cells situated along these nerves. The postganglionic cholinergic parasympathetic fibers originating in these cells reach the pineal gland by way of the nervi conarii. Other preganglionic parasympathetic fibers, however, also reach the pineal, with the nervi conarii, to synapse with either the perikarya or the dendrites of intramural pineal postganglionic parasympathetic nerve cells. The postganglionic acetylcholinergic parasympathetic nerve fibers originating from the intrapineal nerve cells terminate both in the perivascular spaces and essentially in the pineal parenchyma and do not form synaptic junctions with the pinealocytes. Thus, here also, the neurotransmitter released from these terminals reaches the pinealocytes by way of diffusion.

At the ultrastructural level, the endings of the parasympathetic pre- and postganglionic fibers are all acetylcholinesterase-positive, as demonstrated by Romijn (67), and are characterized—at least in the rabbit, and perhaps also in the Djungarian hamster (54)—by clear vesicles measuring 40–50 nm in diameter (Figure 15), intermingled with some dense-core vesicles of about 100 nm in diameter; consequently these can easily be confused with the terminal processes of pinealocytes.

Such parasympathetic innervation has been described only in a few species, and its presence is denied by authors such as Schrier and Klein (68), who assert that the choline-acetyltransferase activity measured by others is in fact due to the presence of carnitine acetyltransferase. Moreover, as it is known that the sympathetic fibers of the pineal have parasympathetic cholinergic characteristics (69–71), most pinealogists are tempted to conclude that the parasympathetic innervation—if present—does not have a profound influence on pinealocyte function. It is true that, to date, little experimental evidence supports this notion (see, however, ref. 72), but it is also true that for most pinealogists, "influence on

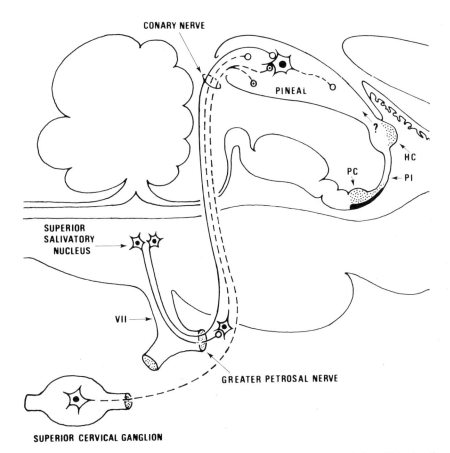

FIGURE 17. Model of sympathetic and parasympathetic innervation of the rabbit pineal gland. **Solid lines** = preganglionic; **broken lines** = postganglionic; ⊙ = noradrenergic; ◯ = cholinergic; **HC** = habenular commissure; **PC** = posterior commissure; **PI** = pars intercalaris. *From Romijn (61), by courtesy, with permission of the publisher.*

pineal function" is erroneously synonymous for "influence on melatonin metabolism." Perhaps nobody has ever looked at the right parameter.

As in the rabbit (Figure 18) (66,67), intramural neurons have been demonstrated in the macaque monkey (65,73), man (74), bat (75), Djungarian hamster (cited in 54), and ground squirrel (76). The number of neurons, however, is very variable. In the rabbit, for example, Romijn (66) found 40 nerve cells, whereas in both bat specimens examined, Kenny (75) was able to find one intrapineal nerve cell only. Until now a distinct intrapineal ganglion has been described in the ferret only (70,77,78). Relatively little is known about these intramural neurons. In the rabbit (61) and the monkey (75), they have been regarded as intra-

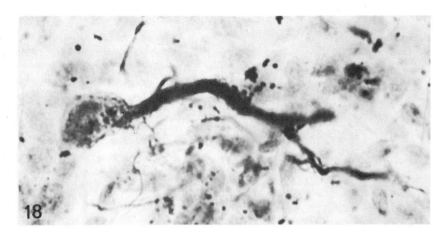

FIGURE 18. Light photomicrograph of an intrapineal neuron in rabbit pineal tissue. A thick offshoot is observed branching between the pinealocytes. Silver staining after Richardson. (× 1200.) *From Romijn (66), by courtesy, with permission of the publisher.*

mural parasympathetic neurons that in the former show axosomatic and axodendritic synapses formed by both postganglionic noradrenergic and preganglionic cholinergic nerve fibers (61). In the ferret, the nerve cells in the ganglion appear to contain acetylcholinesterase (70,71) and do not exhibit a specific amine fluorescence. However, this ganglion, according to Ueck (54), is not part of the parasympathetic system, since the nerve cells project centralward to the brain and are in synaptic contact with fibers originating from the CNS.

Commissural Fibers

In practically all species investigated (details in ref. 9), commissural fibers are present in the pineal. The degree of penetration of these fibers into the pineal, however, varies considerably from one species to another. The fibers, for example, reach the dorsal part of the pineal in some primates (except man, 75) (79,80), the central part in the cat (75,79,80), calf (79), hedgehog (81), and guinea pig (82) and are restricted to the proximal part in the rat (11), horse (79), and rabbit (66). Using silver impregnation, it has been shown that in the monkey (73), rat (11,75), rabbit (66), and hedgehog (81) commissural fibers form loops (Figures 19–22) and leave the organ contralaterally and that in the rat (11), when these fibers are in contact with parenchymal cells, they do not exhibit terminal thickenings. Consequently, for a long time, these fibers have been considered as aberrant.

If it appears evident that, especially in the rat, many of these fibers are really aberrant, it is not evident that all of them are so, especially in species such as the hedgehog (81), in which the number of commissural

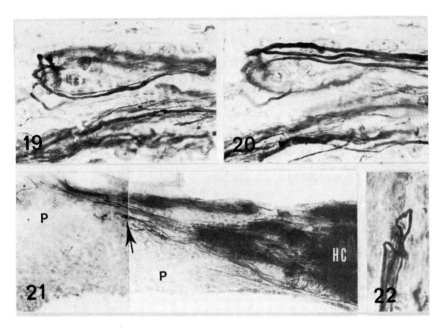

FIGURES 19 and 20. "Aberrant" fibers in the pineal of the hedgehog. By changing the focus of the microscope, it is possible to observe the hairpin-loops made by the fibers. Silver staining after Richardson. (× 610.) *From Pévet (81).*

FIGURE 21. Sagittal section through the dorsal part of the pineal gland **(P)** of the hedgehog. Many nerve fiber bundles are seen after silver impregnation. They originate from the habenular commissure **(HC)**. A nerve fiber (arrow) making a hairpin-loop can be observed. Silver staining after Richardson. (× 240.) *From Pévet (81).*

FIGURE 22. Higher magnification of the aberrant nerve fiber illustrated in Figure 21 (× 830.) *From Pévet (81).*

fibers is very large. Such a possibility has to be taken into consideration because "it is of great interest that, as neuronal impulses are concerned, pinealocyte function may not exclusively depend on stimuli of various physiological significance and origin reaching the gland via its sympathetic innervation" (83).

Hülsemann (84), Møllgaard and Møller (85), Møller (86,87) in the human fetus, Møller et al. (88) in sheep and rabbit fetuses, and Nielsen and Møller (80) in the adult cat and monkey have shown a nervous connection between the pineal organ and the brain. In the cat and monkey, in which commissural fibers penetrate deeply into the parenchyma, some fibers possess end-bulbs close to parenchymal cells (80). Schapiro and Salas (89) have demonstrated that, in the rat, photic stimuli reach the pineal even after complete sympathectomy. Moreover, Dafny and McClung (90), McClung and Dafny (91), and Rønnekleiv et al. (92), after electrical stimulation of the habenular nuclei, noted a clear response in the pineal. Other electrophysiological investigations (93,94) also indicate that stimuli originating in parts of the limbic system of the brain run to the pineal via the medullary striae, the habenular nuclei, and the pineal stalk. Moreover, a direct link between the brain and the pineal has been clearly demonstrated in the ferret, in which lesions in the habenula or the posterior commissure result in degenerative changes in the intra-pineal ganglion (77).

Peptidergic Fibers

Logically, these fibers should be included under the heading Commissural Fibers. However, due to the fact that the discovery of such fibers—not by their own function, which is not known, but because they explain numerous contradictory results reported in the literature (95–97)—is of great physiological importance, the analysis of these fibers is being considered separately.

Such fibers have been called neurosecretory fibers by some authors (see 9). They would be neurosecretory fibers only if the neuropeptides present were released into the general circulation. This is not known at the level of the pineal. We know, at least for vasopressin (98,99), that in the brain neuropeptides might function as a neurotransmitter and not as a neurohormone. We prefer at the present time, for the pineal as for the brain, to call these fibers "peptidergic fibers."

In 1956, Barry (100) described Gömöri-stained fibers in the pineal and the pineal stalk of the horseshoe bat, which, in his opinion, originated from the paraventricular nucleus. Moreover, this author suggested that the substance demonstrated in the extrahypothalamic fibers present in the pineal was probably similar to the secretory substance of the hypothalamo-neurohypophyseal system. This study by Barry, although regularly cited by morphologists, and although not unique, since similar Gömöri-stained beaded fibers were also detected in the hedgehog (1,101,102), rhesus monkey (103,104), and the Mongolian gerbil (105), was completely forgotten by most pinealogists, especially the physiologists. Consequently, when immunoreactive neurophysins I and II were detected in the bovine and human pineal (106–108), and although Reinharz et al. (106) did observe that these two neurophysins behaved similarly to posterior pituitary neurophysins when the same purification procedure was applied, the authors logically explained the presence of one of the neurophysins by the presence of arginine vasotocin (AVT), the only neurohormone so far claimed to be present in the pineal (details in refs. 95–97).

During the past few years, however, it has been demonstrated by immunocytochemistry, at least in rat (109) and bovine pineals (110), that the presence of arginine vasopressin (AVP) and oxytocin (OT), the two neurohypophyseal hormones detected in the pineal by means of radioimmunoassays (111–113), was due to the presence of AVP- and OT-containing extrahypothalamic fibers (Figure 23) originating (in the rat) from the magnocellular AVP- and OT-producing nucleus and running via the subcommissural organ and the deep pineal (when present) or

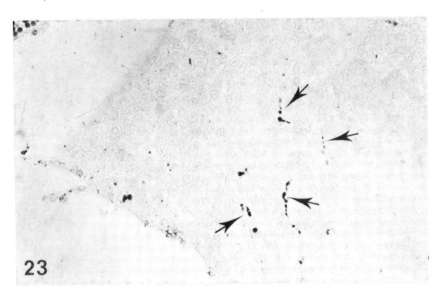

FIGURE 23. Sagittal section through the pineal organ of a Wistar rat. Oxytocin immunoreactive fibers in the anterior part of the pineal organ **(arrows)** × 700. *From Buijs and Pévet (109), with permission of the publisher.*

via the habenular commissure into the pineal stalk, terminating in the rostral part of the pineal gland (109). The presence of such extrahypothalamic fibers in the pineal explains the presence in this gland of neurophysins that are the carrier proteins of OT and AVP, as indeed demonstrated in the bovine pineal (113).

With the development of immunocytochemistry, it seems evident that peptidergic fibers of this type, or another, will soon be observed in the pineal of other mammalian species. In the squirrel monkey, for example, a luteinizing hormone releasing factor (LHRH) reactive perikaryon has been described by Barry (114) in the habenular commissure or in the rostral part of the pineal (not specified by the author). Thus, the presence of peptidergic fibers containing LHRH in the pineal cannot be excluded. Moreover, recently, fibers containing vasoactive intestinal peptide (VIP) have been detected immunocytochemically in the stalk and the anterior part of the pineal of the pig, rabbit (115), and, especially, the cat (115,116), where the VIP-containing fibers penetrate deeply into the posterior pineal gland both from the anterior and posterior commissural areas (116).

HISTOLOGY, HISTOCHEMISTRY, AND CYTOCHEMISTRY

Ontogenetically, the pineal of all vertebrates, including mammals, is formed by an invagination of the neuroepithelium constituting that part of the roof of the diencephalon situated between the habenular and the posterior commissure. The cells of this neuroepithelial proliferation give

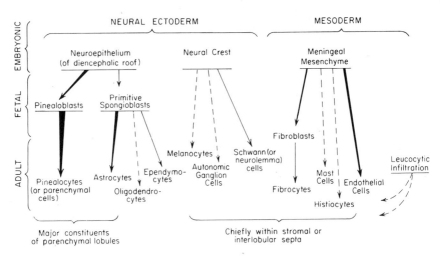

FIGURE 24. Developmental origins of cells found in mammalian pineals. This schematic summary represents a combination of classic views concerning the derivation of various ectodermal and mesodermal cells, with specific views concerning pineal histogenesis. Relative thicknesses of the arrows for cellular descents are intended to reflect approximately the relative number of cells of each kind. Dashed arrows signify origins of cells that are present only variably, according to present knowledge. *From Quay (221), by courtesy, with permission of the publisher.*

rise to the parenchymal cells (or pinealocytes) and spongioblasts of the organ, and the mesenchyma surrounding the neuroepithelial anlage produce, among other elements, connective tissue strands, fibroblasts, and vessels (11). Figure 24 summarizes the developmental origin of these cell types within the mammalian pineal. In this review, we will examine only cells of neuroepithelial origin. For details concerning mesodermal cells present in the pineal, we refer to Vollrath (9).

The Pinealocyte

One population of cells, irregularly shaped and showing a varying number of processes—in the literature called pinealocytes, pinealocytes of population I, light pinealocytes, parenchymal cells, clear pinealocytes, light and dark chief cells (see details and references in 35,117)—is constantly predominant [90% of the parenchymal cells in the rat (118)].

From comparative phylogenetic and ontogenetic studies, it is now apparent that these cells are derived phylogenetically from the neurosensory photoreceptor cells present in the pineal organ of submammalian species (2–4). Several stages in the transformation of photoreceptorlike cells into pinealocytes during ontogenetic development (119,120), which reflect the phylogenetic transformation of the pineal cells, are sometimes visible in the adult pineal of mammals, at least in the mole (121) (Figure 25) and noctule bat (122). In consequence, all

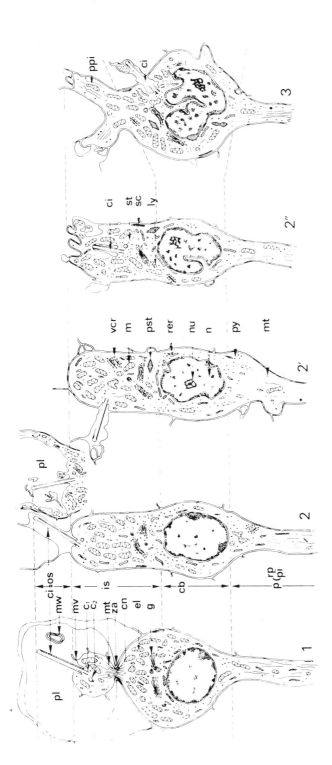

FIGURE 25. Plurality of the derivatives of the photoreceptor cell line in a mammalian pineal organ (adult mole, *Talpa europaea*). **1.** rudimentary photoreceptor cell; **2,2',2".** cells intermediate between photoreceptor cells and pinealocytes; **3.** pinealocyte *sensu stricto*. *Abbreviations:* **c₁** = distal centriole; **c₂** = proximal centriole; **ci** = cilium; **cb** = cell body; **cn** = cellular neck; **el** = mitochondria of "ellipsoid"; **g** = Golgi complex; **is** = inner segment; **ly** = lysosome; **m** = mitochondria; **mt** = microtubules; **mv** = microvilli; **mw** = membranous whorl; **n** = nucleus; **nu** = nucleolus; **os** = outer segment; **pl** = pineal lumen; **p(rp,pi)** = process of a rudimentary photoreceptor cell or an intermediate cell; **ppi** = process of a pinealocyte; **pst** = paracrystalline structure; **py** = polysomes; **rer** = rough endoplasmic reticulum; **sc** = subsurface cisternae; **st** = striated ciliary rootlet; **vcr** = vesicle-crowned ribbon; **za** = zonula adherens. *From Pévet and Collin (121), modified following Vollrath (9), with permission of the publisher.*

these cells can be regarded as pinealocytes. Because some authors referred to all cells of the pineal organ as pinealocytes, Wolfe (123) has termed them "pinealocytes *sensu stricto*," a term that has subsequently been widely adopted by many authors. However, although this designation is appropriate when only one population of pinealocytes is present, it cannot be used for species in which two distinct populations have been observed (see later). Consequently, in the mole rat (124), noctule bat (122,125), and the pipistrelle bat (126), we have termed these cells "pinealocytes of population I." It should be realized that the terms "pinealocyte *sensu stricto*," used when only one population of pinealocytes is present, and "pinealocyte of population I," used when more than one population of pinealocytes is present, characterize the same cells—cells homologous to the photoreceptor cells of lower vertebrates and containing granular vesicles. The question arises as to whether different types of pinealocytes *sensu stricto* (or of population I) can be distinguished. The answer to this question depends on the direction of research of the authors (morphology, functional aspects, phylogeny, etc.). For example, in the rat pineal gland, Arstila (127) morphologically distinguished two different types of pinealocytes *sensu stricto* (light chief cells and dark chief cells) that, according to this author, would also show different functions. Karasek (118) and Gusek (128), however, interpret this difference in morphological aspect as the result of differences in the functional state of the same cell type.

Light and dark pinealocytes *sensu stricto*/population I were also observed in many other mammals. In many species, such as the dog, gerbil, golden mole, hamster, hedgehog, mole, pipistrelle, pocket gopher, and rat, the ultrastructure of the two cell types is not basically different, their differentiation being based only on different shades of the cells. Moreover, in the hedgehog (81) and the gerbil (129), the relative number of dark and light pinealocytes was demonstrated to depend on the choice of the fixative. This observation strongly supports the hypothesis that this difference in morphological aspect is the result of a difference in the functional state of the same cell type. Moreover, it can be stated that a specific secretory process, characterized by the formation of granular vesicles (GV), is common to all cells of this category. This is in favor of the physiological unity of this population.

PROBLEM OF THE PRESENCE OF TWO POPULATIONS OF PINEALOCYTES

As already discussed (35,117), the category of cells differing from pinealocytes *sensu stricto* (or population I) represents a heterogeneous group, most often identifiable as interstitial, glial, or gliallike cells (see the section on The "Glial" Cells). In numerous animals, however, another group of cells distinguishable from both glial cells and pinealocytes *sensu stricto* or population I is present. These cells have been named pigment-containing cells in the chinchilla (130) and pocket gopher (131), dark pinealocytes (not related to pinealocytes *sensu stricto* or population I) in the rabbit (51,132), guinea pig (133), macaque (134), and mouse (135), and pinealocytes of population II in the mole rat (124), noctule bat (122,125), and pipistrelle (126). In the chinchilla (130) and the pocket gopher (131), they have been termed pigment-containing cells because of their content of pigment granules. In rabbits (51), numerous pigment granules were observed in dark pinealocytes. In some pinealocytes of population II of the noctule bat, granular pigment has also been described (125). In this animal, the pinealocytes of population II are, moreover, characterized by the presence of an extraordinarily large amount of glycogen granules. This is also true for the dark pinealocytes in the rabbit (136). Although at present it is very difficult to establish whether these cells belong to the same functional group, it can be suggested, on the basis of the previously mentioned characteristics, that all these cells most probably belong to the same functional group.

Pinealocytes are phylogenetically derived from photoreceptor cells. It remains to be established whether these peculiar cells can be considered to be true pinealocytes or whether they are of a different phylogenetic origin. So far, it can only be stated that, in the mole-rat, noctule bat, and pipistrelle bat, ciliary derivatives characterized by a 9 + 0 tubular pattern have been observed in this group of cells. In addition, in the noctule bat a certain polarity in the distribution of cell organelles resembling that described in the rudimentary photoreceptor cells of nonmammalian vertebrate pineal organs has also been reported. Moreover, in the mole-rat, noctule, and pipistrelle, these cells are characterized by the presence in their cytoplasm of vacuoles containing flocculent material of moderate electron density, originating from cisternae of the granular endoplasmic reticulum. In species having only a single population of pinealocytes (garden dormouse, hedgehog, mole, American mole, rat), a similar "ependymallike" secretory process is present in the pinealocytes *sensu stricto*. On the basis of these observations, we have called these cells of the mole-rat, noctule bat, and pipistrelle "pinealocytes of population II." "Pinealocytes" because we believe that they are true pinealocytes (homologous to photoreceptor cells in lower vertebrates) and "population II" to differentiate them from pinealocytes of population I. The existence of two populations of true pinealocytes in some mammalian species is strongly supported by data in the literature. Flight (137), Meiniel (5,6,138), and Vivien-Roels and Meiniel (139), for example, have described two different populations of photoreceptor cells in the pineal gland of *Diemyctylus viridescens viridescens* (Amphibia: Urodela) and *Lampetra planeri* (Agnatha: Petromizontidae) and of the rockling (Fish: Teleostei). The presence in the same pineal organ of two morphologically as well as biochemically different populations of photoreceptors (5,6,138–140) may point to the existence of two different lines of sensory cells (5,6). This new concept of the phylogenetic evolution of the vertebrate pineal cells (for more details, see 6) would explain the presence of the two different populations of pinealocytes observed in some mammalian species.

Additional evidence, however, does not support this concept. Petit

(141) and McNulty (142–144) described the presence of sensory cilia (9 + 0) in the pineal supportive cells of some fish and reptiles. Moreover, McNulty (143) described in such cells an organellelike specialization (glycogen-bound vacuoles) and noted that this situation was strikingly similar to that observed in the pinealocytes of population II of the noctule bat. However, such glycogen-bound vacuoles have also been observed in pinealocytes *sensu stricto*; for example, in the golden mole (145) and in the pipistrelle (126). This structure is observed in both populations of pinealocytes. Moreover, looking at the illustration presented by McNulty (Figures 9 and 10, ref. 144), it seems that the two cell types possessing a ciliary derivative with a 9 + 0 arrangement of paired tubules, one of them being identified as supportive cell by this author, could correspond to the two types of photoreceptors identified by Meiniel (5,138) and Vivien-Roels and Meiniel (139) in *Lampetra planeri* and the rockling, respectively.

Some recent studies on the glial cells, strongly suggesting that both "true glial cells" and "not true glial cells" could be present close to the pinealocytes and confused with each other, indicate that this problem is yet more complex (see in the section on The "Glial" Cells).

SECRETORY ACTIVITIES

Two different groups of compounds considered responsible for its endocrine capabilities are elaborated by the pineal gland: indoleamines, especially melatonin, and peptidergic compounds. We will examine the cytological aspect of these two pineal productions and the possible relationship between them.

Cytological and Cytochemical Aspect of Indoleamine Secretion. In indole metabolism, the amino acid tryptophan is converted to 5-hydroxytryptophan (5-HTP) by hydroxylation. Decarboxylation of this indole derivative leads to the formation of 5-hydroxytryptamine (serotonin, 5-HT).

Using the histochemical procedure of Falck and coworkers (146), combined with microspectrofluorometric analysis for adequate identification of the fluorogenic compounds, 5-HTP and/or 5-HT (which cannot be differentiated by this technique) have been found in the pineal of numerous mammalian species. The intensity and the localization of the reaction is, however, greatly variable. 5-HTP/5-HT fluorophores are absent or very weak in numerous species, such as the cat, cow, dog, hedgehog, man, and sheep (references and details in 147). In some other species, such as the gerbil, 5-HTP/5-HT is present only in the pinealocytes, whereas in the dormouse, ferret, hamster, monkey, mouse, and rat, fluorescence was observed in all parenchymal cells (details in 147). Presence of 5-HTP/5-HT was also detected in the sympathetic nerve endings of the pineal of numerous species (see earlier under Innervation).

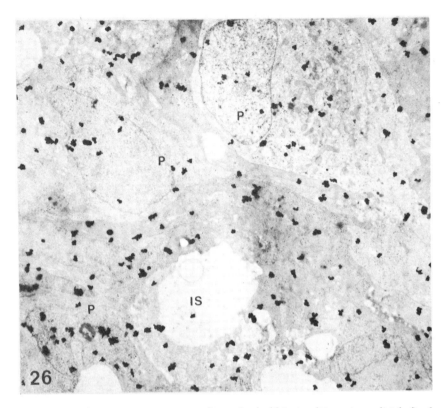

FIGURE 26. Electron microscope autoradiograph of rabbit pineal tissue immediately fixed after incubation for 1 hour in medium containing ^{3}H-5-hydroxytryptophan. A moderate and diffuse labeling of the pinealocytes **(P)**, including the cell nuclei, can be observed. Note that silver grains are scarce over intercellular spaces **(IS)**. (× 2800.) *From Romijn et al. (149), by courtesy with the permission of the publisher.*

These different results on the localization and relative amounts of 5-HTP/5-HT are probably due to a number of factors such as animal species, age of animals, and technical procedures used. In our opinion, the time of day, the season, and the physical environment must be taken into consideration, especially because it is well known that pineal 5-HT in all vertebrates is subject to circadian and circannual rhythms.

In order to provide information concerning the site of indoleamine metabolism, tritiated 5-HTP and 5-HT were used as precursors. Experiments in vivo or in vitro were developed by different teams. The results obtained that support those previously obtained by Falck and coworkers' technique permit a much more refined analysis of the distribution of tritiated indoleamines.

In the hamster, mouse, rabbit (Figure 26), rat, and rhesus monkey, (^{3}H)-5-HTP or (^{3}H)-5-HT were taken up by all the parenchymal cells.

Using tritiated 5-HTP, a diffuse labeling of pinealocytes was observed in the monkey, mouse, rabbit (Figure 26), and rat. This would suggest that the synthesis of serotonin and other pineal indoleamines may not necessarily happen in membrane-limited organelles, but in the cytosol.

Subcellular fractionation of pineal tissue has shown that the enzyme 5-hydroxylase, which converts tryptophan into 5-HTP, is restricted to the mitochondrial fraction (148), and that treatment with parachlorophenylalanine (p-CPA), an inhibitor of this enzyme, did not cause any alteration in rabbit pinealocyte ultrastructure, except for an enlargement of the mitochondria and an increased number of their cristae (149). These observations suggest that hydroxylation of tryptophan to 5-HTP happens at the mitochondrial membranes, whereas the conversion of 5-HTP to 5-HT by aromatic L-amino acid decarboxylase may occur freely in the cytosol (149). In some nonmammalian species such as the parakeet and the lizard, however, the labeling appears to be preferentially related to the rudimentary photoreceptor cells—the homologues of pinealocytes in nonmammalian species—especially to cell zones containing granular vesicles (GV), which are very abundant in these two species. On a cellular basis, the significance of this labeling is not clear and the interpretation of such autoradiographical results requires combination with other techniques (pharmacology, ultracytochemistry, etc.).

The most complete study on this problem has been performed in two nonmammalian species, the common lizard (150,151) and the parakeet (152). Although this review is devoted exclusively to mammals, we think it necessary to report these results, especially because they can give important information also applicable to mammals. In these species, the radioautographic reactions were regularly found in rudimentary photoreceptor cells, especially in the inner segment, the cell body, and its process. Silver grains were mainly observed in the regions of the perikaryon and the perivascular processes in which granular vesicles are found. Using (³H)-5-HTP as a precursor, after inhibition of the decarboxylation step or reserpine-induced depletion of 5-HT, the number of silver grains was significantly reduced and their distribution was diffuse in the cell. After inhibition of the oxidative deamination step with nialamide, the labeling was, on the contrary, considerably increased. The autoradiographic reaction in these two species is essentially located in cell zones containing GV. The argentaffin and chromaffin reactions (63,153) of certain neurons and endocrine cells reflect a high content of strong reducing compounds, such as catecholamines or serotonin. Depending on the fixative solution used, this cytochemical technique permits a study of the total amines or of indoleamine alone. Using this cytochemical reaction in the lizard and parakeet, a heavy silver precipitate occurs selectively over the GV in the pineal secretory rudimentary photoreceptor cells. A weak background staining was also seen in the form of small silver grains scattered diffusely in the remainder of the cytoplasm and the nucleus of the secretory rudimentary photoreceptor cells, as well as in all cellular components of adjacent cells. The presence of precipitates over GV reflects the presence of reducing compounds. As, using the

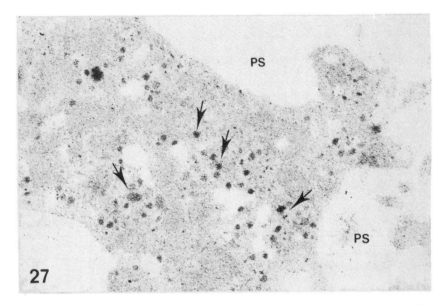

FIGURE 27. Nialimide-treated mouse. Positive argentaffin reaction over granular vesicles **(arrow)** in a pinealocyte process facing a perivascular space **(ps). mit** = mitochondria. (× 36,000.) *From Juillard and Collin (155), by courtesy, with permission of the publisher.*

technique of Falck and coworkers, Meiniel et al. (154) and Juillard and Collin (152) have observed that noradrenaline was present in sympathetic nerve fibers only, it is very probable that the results obtained indicate the presence of 5-HT in the GV. The use of drugs known to increase or decrease the level of 5-HT confirms this indication. After p-CPA treatment (inhibition of 5-HT synthesis), no selective accumulation of electron dense precipitates over GV was observed. On the contrary, nialamide treatment markedly increased the reducing capacity of GV, since they became more argentaffin- or chromaffin-positive than the controls. Also, after this treatment, the electron-dense precipitates accumulate selectively only over the GV.

Combining histochemical, autoradiographic, ultracytochemical, and pharmacological investigations, as previously outlined, Collin (147) arrived at the conclusion that in the pineal of at least the lizard and the parakeet, 5-HT is synthesized in the rudimentary photoreceptor cells and that the major part of the pool of 5-HT is stored in the GV. This 5-HT pool in the GV would be the consequence of a secondary local storage following its synthesis in the cytosol.

Although Juillard and Collin (155) have recently demonstrated that in the mouse part of the 5-HT present in the pinealocytes was located in the GV (Figure 27), it is difficult to generalize the findings obtained in the lizard and the parakeet to other nonmammalian species because of the lack of information relating to this problem. Moreover, it is necessary

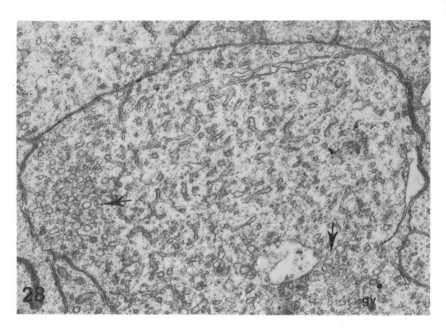

FIGURE 28. Club-shaped terminal of an offshoot of a pinealocyte. The branched tubular smooth endoplasmic reticulum and the accumulation of vesicles **(arrow)** pinched off from these tubulae have gray contents. **GV** = granular vesicle. (× 22,000.) *From Romijn (51), by courtesy.*

to be especially careful, because in most of the nonmammalian and mammalian species, GV are very scarce elements in the pinealocytes and because Sheridan and Sladek (156) observed that in the monkey serotonin is not GV-related. Possibly, the trapping of 5-HT by the GV depends on the number of GV in the cell and on the number of agranular binding sites of this indole (147). The finding of the presence of 5-HT in the GV of some species raises the question of the role of serotonin in the pineal. This will be examined in a subsequent section.

Concerning the other 5-HT derivatives, especially melatonin, until now very few results have been obtained and no sound proof has been given for the assumption that derivatives of 5-HT such as melatonin would be present in the GV (12,157–159). It should be mentioned, however, that Romijn (160), on the basis of pharmacological experiments in the rabbit, hypothesized that the smooth endoplasmic reticulum (Figure 28) would somehow be involved in indoleamine synthesis. Lin et al. (159) arrived at a similar conclusion in the hamster, noting that the enzyme HIOMT would be present in the smooth endoplasmic reticulum.

Using antibodies against melatonin, Freund et al. (161) obtained an immunoreaction that was restricted exclusively to some rat pineal cells in the cortical area of the pineal and that appeared only during the dark phase. This result, however, which was contradictory to that already

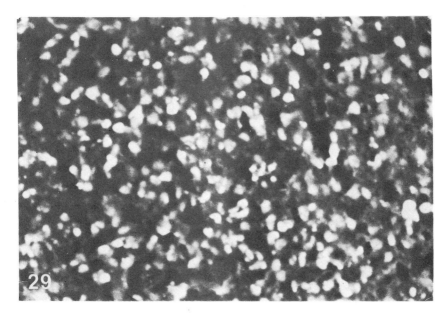

FIGURE 29. Immunohistochemical demonstration of melatonin in the mouse pineal. Most of the pinealocytes are fluorescent. (× 560.) *From Vivien-Roels et al. (163), by courtesy, with permission of the publisher.*

published by Bubenik et al. (162), was also not confirmed by Vivien-Roels et al. (163), who found immunoreactive cells throughout the gland in many mammalian species (Figure 29) during both the light and dark phases. As yet, the immunotechniques used do not permit us to identify exactly the cell population implicated in the formation and storage of melatonin. However, looking at the number of immunoreactive cells in the pineal of the different species studied (mouse, hamster, and rat), it is—in our opinion—very probable that these cells are pinealocytes.

Peptide/Protein Secretion in the Pineal Cells. *Fluorescence Histochemical Aspect.* Smith (164) and Smith et al. (165,166) reported that some rabbit and rat pinealocytes contain a yellow autofluorescent substance that was demonstrated to be a protein containing much tryptophan and that, according to Smith, could possibly be a carrier protein of pineal hormone(s). Later, a similar autofluorescent substance was also described in the hedgehog (81) and the mole (81,167). In this last mentioned species, compared to that in the rat, rabbit, and hedgehog, the quantity of autofluorescent material was very large (Figure 30). A comparison of the fluorescence histochemical observation with the ultrastructural one (81,167,168) suggests that this autofluorescent material could be identical with the proteinaceous material, or with a part of it, that is located in the cisterns of the granular endoplasmic reticulum (the "ependymallike"

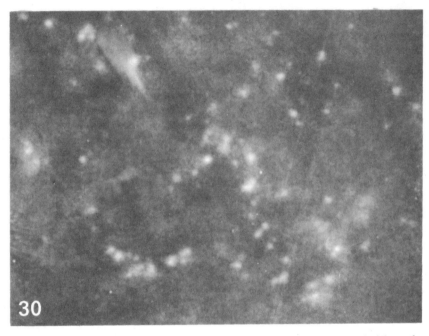

FIGURE 30. Autofluorescent material regularly dispersed in the pineal gland of the mole. (× 460.) *From Pévet et al. (167), with permission of the publisher.*

secretory process; see the following section). This view is supported by the fact that in the rat, after castration or injection of gonadotropins, both experiments that provoke an increase in number of vacuoles characteristic of the ependymallike secretory process (169–171), an increase in number of pinealocytes containing autofluorescent material has been described (81,172,173). However, this suggestion has to be verified.

Immunocytochemical Aspect. Using antibodies against vasotocin, α-melanocyte-stimulating hormone (α-MSH), LHRH, and somatostatin (174–177), a distinct population of stained cells are seen diffusely distributed throughout the gland (Figures 31 and 32). They are irregular in shape, showing long perivascular and intercellular processes. The morphological appearance and the distribution of the stained cells are similar after using all antibodies, suggesting that the latter stained a compound or compounds in the same cells; a suggestion proved to be true by means of serial sections (176). The nature of the immunocytochemically stained cells has not been determined, but the authors (176,178) consider the cells to be pinealocytes.

A comparison of the staining potentialities of different antibodies led us to the conclusion (95–97,175,176) that the immunoreaction obtained

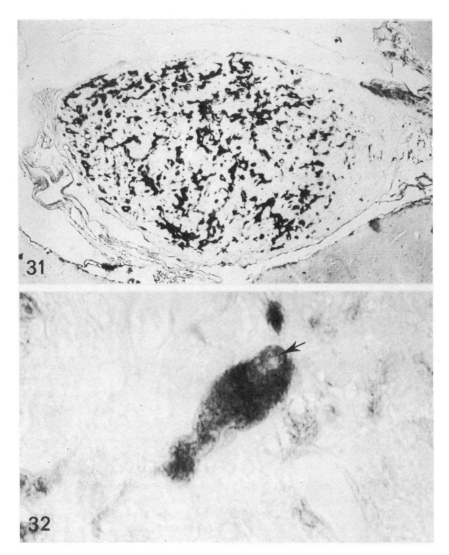

FIGURE 31. Sagittal section through the pineal gland of an adult Wistar rat immunocytochemically stained with an antiserum to AVT. The dark reaction product indicates the cells containing the AVT-like compound. (× 95.) *From Pévet et al. (176), with permission of the publisher.*

FIGURE 32. High magnification of an immunocytochemically stained cell body using an antibody against AVT. **Arrow** = nucleus. (× 800.) *From Pévet et al. (176), with permission of the publisher.*

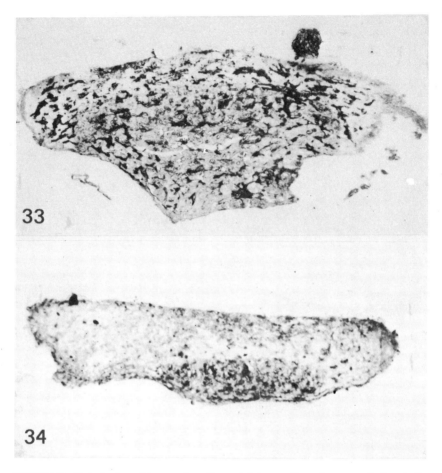

FIGURE 33. Pineal cultured in noradrenalin containing medium, immunocytochemically stained with an antibody against AVT. (× 125.) *From Pévet et al. (176), with permission of the publisher.*

FIGURE 34. Cultured pineal explant immunocytochemically stained with an antibody against AVT. Noradrenalin was not present in the medium. (× 125.) *From Pévet, unpublished data.*

was not due to either AVT, α-MSH, LHRH, or somatostatin, but to the presence of unidentified compounds with which the different antibodies would cross-react.

Using the organ culture technique, it could be demonstrated that this (these) unidentified compound(s) was (were) really synthesized by, and not concentrated in, the pineal (Figure 33) (176). This technique also showed that the synthesis of the compound was under the control of noradrenaline, the presence of this amine in the medium provoking an increase in the number of immunoreactive cells (Figures 33 and 34) (110). Interestingly, a preliminary ultrastructural study of culture explants under exactly the same conditions seems to indicate an increase in activity of the "ependymallike secretory" process (110).

Cytological Aspect. Glial cells and pinealocytes are the two types of cells present in the pineal of mammals. To date, however, cytological evidence for any secretory activity of the latter cell type has not been described. The observations made in this chapter thus exclusively concern the pinealocytes.

In most secretory processes involved in the production of peptidergic/proteinaceous substances, a common scheme is generally accepted. Protein biosynthesis takes place within the cisterns of the granular endoplasmic reticulum (GER), whereas the products of the synthesis are transported and packed in the Golgi saccules. Such a secretory process is also characteristic of the pinealocyte.

Another mechanism in the biosynthesis and release of proteinaceous material termed "ependymal secretion" has been described by many authors. Ependymal secretion is essentially characterized by the production of vacuoles by the cisterns of the granular endoplasmic reticulum (GER) without apparent intervention of the Golgi complex; the content of the vacuoles is released directly into the pericapillary or pericellular spaces or into the third ventricle. A similar mechanism—therefore also

FIGURE 35. Granular vesicles **(arrows)** in a pinealocyte process of an equatorial mammal, the Malaysian rat *(Rattus sabanus).* (× 25,000.) *From Pévet and Yadav (180), with permission of the publisher.*

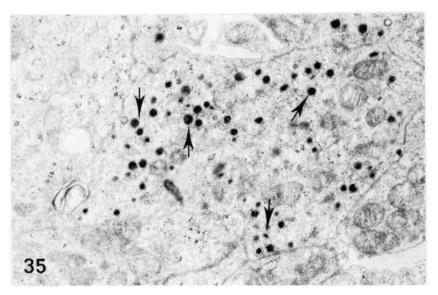

35

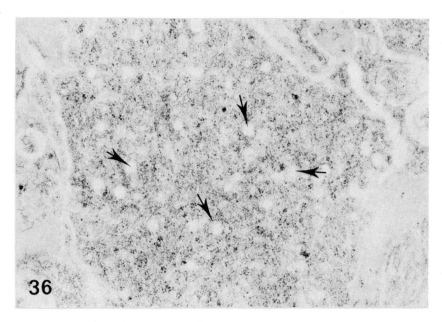

FIGURE 36. Ending of a mouse pinealocyte process after pronase treatment. Note the total extraction of the dense core of the granular vesicles **(arrows).** (× 22,000.) *From Juillard (179), by courtesy, with permission of the publisher.*

termed ependymallike secretory process (34)—is present in the pinealocyte (see details and references in ref. 35).

We will deal now in detail with these two different secretory processes, which can be closely related, at least in some species (35), and their regulation.

Granular vesicles (GV) have been observed in the pinealocytes of practically all mammalian species studied (34,35). After their formation, the GV migrate to the endings of the pinealocyte processes (Figure 35) to release their content into the perivascular space. Generally, excretion of the compound stored in the dense core, which is proteinaceous in nature as demonstrated in the hamster and the mouse (Figure 36) (179), appears to occur in situ by dissociation of the content of the GV (Figures 38–40). A release by exocytosis was, however, also clearly observed (Figure 37) (180,181). It is probable that, as with some other peptide-producing endocrine glands, such as the pancreas (182), both mechanisms are present, one being used for a continuous slow release and the other for an immediate and rapid one. The identification of the compounds (indoleamines?) implicated in the regulation of such a mechanism would be important.

The Golgi production of the GV (Figure 41) appeared to depend on different physiological conditions and on the integrity of the pineal sympathetic innervation. In cultured pineal of the hamster (183), rat (158,183), and rabbit (184), and in rat pineal tissue grafted under the kidney capsule (185)—experiments in which the pineal is evidently denervated—a drastic decrease in number of GV was observed in the pinealocyte. In contrast, Karasek (158), Romijn and Gelsema (184), and Haldar-Misra and Pévet (183) showed that addition of noradrenaline (NA) to the culture medium caused a marked numerical increase of GV. These observations have been confirmed in vivo by Lin et al. (159), who described a decrease in number of GV after pineal denervation by superior cervical ganglionectomy in the hamster, a result that was contested by Sheridan (186). Sheridan observed, in the same species and under the same experimental conditions as well as after destruction of the noradrenergic innervation by 6-hydroxydopamine injections, an increase in number of GV. Moreover, contrary to the observations in the hamster, rat, and rabbit, in the mouse pineal in vitro addition of NA to the medium provokes a drastic decrease in number of GV (187). From this it can be concluded that the formation of GV in the pinealocytes and, thus, the activity of the process of protein secretion characterized by the formation of GV are controlled by sympathetic innervation. The results obtained, however, indicate that this control is species-dependent and that, as in mice, activation of adrenergic innervation provokes an inhibition of this protein secretory process, whereas in the hamster, rat, and rabbit it provokes an activation. This difference in the effect of the sympathetic innervation could possibly explain some of the contradictory observations reported in the literature when relationships between light/dark periodicity and pineal function are considered.

Blinding or constant darkness is considered a prime stimulus for pineal activity, especially because such experimental procedures, via an activation of the sympathetic nervous system, provoke an increase in melatonin synthesis. Considering the protein secretory process as characterized by the formation of GV, after such treatment some authors (186,188) observed an increase in number of GV in the hamster, whereas others (135) described a decrease in the mouse. These opposite results agree with the in vitro observations described earlier. The results described in naturally blind animals are also contradictory. In the mole (168) and the mole-rat (124), GV are very rare, whereas in the golden moles *Amblysomus hottentotus* (145) and *Chrysochloris asiatica* (189) their number is exceptionally large. After constant illumination, a treatment that provokes inhibition of indoleamine formation by inhibition of sympathetic activity, a decrease in number of GV was clearly observed in the mouse (190) and rabbit (160), two species that react differently in the in vitro situation. According to Romijn (160), this decrease would be provoked by lack of free NA, the pinealocytic neurotransmitter. Continuous illumination would cause a sympatholysis by "photoinhibition," a result that is in accordance with the in vitro observation of the same author (184). Matsushima et al. (190) give a similar explanation for the results obtained in the mouse. This explanation, as well as this result, is in contradiction to the in vitro observations described previously (187). This contradiction, however, is perhaps more apparent than real. Matsush-

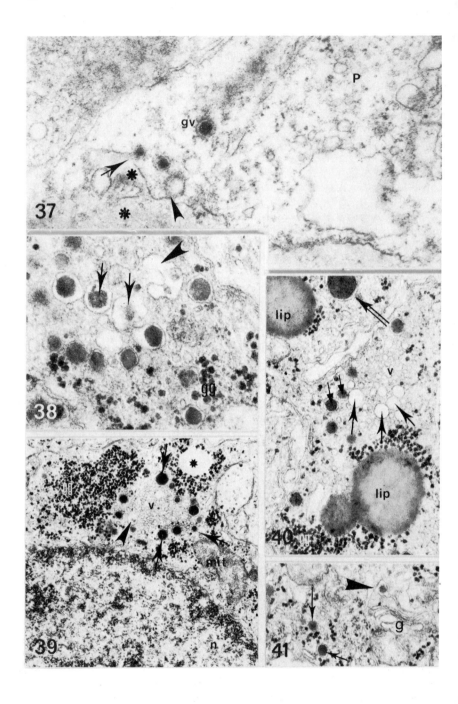

FIGURE 37. Malaysian rat *(Rattus sabanus)*. Micrograph suggesting that granular vesicles can be released (arrow) by exocytosis into the perivascular space (*). **Arrowhead** = image-indicating release of a large, clear vesicle; **GV** = granular vesicles; **P** = pinealocyte ending. (× 37,800.) *From Pévet and Yadav (180), with permission of the publisher.*

FIGURE 38. Granular vesicles in the golden mole *(Amblyosomus hottentotus)* pinealocyte. Note the apparent dissolution of the matrix **(arrows)** and the fragmentation of a vesicle after the dissolution of the matrix **(arrowhead)**. **gg** = glycogen granules. (× 59,500.) *From Pévet and Kuypers (145), with permission of the publisher.*

FIGURE 39. Part of a golden mole pinealocyte. Numerous small clear vesicles **(v)** are present between granular vesicles **(small arrows)**. The vesicles are associated with an accumulation of glycogen granules **(gg)** and a vacuole (*). Note also the presence of a granular vesicle, the matrix of which has almost completely disappeared **(arrowhead)**. **n** = nucleus. (× 22,100.) *From Pévet and Kuyper (145), with permission of the publisher.*

FIGURE 40. Golden mole pinealocyte. The clear vesicles **(large arrows)** seem to correspond to the granular vesicles **(small arrows)** after complete dissolution of their core. Note also the presence of numerous small clear vesicles **(v)** and of a very large granular vesicle (double arrow). **gg** = glycogen granules; **lip** = lipid droplet. (× 33,600.) *From Pévet and Kuyper (145), with permission of the publisher.*

FIGURE 41. Granular vesicle (arrowhead) visibly produced by a Golgi saccule in a golden mole pinealocyte. **Small arrow** = granular vesicles; **g** = Golgi complex. (× 28,000.) *From Pévet and Kuyper (145), with permission of the publisher.*

---

ima (190) indeed observed a decrease in number of GV after 35 days of continuous illumination, but an increase during the first 3 days of the experiment. This last result is in accordance with that obtained in the in vitro situation.

These data, obtained under various experimental conditions, seem to demonstrate that, if noradrenergic innervation of the pineal is implicated in the control of protein secretory processes, at least in those character-ized by the formation of GV, it is also evident that this control is a complicated one. Some of the contradictory results obtained could be explained by the fact that NA not only controls this process but also indoleamine metabolism in the pineal and that these indoles may reg-ulate this process (see following). Thus, a regulatory mechanism at dif-ferent levels may exist, a mechanism that may be complicated by the fact that other factors influence the formation of GV by the pinealocytes. For example, administration of gonadotropic hormones in the rat in vivo (170,171) or stimulation of cultured rat pineal explant by gonadotropic hormones or dibutyryl cAMP—a compound known to increase pineal activity (158,191)—provokes an increase in number of GV. All these results, although contradictory, suggest that the GV represent a major secretory product in packaged form, an idea that has now been accepted by most authors.

As already mentioned, blinding provokes a decrease in the number of GV in mice and an increase in the hamster. These opposite results were both interpreted as a consequence of the increase of the antigonadotropic activity of the pineal provoked by blinding, whereas the authors (186,192) suggested that GV could contain an antigonadotropic compound. Such a hypothesis, however, although attractive, does not explain most of the results reported in the literature.

Pineal grafted under the kidney capsule is always able to nullify the effect of pinealectomy on the estrous cycle (193); but under these conditions pinealocytes do not contain GV. A large amount of GV have been observed in the pinealocytes of the golden mole and of the Malaysian rat *(Rattus sabanus)*, species breeding throughout the year and in which antigonadotropic activity of the pineal cannot be envisaged (see details in 34,35,145,180). Moreover, in two seasonally breeding animals, the garden dormouse (194) and the cotton rat (195), an increase in the number of GV has been observed just during the period of sexual activity. These results do not fit with the idea that the GV would contain an antigonadotropic compound. It is evident that the GV contain a hormonal proteinaceous compound; but if this compound is involved in the antigonadotropic activity of the gland at all, its involvement is probably indirect. Another problem related to the possible presence of an antigonadotropic hormone in the GV is the fact that these cellular elements are rare in most of the species studied to date. With the exception of the hamster and the mouse—both animals living under artificial laboratory conditions—the golden hamster *(Amblysomus hottentotus* and *Chrysochloris asiatica)* and the Malaysian rat *(Rattus sabanus)*, in which their number is considerable, the GV are scarce elements in mammalian species. Most authors hold that this is due to a rapid turnover of the synthesis and release of the compound stored in the GV. It seems, however, difficult to accept (Pévet, 34,35,97) that the high turnover mentioned would be present in some animals but not in others.

In our opinion, the presence or absence of a large amount of GV has to be related to their physiological function. As already explained, it is now well known that the pineal gland participates in the control of seasonal reproduction, being an endocrine synchronizer between the annual variations of the environmental conditions and the gonadal axis. In all mammalian species living under natural conditions in temperate and polar regions so far examined—species that are seasonal breeders— the GV in the pinealocytes are rare. On the other hand, in three of the few equatorial/tropical mammalian species electronmicroscopically examined (the golden moles and the Malaysian rat)—species that are not subjected to large annual variations in daylength—numerous GV were observed in the pinealocytes. Until now, of all animals studied and living under natural conditions, the GV are most numerous in these three species only. These animals are constantly sexually active, as are the hamster and the mouse, two laboratory animals likewise characterized by a large amount of GV in the pinealocytes. Possibly, a relationship exists between the presence of a large number of GV in the pinealocytes

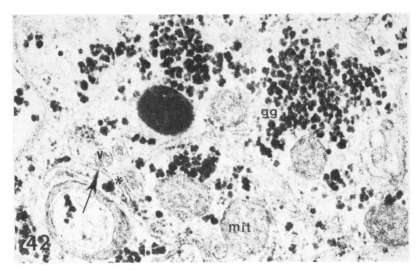

FIGURE 42. Formation **(arrow)** of a vacuole containing flocculent material **(v)** directly by a cistern of the granular endoplasmic reticulum **(*)** in the noctule bat *(Nyctalus noctala* pinealocyte. **mit** = mitochondria; **gg** – glycogen granule. (× 51,300.) *From Pévet et al. (125), with permission of the publisher.*

and the "lack of necessity" of the gland to synchronize the variation in daylength and sexual activity (34,180). Only a thorough knowledge of the biochemical nature of the content of the GV will enable us to verify the correlations observed. To date, however, the exact chemical nature of the substance present in the GV is unknown.

In the American mole, garden dormouse, hedgehog, mole, mole-rat, noctule bat, pipistrelle bat, and rat, a peculiar activity of the GER, leading either to the formation by the cisterns of vacuoles containing flocculent material of moderate electron density (Figures 42 and 43) or to an accumulation of material in its cisterns (Figures 44–47), has been observed (34,35). The proteinaceous nature of the content of these vacuoles has been demonstrated, at least in the mole (Figure 46) (196). As explained in detail earlier (34,35,96,97,117,197), the accumulation of proteinaceous material in the cisterns of the GER, which were observed in all fossorial blind mammals living in temperate zones, is probably the result of an exacerbation—provoked by the life in continuous darkness of these animals—of the secretory process characterized earlier and termed "ependymallike."

The observations made in the mole demonstrate that this process is complicated. In the pinealocytes of the adult mole, two types of accumulations of proteinaceous material (APM) occur in the cisterns of the GER: (1) lozenge-shaped APM, paracrystalline in structure, and (2) spherically shaped APM in which a crystalline organization is not apparent (168). These two types of APM are also present in the mole fetus

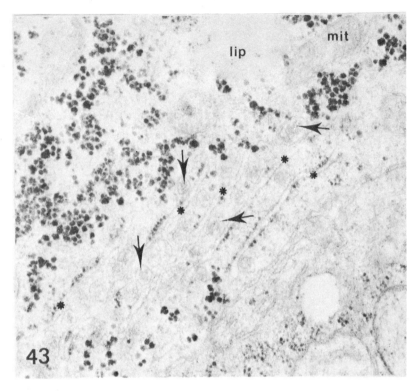

FIGURE 43. Parallel cisterns of the granular endoplasmic reticulum (*) between which many vacuoles containing flocculent material of a moderate electron density **(small arrows)** are present, in a noctule bat pinealocyte. **lip** = lipid droplets; **mit** = mitochondria. (× 45,000.) *From Pévet et al. (125), with permission of the publisher.*

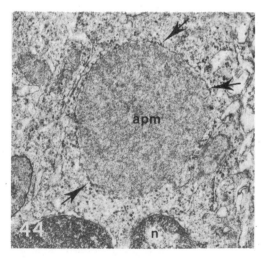

FIGURE 44. Accumulation of proteinaceous material **(apm)** completely occupying a cistern of the granular endoplasmic reticulum in a mole-rat pinealocyte. Ribosomes **(arrows)** on the membrane of the cistern. **n** = nucleus. (× 35,000.) *From Pévet et al. (124), with permission of the publisher.*

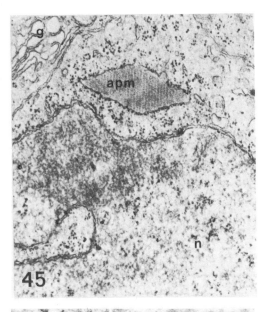

FIGURE 45. Accumulation of proteinaceous material presenting a typical paracrystalline aspect **(apm)** in a mole pinealocyte. **g** = Golgi apparatus. (× 27,680.) *From Pévet (168), with permission of the publisher.*

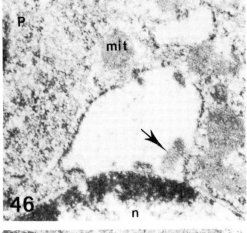

FIGURE 46. Mole pinealocyte after pronase treatment. In the material located between the two layers of the nuclear envelope, hydrolysis of the paracrystalline structure is incomplete **(arrow).** **mit** = mitochondria; **n** = nucleus; **p** = pinealocyte. (× 39,000.) *From Pévet (196), with permission of the publisher.*

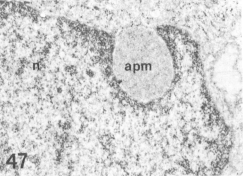

FIGURE 47. Accumulation of proteinaceous material **(apm)** between the two layers of the nuclear envelope in a mole-rat pinealocyte. **n** = nucleus. (× 17,500.) *From Pévet et al. (124), with permission of the publisher.*

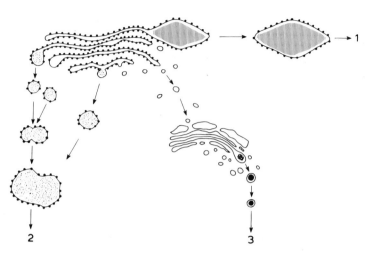

FIGURE 48. Schematic representation of the different secretory processes involved in the secretion of the proteinaceous compounds observed in the pinealocytes of the mole fetus. **(1)** Formation of an accumulation of proteinaceous material, with characteristic lozenge shape and paracrystalline structure, in a dilated ending of a cistern of the granular endoplasmic reticulum. **(2)** Vacuoles containing material budding off the cisterns of the granular endoplasmic reticulum and forming, by fusion or by increase in size, the second type of accumulation of proteinaceous material. **(3)** Concentration in the Golgi apparatus of material originating from the cistern of the granular endoplasmic reticulum and formation of granular vesicles by a budding-off process. In the mole fetus, these three morphological aspects of protein synthesis can be observed in the same pinealocyte. *From Pévet (197), with permission of the publisher.*

(197). The study in the fetus, however, demonstrates that these two types of APM differ in origin. This may indicate that the just mentioned two types of APM do not consist of the same kind of material. This is supported by the fact that paracrystalline APM, commonly found in the adult mole, was occasionally observed in the fetus, the noncrystalline APM being dominant. As the pinealocytes also contain GV, the fetal mole appears to release three fractions (Figure 48) (197). This raises the question of the possible relationships between the process characterized by the formation of GV and the "ependymallike" secretory process. In the garden dormouse, hedgehog, and rat, as in the mole, both processes are present in the same cell population and even in the same cell.

Recently, it has been suggested that the different biological activities of the mammalian pineal would depend on an unknown compound, a large-molecular common precursor that is cleaved to give rise to a number of small-molecular, biologically active peptidic compounds (95,176). It could be that these different secretory processes represent the morphological basis of this phenomenon. Such a system does not exist in some species such as the mole-rat, the noctule bat, and the pipistrelle bat, since each of the two secretory processes is specific for a special population of pinealocytes. The activities of this "ependymallike" secretory process in pinealocytes seem to be specifically influenced by the endocrine activities of the gonadal axis.

In the mole, a parallelism between this synthetic activity of the pinealocytes and the hormonal production of the gonadal axis has been established (198). Accumulation of proteinaceous material in the pinealocytes of the garden dormouse has been observed during the natural period of anestrus (winter, during hibernation) and also during experimentally induced anestrus (194,199). In the hedgehog, vacuoles containing such material have been described between the cisterns of the GER, both at the beginning of the period of sexual quiescence (81,200,201) and at the beginning of the period of an experimentally provoked decrease in sexual activity (202). After administration of gonadotropic hormone—human chorionic gonadotropin (HCG) and Pregnant Mare Serum Gonadotropin (PMSG), formation by the cisterns of the GER of a large amount of vacuoles containing flocculent material has been observed in rat pinealocytes (169). A similar observation was made in rat pinealocytes after castration (170,171). According to Karasek and Marek (169), this activation could also be due to enhanced gonadotropic hormone levels provoked by the operation. Under natural conditions, the secretory process of such pinealocytes appears to be enhanced in the European mole, the American mole, and the Yugoslavian and Israeli mole-rats, whose pineal activity, which is probably antigonadotropic (81), is stimulated by their subterranean life. An "ependymallike" secretory process has also been observed in the noctule bat and pipistrelle bat, which, being nocturnal animals, can be supposed to have a very active pineal gland. It thus seems that the "ependymallike" secretory process, by which material of a proteinaceous nature is produced, plays an important role in pineal physiology. However, in this case also, only chemical identification of the proteinaceous content of these vacuoles will permit a determination of its exact function.

Relationships Between Indoleamines and the Protein Secretory Processes. The pineal is engaged in both the metabolism of indoleamines and the production of proteinaceous material (147,203). A possible relationship between these two pineal products thus has to be considered. The indoleamines produced in the pinealocytes may intracellularly influence the formation, storage, and/or release of pineal peptide effector compounds as could the indoleamines released from the retina, Harderian gland, and intestines (see details in refs. 16,204–206), which may reach the pineal via the general circulation.

Very few data related to this problem have been reported, and most of them concern melatonin and serotonin. Experimentally, it has been demonstrated that injection of 5-HT during the period of sexual activity in the hedgehog provokes, next to an inhibition of sexual activity, the formation in the pinealocytes of vacuoles containing flocculent material as characterized by the "ependymallike" secretory process (202). Melatonin chronically administered in the hamster causes an increase in the number of GV (207). A single injection of 25 µg of melatonin provokes a decrease in the number of GV in the endings of the mouse pinealocyte processes. Melatonin, administered in daily intraperitoneal doses of 50 µg over a period of 5 days was observed to increase markedly the number of GV in the terminal endings of pinealocyte processes during the light period, but led, during the dark period, to a decrease in their number to a level below that of diluent-treated controls (208). Pinealocytes of melatonin-treated rats are characterized by an increased number of microtubules, structures that are involved in secretory processes in a variety of cells (209). The ultrastructural results all suggest that exogenously administered melatonin or 5-HT, which reach the pineal via the general circulation, influences the pineal secretory process involved in protein synthesis.

The intracellular relationship of indoleamines with protein synthesis in pineal cells has been studied mainly in nonmammalian species. Autoradiographical, histochemical, ultracytochemical, and pharmacological investigations have shown that in the parakeet and the lizard 5-HT coexists with a proteinaceous compound in the GV (see earlier). In mammals, Juillard and Collin (155), combining different techniques, concluded that GV in mouse pinealocytes also contain 5-HT. However, in contrast to the parakeet and the lizard, in which most of the 5-HT is concentrated in the GV, in the mouse only a small part of the 5-HT pool is taken up by these vesicles (155). After an ultracytochemical study, Lu and Lin (210) also concluded that in the hamster 5-HT is present in the GV of pinealocytes.

The obvious presence of 5-HT in the GV of some species raises the question of the role of 5-HT in the pineal. Clearly, possible relationships between 5-HT and proteinaceous compounds (hormones?) have to be examined. In numerous cells that produce a polypeptidergic hormone, such as calcitonin by the thyroid parafollicular cells, there is a concomitant presence of the hormone and of 5-HT in the GV, whereas a functional interrelationship has been proved to exist between the two compounds. It can be suggested, also, that in the GV of pinealocytes or of rudimentary photoreceptor cells, at least in some species, 5-HT is linked with a proteinaceous hormone, both compounds being released together into the circulation, or that 5-HT would be implicated in some stage in the process of synthesis, storage, or release of the proteinaceous hormones. This situation recalls the case present in some endocrine cells, APUD cells, or paraneurons (see details in ref. 211).

Serotonin having been detected in the GV of the pinealocytes in some species, it is logical to assume, as was indeed suggested by many authors, that derivatives of 5-HT, such as melatonin, would also be present in the GV and would also be implicated in the synthesis and release of proteinaceous hormones. No sound proof for the presence of any 5-HT derivatives in GV has been given to date, but some experiments (212) demonstrate that melatonin, 5-methoxytryptophan, and 5-methoxyindole-3-acetic acid could also be implicated in the control of the release process of the GV content.

OTHER CELL ORGANELLES

Many cell organelles, such as smooth and rough endoplasmic reticulum, subsurface cisterns, annulate lamellae, mitochondria, ribosomes, Golgi apparatus, multivesicular bodies, centrioles, cilia, microtubules, microfilaments, vesicle-crowned rodlets, lipid inclusions, glycogen granules, and pigment granules have been described in the pinealocytes of many species. Evidently, all these organelles are involved in pinealocyte activity. However, it is difficult, if not impossible in the frame of the present chapter, to review all the information accumulated in recent years. Details on granular endoplasmic reticulum and Golgi apparatus, as well as on their production have been given in the preceding section. We will concentrate our analysis on those cell organelles that, to us, seem of primary importance for the secretory or physiological activity of the pinealocyte. For details concerning the other structures, such as accumulations of material between two cisterns of the GER, annulate lamellae and related structures, centrioles, ciliary structures, microfilaments, microtubules and subsurface cisterns, we refer to Pévet (34,35) and especially to Vollrath (9).

Concentric Lamellae. Concentric lamellae, or membrane whorls (Figure 49), are observed in some mammalian species, both under natural and experimental conditions. Similarly organized reticular formations have been described in many cell types, particularly in endocrine glands (details and references in refs. 34,35). Although the function of these structures in the endocrine cells is enigmatic, most authors (213–215) infer that their formation is in some way related to secretory activity. That such membrane whorls are rather abundant in animals living under natural conditions, especially in nocturnal or fossorial ones (124,125), and that the same holds for the infertile diabetic mutant mouse, but not for the littermate controls (216), suggests that these structures occur in pinealocytes that display increased secretory activity. Their formation in the hedgehog supports this opinion. During the period of progressive decrease of sexual activity at the end of September until the middle of December (western part of France), the pinealocytes show the formation and differentiation of a peculiar reticular structure that is composed of membranous lamellae consisting of granular endoplasmic reticulum and of many vacuoles containing flocculent material (Figure 50) (81,201). The membranous whorls are the final stage of the development of this system. The first stages of this development, which are also experimentally reproducible (202), are characterized by the formation of vacuoles containing flocculent material. Such vacuoles are typical of the "ependymallike" secretory processes described earlier. These observations prove, at least in the hedgehog, that the whorl structures correspond to an increase of pinealocyte synthetic activity.

If, as earlier suggested, the "ependymallike" secretory process is, indeed, involved in the production of a hormonal compound by the pinealocytes, the whorllike transformation of the endoplasmic reticulum

48

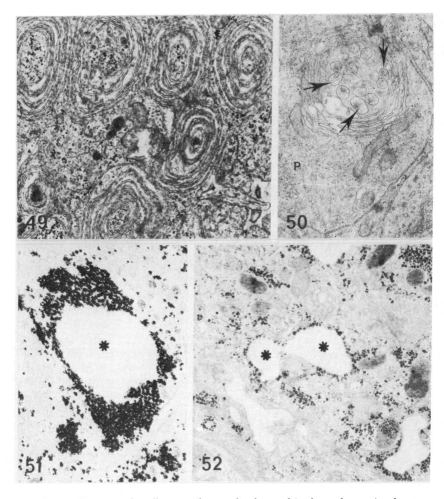

FIGURE 49. Concentric lamellae very frequently observed in the mole rat pinealocytes. (× 22,000.) *From Pévet et al. (124), with permission of the publisher.*

FIGURE 50. Numerous vacuoles containing flocculent material **(arrow)** in the middle of a system composed of circular cisterns of granular endoplasmic reticulum in a pinealocyte of a hedgehog, sacrificed during the period of decrease of sexual activity. **P** = pinealocyte. (× 24,600.) *From Pévet and Saboureau (201), with permission of the publisher.*

FIGURE 51. Part of a noctule bat pinealocyte stained for glycogen (periodic acid–thiocarbohydrazide–silver proteinate staining). A vacuole **(*)** lies in the center of an accumulation of glycogen granules. (× 20,000.) *From Pévet, unpublished data.*

FIGURE 52. Two vacuoles probably fusing **(*)** in the cytoplasm of a noctule bat pinealocyte. (× 21,000.) *From Pévet et al. (125), with permission of the publisher.*

could be the consequence of antigonadotropic secretory activity of the pinealocytes, as was earlier suggested (81,200). This is supported by some literature data. Roux et al. (217) observed an increase in number of whorllike structures in the pinealocytes of the dormouse during sexual quiescence. In hamsters, blinded for 6 weeks, the pineal manifests antigonadotropic effects (218,219), whereas in similar conditions an increase of whorllike structures in hamster pinealocytes has been observed (220). It is thus probable that the whorllike structures in mammalian pinealocytes are involved in the synthesis or secretion of an active compound. A time study of the formation of these peculiar elements has been realized only in the hedgehog (see earlier). Although some profiles in the noctule bat (figure 22 in Pévet et al., 125) and in the rat (figure 2 in Karasek and Marek, 169) resemble those observed in the hedgehog, a similar process has never been described in other mammalian species.

Glycogen and Vacuolar System. Histochemical and ultrastructural studies on the distribution of glycogen granules in the pineal have been made in numerous species, including the goat, horse, mouse, pig, noctule bat (Figure 51), human, monkey, golden mole, mole-rat, and rabbit (see details and references in 34,35,221). The exact function of glycogen metabolism and its relationship with other pinealocyte biochemical activities remain, as yet, unknown, but these appear to depend on different physiological conditions. Circadian level changes, showing a peak at the beginning of the dark period, have been found in mice (222–224). Continuous darkness and short- and long-term continuous illumination are all experimental conditions under which the glycogen content in the mouse (225,226), as well as the rat (227), is modified. The nocturnal decrease of glycogen concentration in the pineal of mammals appears also to be controlled by noradrenergic innervation (228). In species exposed to low environmental lighting, such as the mole-rat, golden mole, and noctule bat, glycogen was found to be especially abundant. A similar observation has also been made in some nocturnal blind mammalian and nonmammalian species (142–144). Glycogen granules in the noctule bat (122,125) and the golden mole (145) morphologically appear to be involved in the formation of intracellular vacuoles (Figures 52 and 56), which are formed by dilations of cisterns of the GER. Such dilation seems to be preceded by a morphological association between glycogen and the cisterns of the GER, at least in the golden mole (145). Lipids also seem of basic importance in this vacuolar formation, as suggested by the integration of some lipid droplets in the vacuoles observed in the golden mole (Figure 56) (145). Perhaps these large vacuoles in the pinealocytes represent the site of storage and of maturation of some secretory products.

A different vacuolar system has been described in some other mammals such as the garden dormouse, golden mole, hamster, hedgehog, noctule bat, and pipistrelle bat (see references in ref. 34). This is characterized by the formation of a single, very large vacuole that occupies

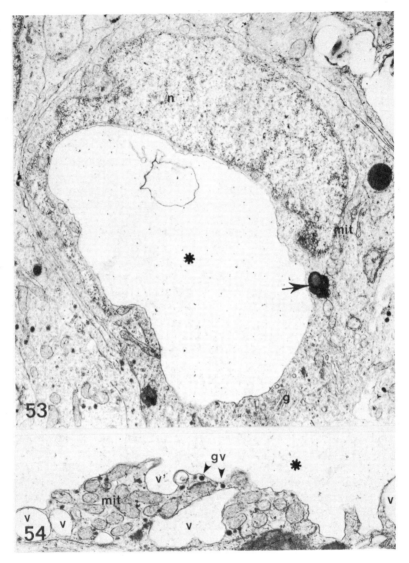

FIGURE 53. Vacuolated pinealocyte of a male hedgehog. The vacuole is large **(*)** but does not occupy the cell completely Lipids **(arrow)**, Golgi complex **(g)**, mitochondria **(mit)** are present in the remaining cytoplasm. **n** = nucleus of vacuolated pinealocyte. (× 15,300.) *From Pévet (229), with permission of the publisher.*

FIGURE 54. Larger magnification of part of the cytoplasm in a vacuolated pinealocyte from a male hedgehog. Many small vacuoles **(v)** and granular vesicles **(gv)** are present in the cytoplasm. The small vacuoles appear to fuse **(v')** with the large vacuole **(*)**. mit = mitochondria. (× 17,800.) *From Pévet (229), with permission of the publisher.*

the cell almost completely (Figure 53). These vacuoles appear to be formed by an increase in size of a primary vacuole originating from a cistern of the GER, due to its confluence with smaller vacuoles often observed next to the large one (Figure 54) (details in ref. 229). The nature and function of these vacuoles cannot easily be explained.

The scarcity of such vacuoles in the majority of the animals studied might suggest that they are due to cell degeneration. However, the presence of many vacuolated pinealocytes in the female mole during the proestrous phase (198) points to a physiological relationship between changes at the level of the pituitary-gonadal axis and this vacuolization. The observation of Welsh and Reiter (230) that the number of vacuolated pinealocytes increases with age, and that their formation is prevented by superior cervical ganglionectomy at 1 month of age, also demonstrates that their importance in the physiological activity of the pineal is beyond doubt. Further investigations are necessary, however, to understand completely the formation and function of this vacuolar system.

Mitochondria. Mitochondria are structures present in all eukaryotic cells. Their significance in cellular metabolism is well known. They are energy-transducing systems. Beside this "classic" function as "energy centers," mitochondria are also known, depending on the cells concerned, to contain numerous enzymes. In the pinealocyte, for example, the conversion of tryptophan to 5-hydroxytryptophan, due to the presence of the enzyme tryptophan 5-hydroxylase, takes place in the mitochondria (148).

Mitochondria are generally considered randomly dispersed within the cell body. However, a distribution of mitochondria in what could be called the supranuclear region of the pinealocytes, reminiscent of the situation in photoreceptor cells, has been clearly depicted in the pinealocytes of the mole (Figure 25) (121) and noctule bat (Figure 55) (122). A similar distribution of mitochondria in some pinealocytes seems evident in the rat (123) and the guinea pig (133), when looking at the illustrations presented by the authors. This nonrandom distribution of the mitochondria in some pinealocytes points to the phylogenetic relationship of the mammalian pinealocytes to pineal photoreceptor cells of lower vertebrates.

Different types of mitochondria observed in the pinealocytes, and their internal structure, have been described in detail by Vollrath (9). We refer the reader to this work for more details, and we will concentrate our analysis on the changes described after experimental procedures. Romijn et al. (149), for example, observed, in vitro, a spherical enlargement of the mitochondria in the "light" pinealocytes of the rabbit after addition of p-chlorophenylalanine, an inhibitor of tryptophan-5-hydroxylase. According to these authors, and comparing the observations of Hori et al. (148) cited earlier, this enlargement suggests that mitochondria are somehow involved in 5-HT synthesis. The authors (149) hypothesize that hydroxylation of tryptophan to 5-hydroxytryptophan takes place in the

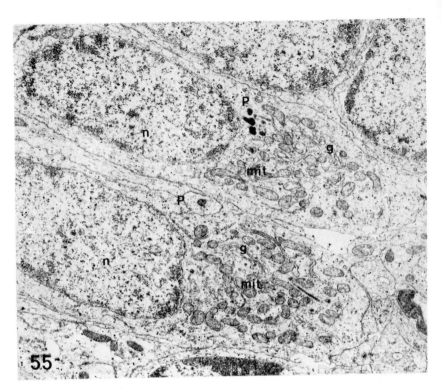

FIGURE 55. Pinealocytes **(P)** of noctule bat characterized by a polarity in the distribution of mitochondria **(mit). n** = nucleus; **g** = Golgi apparatus. (× 10,500.) *From Pévet et al. (122), with permission of the publisher.*

mitochondria, whereas the conversion of 5-hydroxytryptophan to 5-HT occurs freely in the cytosol. The enlargement of the mitochondria after such treatment could be explained as a compensatory reaction to inhibition of tryptophan-5-hydroxylase located on the mitochondrial membrane. Clementi et al. (231) observed a decrease in the number of mitochondria in the pinealocytes of rats treated systematically with estrogen and an increase after implantation of estrogen in the median eminence. The same authors also described an increase in size of the mitochondria after castration. This last-mentioned result was confirmed by Karasek et al. (170) who observed, moreover, an increase in the number of mitochondria, especially evident as regards tigroidlike mitochondria. Similar observations were made after gonadotropic hormone treatment either in vivo or in vitro (169,191). Despite this information, we should realize that nothing substantial from a functional point of view has been reported. Evidently, mitochondria in pinealocytes need more attention.

Lipid Droplets. Lipid droplets are present in most animal cells. Like mitochondria, they are probably involved in the general cell metabolism.

No lipid compounds characteristic of pineal tissue have been chemically isolated or identified (221).

In the majority of species examined by means of histochemistry and cytology, the number of lipid droplets was small (see list and references in ref. 9). Large amounts of lipid droplets, however, were observed in rat and ground-squirrel pinealocytes (232). They have been considered "secretory products" by earlier investigators (see references in Quay, 221).

Histochemical, histological, and ultrastructural studies have shown that the lipid content of the pineal shows changes under various physiologic conditions. Fluctuation in number of lipid droplets occurs in mammalian pinealocytes under various conditions of illumination (233), during different phases of the estrous cycle (234), and under certain hormonal conditions (235). This observation has been confirmed at the ultrastructural level by Karasek's group. After injection of gonadotropic hormones (169) or after orchidectomy, followed or not by administration of LHRH (170), an increase in number of lipid droplets was observed, whereas after hypophysectomy their number decreased (118). Administration of p-chlorophenylalanine, a 5-HT-depleting agent, led to a distinct reduction in the electron density of the lipid inclusions (236). This result is interesting, because it supports the earlier concept that lipid droplets may contain 5-HT and melatonin (237), two lipid-soluble substances. This concept has recently been revived by the observation of Roux and collaborators that liposomes are very abundant in the female garden dormouse during sexual quiescence, either naturally or experimentally induced (194,199,238,239) and that they are reduced in size and number in sexually active animals. The same group (240) observed that during winter the development of liposomes paralleled the increase in indoleamine content, an observation that led these authors to suggest that liposomes might be involved in an indoleaminergic, antigonadotropic pineal secretory process.

All these observations indicate that lipid droplets could be either directly or indirectly involved in the process of synthesis and/or secretion by the pinealocytes. This opinion is supported by the observation that liposomes are morphologically involved in the formation of a vacuolar system as described in some mammals (Figure 56) and occasionally associated with membranes of the GER or mitochondria (123,127,241).

Vesicle-Crowned Rodlets. Vesicle-crowned rodlets (VCR) have been observed in practically all species investigated. They consist of an electron-dense rod surrounded by a single layer of small vesicles and lie singly or in groups, very often close to the cell membrane (Figures 57 and 58). In analogy to the synaptic ribbons present in the photoreceptor cells of the retina and the pineal of lower vertebrates, most authors (9) logically call these organelles "synaptic ribbons." In photoreceptor cells, synaptic ribbons, which show generally an axodendritic orientation, form part of a complex of other morphological features characterizing a true synaptic junction, such as a pre- and postsynaptic thickening and fila-

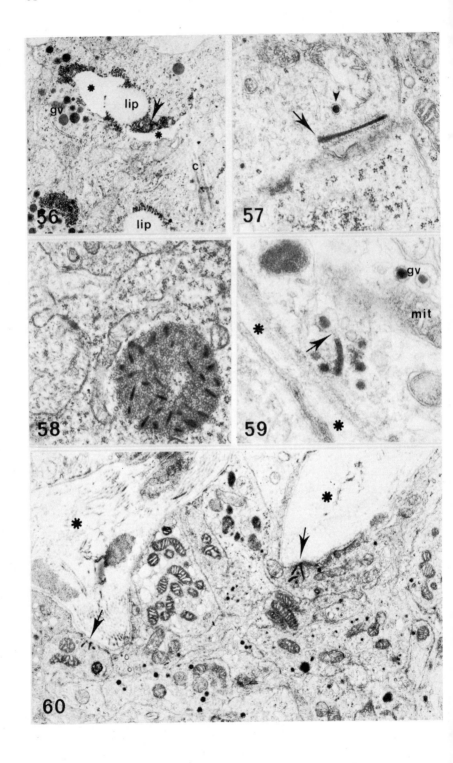

FIGURE 56. Complex formed by two vacuoles (dilated cisterns of the granular endo-plasmic reticulum) (*), accumulation of glycogen granules (arrow), granulated vacuoles (gv), and lipid droplet (lip) in a golden mole pinealocyte. c = ciliary structure. (× 21,000.) *From Pévet and Kuyper (145), with permission of the publisher.*

FIGURE 57. Vesicle-crowned rodlet (arrow) lying parallel to the plasma membrane in a Malaysian rat pinealocyte. **Arrow head** = granular vesicle. (× 31,000.) *From Pévet and Yadav (180), with permission of the publisher.*

FIGURE 58. Concentration of vesicle-crowned rodlets observed in the pinealocytes of the baboon *(Papio ursinus)* during the dark phase of a circadian light-dark cycle. (× 27,000.) *From Theron, unpublished data, by courtesy.*

FIGURE 59. Probable attachment of a granular vesicle (arrow) to the rodlet of a vesicle-crowned rodlet structure in a Malaysian rat pinealocyte. * = perivascular space; **gv** = granular vesicles; **mit** = mitochondrion. (× 42,000.) *From Pévet and Yadav (180), with permission of the publisher.*

FIGURE 60. Pinealocyte processes in the Malaysian rat. Note the large number of granular vesicles and, especially, the vesicle-crowned rodlets (arrows) close to the perivascular space (*) (× 15,500.) *From Pévet and Yadav (180), with permission of the publisher.*

---

mentous material present in the synaptic cleft. In mammals, an asso-ciation with other structures typical of a true synaptic connection has never been observed. Due to this fact, we prefer not to use the term "synaptic ribbons," which implies a physiological role similar to that of true synaptic ribbons that, although possible, is not demonstrated. In accordance with Arstila (127) and Collin (3,4) we use the term "vesicle-crowned rodlet," by which a specific function a priori is not implied.

In the past years, vesicle-crowned rodlets have attracted special at-tention, not only because they are possibly phylogenetic relics (4), re-minders of the original neurosensory function of the cells, but also be-cause they have been shown to react under various experimental and physiological conditions. Their number, as well as their size and location in the cell, seems to depend on environmental lighting conditions. Pineal glands of the guinea pig (242), gerbil (129), and rabbit (160), kept under continuous illumination, showed a large increase in number of VCR. Moreover, in the guinea pig, Vollrath and Huss (242) observed that, in continuous light, a higher percentage of VCR is found bordering the cell membrane than in animals kept under a lighting schedule of 14-hours illumination and 10-hours darkness. In mammals subjected to a lighting schedule of 12L/12D, different results concerning the VCR have been described. In the pinealocytes of the guinea pig, a decrease in number of VCR was observed during the first two-thirds of the light period, and an increase in the last third of the light period and during darkness (243). A similar circadian rhythm has also been demonstrated in the baboon (244) and the rat (245,246). Such a rhythm, however, does not persist in in vitro conditions, as demonstrated by Karasek and Vollrath (247). In the rat, Vollrath et al. (248) have also described an additional 7-day-cycle, whereas in the dormouse, Richoux et al. (138) observed an annual cycle in the number of VCR. The observation that VCR numbers are small during the day and large during the night suggests that the rhythm of the VCR is cued by environmental lighting mediated by the amount of noradrenaline released from sympathetic nerve fibers known to regulate pineal function (11,64). It appears, however, that VCR are only partly dependent on environmental factors such as photic stimuli. This is indicated by the fact that in guinea pigs (243) VCR increased in number prior to the onset of darkness, whereas the noradrenaline content of the gland is directly related to the period of environmental lighting, increasing throughout the dark period and decreasing throughout the light period (249). In the blinded rat, a regular circadian rhythm in the number of VCR has been observed after a period of readjustment (250). As noted by Vollrath (243), it thus appears that the amount of VCR varies according to an endogenous rhythm that, perhaps, is synchronized by environmental lighting conditions.

The number of VCR also seems to be controlled by various other factors. After orchidectomy (251) or orchidectomy followed by administration of LHRH (170), a considerable increase in number of VCR was observed in rat pinealocytes. A similar increase occurs in the gerbil (129) and in the rabbit (160) after sympathectomy. This last-mentioned observation, however, is in contrast to earlier findings in the rat (127) in which no change in number of VCR was observed after ganglionectomy. Arstila et al. (252) also found a disappearance of VCR in rat pinealocytes in vitro. This result was not confirmed by Karasek (251) who, on the contrary, observed a large increase in number of VCR under, apparently, the same conditions.

Pregnancy (133,253), immobilization stress (254), naturally occurring sterility (253), and cold (255) have also been shown to increase the number of VCR in mammalian pinealocytes.

All these observations suggest that the VCR of the mammalian pinealocytes represent cell organelles of a definite, but as yet unrevealed, functional significance. The fact that (1) in most mammalian species the VCR are located close to the cell membrane of one pinealocyte and almost exclusively face the cell membrane of an adjacent pinealocyte, that (2) in most mammalian species they are not topographically related to blood vessels, and that (3) nerve fibers responsible for the regulation of pinealocyte function do not contact all of the pinealocytes, has induced Vollrath and Huss (242) to suggest that the VCR are involved in the intercellular communication between adjacent pinealocytes. In another paper, Vollrath (243) elaborated on his concept, stating that the VCR could possibly be excitatory structures, altering the physicochemical properties of neighboring pinealocytes. As a result, the secretory activity of the pineal gland as a whole would be increased. The VCR might induce changes in the activity of enzymes involved in melatonin synthesis (details in ref. 243). Since pinealocyte activity is closely related to environmental lighting conditions, and since the VCR increase in number prior to the onset of darkness (at least in the guinea pig, 243), and darkness enhances pineal activity (18,64), it seems that VCR are an essential prerequisite for enhancing the secretory activity of the gland. Vollrath and Huss (242) also thought that the VCR cell-membrane complex could represent part of a true synapse and that the pinealocytes possessing VCR would not, or would not exclusively, be endocrine in nature but neuronal or neuroendocrine, in the sense that they would combine neuronal and endocrine properties (256). The VCR could establish circuits between adjacent pinealocytes, similar to neuronal circuits, and play a role in neuroendocrine integration. Vollrath's general concept appears very attractive and is generally accepted by other authors. Some results reported in the literature, however, apparently do not fit with this concept and indicate that the problem is more complicated.

In the Malaysian rat *(Rattus sabanus)* (180), for example, most of the VCR observed in the pinealocytes lie perpendicular to portions of the cell membrane in direct contact with the perivascular space (Figure 60). So far, *Rattus sabanus* is the only mammalian species in which such a location of the VCR has been found. However, it should be noted that in a nonmammalian species, the turtle *(Podocnemys unifilis)*, VCR have also been "extremely frequently" observed in such a close proximity to the perivascular space (257). This special location suggests that, rather than being implicated in intercellular contacts, VCR might release substances into the systemic circulation, thus supporting the supposition of Karasek (251) that VCR possibly play a role in the secretory activity of pinealocytes. The VCR located close to the perivascular space are also very often associated with GV (Figure 59). This suggests that VCR may also be implicated in some way in the release mechanism of the contents of the GV.

For a complete understanding of the function of the VCR, it would be important to know their origin, formation, and chemical composition. According to Vollrath (243), "the absence of any structure which could be regarded as a precursor of synaptic ribbons (VCR) suggests that the actual process of formation, as far as the morphological side is concerned, is very rapid and inconspicuous." Negative reactions for glucose-6-phosphate and thiamine pyrophosphate at the level of the vesicles of the VCR, with positive reactions obtained in the smooth and rough endoplasmic reticulum (258), indicate that the VCR do not originate from either of these reticula. However, in the baboon (244) it appears as though the vesicles of the VCR originate from the smooth endoplasmic reticulum. In rat pinealocytes, microtubules and microtubular sheaths were not infrequently found in the vicinity of the VCR (251). The author feels that microtubular sheaths arising from centrioles may be precursors of VCR.

Concerning the chemical composition of the VCR, it appears that they do not show acetylcholinesterase activity, which proves that they are not cholinergic (69,127). According to Krštić (258), in mammals the vesicles associated with the ribbons yield a negative reaction to biogenic amines. This suggests that they are also not adrenergic. Krštić (258) observed that the vesicles give a negative reaction for thiamine pyrophosphate and were not found to be associated with detectable concentrations of sodium (Na) or calcium (Ca). Since, in true synaptic vesicles, a clearly positive thiamine pyrophosphate reaction (259) and the presence of Na or Ca can be demonstrated, the results of Krštić (258) prove that the VCR possess a functional mechanism that differs from that of true synaptic vesicles. This justifies our terminology, vesicle-crowned rodlets (VCR), instead of synaptic ribbons.

Although the true nature and function of the VCR have not yet been determined, it is clear that they are, physiologically speaking, very important cell organelles. However, although they have been observed in practically all mammalian species studied, it should be realized that these cellular elements are rare in most pinealocytes. With the exception of the guinea pig, baboon *(Papio ursinus)* (Figure 58), and Malaysian rat *(Rattus sabanus,)* in which their number is very considerable, and the rat and rabbit, in which it is less but still rather large, the VCR are scarce elements. In some mammals, such as the hedgehog and the mole, their number is so small that it is difficult to ascribe a role to these structures (81,168,201).

Is the presence or absence of a large amount of VCR related to a physiological process? To date it is not possible to answer this question. However, looking at the species characterized by the presence of a large amount of VCR, it appears that both the baboon and the Malaysian rat are tropical/equatorial species and that the third one, the guinea pig, is a domestic species obtained from a wild species originating from the tropical/equatorial zone of South America. The number of equatorial/tropical species studied is still too small to draw any conclusion from this possible correlation, but, again, this demonstrates the importance of comparative studies on the organ in different biotopes.

Calcareous Concretions (Corpora Arenacea). The presence of calcareous concretions (Figures 61 and 62) in the mammalian pineal is a well-known feature. They are found in a number of species such as the fruit bat *(Eidolon helvum)* (110), gerbil (260), goat, horse, gnu, mink, mule, ox, pig, and human (9,221). In the literature, these pineal concretions have a long history. For a long time they have been held as signs of pineal atrophy and involution in man and have been related to age changes and states of disease (221). It is now evident, although not always accepted, that calcification is a normal, rather than a pathological, process and that neither the morphology nor the activity of several enzymes (249) of the pinealocytes is altered by the presence of calcified inclusions.

In the gerbil, the formation of calcareous concretions and their increase in number appear to run exactly parallel to those of the vacuoles in the pinealocytes as earlier described. According to Welsh and Reiter (230) and Japha et al. (260), these concretions originate from vacuolated pinealocytes. During the secretory process, the pinealocytes could release

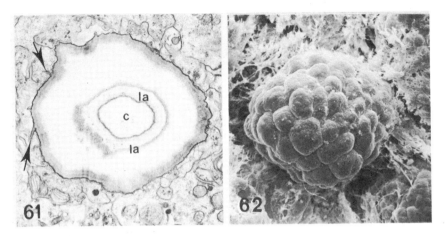

FIGURE 61. Gerbil pinealocyte large extracellular pineal concretion (c) consisting of several lamina (la). The concretion is surrounded by numerous pinealocyte and glial cell processes. In many cases, the concentration and the processes are closely associated, with the concretion actually extending into invaginations of the cell membranes (arrows). (× 7400.) *From Welsh and Reiter (230), by courtesy, with permission of the publisher.*

FIGURE 62. Scanning electron microscopic survey of a calcareous concretion within a human pineal gland. (× 140.) *From Krštić (266), by courtesy, with permission of the publisher.*

a carrier protein intracellularly into the vacuoles; this protein, together with calcium, could be deposited as multilayered pineal concretions (Figure 61). After the concretion has developed to a certain point, the pinealocyte could break down and release the concretion into the extracellular space (104,261). This idea, however, is not accepted by all authors. Diehl (262), for example, observed that most of the intrapineal concretions in the rat lie intracapsularly and, hence, are not directly related to the pineal parenchyma. This author, noting the occurrence of calcareous concretions in the immediate and more distant vicinity of the pineal body, feels that the widespread occurrence of such structures may be related to processes other than secretion, attributing their formation to a reduced drainage of tissue fluid in the pineal (for more details on the calcareous concretions, refer to ref. 9).

The "Glial" Cells

Beside pinealocytes, a varying number of elements occur in the mammalian pineal gland. Some authors termed these cells interstitial or supportive cells, others glial cells, gliallike cells, or astrocytes. It should be realized that, as is so often the case, this difference in terminology masks a physiological problem. In the rat, for example, Wolfe (123) called these cells interstitial cells because of their apparent ultrastructural dissimilarity to true glial cells. Milofsky (263), however, considered them to be typical glial cells, whereas Arstila (127) concluded that the interstitial cells apparently form a specialized parenchymal cell type with features in common with the glial cells of the central nervous system.

According to Collin (3,4), the mammalian pineal is composed of two populations of intrinsic cells, pinealocytes and interstitial cells. Collin (3) suggests that these two populations are unique, due to their peculiar phylogeny. Pinealocytes would be derived from photoreceptor cells, and interstitial cells would originate from the so-called supportive cells of the pineal of lower vertebrates. Consequently, according to Collin, all cells of the mammalian pineal gland that are not pinealocytes are classified as interstitial cells. Accepting Collin's concept, it is evident that it would be better to call these cells—which, in this concept, are not true glial cells—interstitial cells, as did Wolfe (123) and Arstila (127). However, many authors, including ourselves, although appreciating Collin's idea, nevertheless always preferred to call these elements glial or gliallike cells. The reason is that, although structurally insufficiently similar to any of the known glial cells, they always present a general gliallike aspect and especially because, as compared with other endocrine glands, such as testis and ovary, the term "interstitial" implies an endocrine function.

The recent use of immunocytochemical techniques seems to further complicate this problem. Møller et al. (264) demonstrated that two glial marker proteins, GFA and S-100, are present in certain cells of the rat pineal, which would thus be macroglial cells, or cells of macroglial origin. These results have been confirmed in the hedgehog, using a different antibody against GFA (110). Several factors indicate that these GFA or S-100 positive cells are in the rat the so-called interstitial cells of Wolfe (123) and in the hedgehog the so-called glial cells of Pévet (81). All these observations strongly suggest that, possibly, cells homologous to the interstitial cells of lower vertebrates, and called glial or gliallike cells, but also "true glial cells" or at least cells of macroglial origin, could be present in the pineal parenchyma and confused by investigators. In our opinion, this possibility of confusion, if true, needs thorough examination, especially when the problem of the presence of two different populations of pinealocytes is envisaged (see previously).

Glial cells and their processes in the pineal present great interspecies variations. For a detailed analysis, we refer to Vollrath (9). At the ultrastructural level, these cells are easily differentiated from the pinealocytes because they are essentially characterized by an abundance of microfilaments running parallel in the cell processes. These glial processes terminate among pinealocytes, either on other glial cells or near the perivascular space where they may form glial barrier membranes separating the pinealocyte process endings from the perivascular space (Figure 63).

To date, no function can be attributed to these glial cells. In 1976, Bowie and Herbert (174) suggested that, in the rat, they may contain arginine vasotocin. Later, however, these authors reevaluated this opinion and concluded that the immunoreaction obtained—which was due to a cross-reaction of anti-AVT with an albuminlike substance (265)—

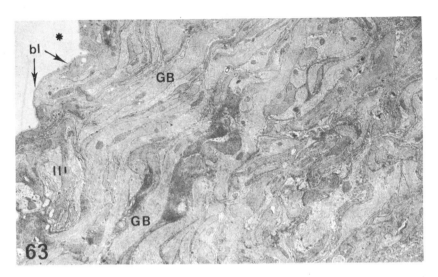

FIGURE 63. Hedgehog pineal gland. Numerous glial cell processes forming a glial barrier **(gb)** near the perivascular space **(*)**. **bl** = basal lamina. (× 5000.) *From Pévet (200).*

FIGURE 64. Ependymal cell **(EP)** of a hedgehog pineal gland in direct contact with the cerebrospinal fluid present in the third ventricle **(IIIv)**. Note below the ependymal cell the numerous glial processes forming a barrier **(GC)** and the pinealocyte **(P)**. **NE** = myelinated nerve fibers. (× 6,500). *From Pévet (200).*

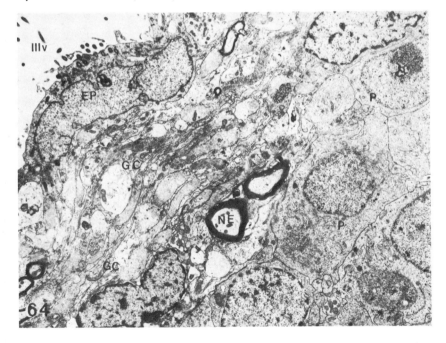

was probably located in pinealocytes (178), an observation that has been confirmed by another group (175).

Ependymal Cells

In view of the concept that functional interrelationships may exist between the pineal gland and the cerebrospinal fluid, and that vasotocin could possibly be synthesized in them (22,23), ependymal cells are important to consider. These cells, lining the pineal recess (Figure 64), are in direct contact with the third ventricle. They might, thus, not only release a hypothetical hormonal compound directly into the third ventricle but could also be implicated in the transport of substances from the cerebrospinal fluid into the pineal (see earlier).

Unfortunately, the ependymal cells of the pineal recess have been neglected by cytologists and available information is very scarce. These cells are generally characterized by a well-developed Golgi apparatus and granular endoplasmic reticulum and by the presence of a deeply invaginated nucleus. The apical cell surface is also most often packed with microvilli and cilia (Figure 64). Ependymal cells arranged in rosettes are also seen in the pineal parenchyma, but most often near the pineal recess (for details see ref. 9). To date, none of the immunocytochemical studies related to the problem of vasotocin in the pineal (95–97,174,176) support Pavel's hypothesis that these cells produce vasotocin.

GENERAL CONCLUSION

The morphological, histological, ultrastructural, histochemical, and cytochemical observations reported in this review clearly indicate that the pineal gland is a highly active organ synthesizing different compounds, either indolic or protein in nature.

In light of the different concepts dealt with and because it is evident that only chemical identification of the different pineal hormones produced by this gland will permit a determination of its function, it appears that only gradually will pineal function become more understandable. From comparative morphological, histological, and ultrastructural studies, it seems evident that, if the pineal is involved in long-term adaptation of reproduction to environmental lighting conditions (32,219), other external factors should also be considered. The pineal of mammals—and probably also that of nonmammalian species (38)—probably integrates not only information on the daylength, but also other information such as temperature, rainfall, and food, separately or in association, depending on the ecological situation in which the species lives, thus allowing for specific seasonal functions, such as breeding (34–36).

ACKNOWLEDGMENTS

The author wishes to thank Prof. Dr. J. Ariëns Kappers for his stimulating interest in this study and for critically reading the manuscript and Miss J. Sels for secretarial aid.

REFERENCES

1. Oksche A. Survey of the development and comparative morphology of the pineal organ. Prog Brain Res 10:3–29, 1965.
2. Oksche A. Sensory and glandular elements of the pineal organ. *In* The Pineal Gland, ed G E W Wolstenholme, J Knight. Churchill, Livingstone, London & Edinburgh, 1971, pp 127–146.
3. Collin J P. Contribution à l'étude de l'organe pinéal. De l'épiphyse sensorielle à la glande pinéale: modalités de transformation et implications fonctionelles. Ann Stat Biol de Besse-en-Chandesse Suppl 1:1–359, 1969.
4. Collin J P. Differentiation and regression of the cells of the sensory line in the epiphysis cerebri. *In* The Pineal Gland, ed G E W Wolstenholme, J Knight. Churchill, Livingstone, London & Edinburgh, 1971, pp 79–125.
5. Meiniel A. Ultrastructure of serotonin-containing cells in the pineal organ of *Lampetra planeri* (Petromyzontidea). A second sensory cell line from photoreceptor cell to pinealocyte. Cell Tiss Res 207:407–427, 1980.
6. Meiniel A. New aspects of the phylogenetic evolution of sensory cell lines in the vertebrate pineal complex. *In* The Pineal Organ. Photobiology-Biochronometry-Endocrinology, ed A Oksche, P Pévet. Elsevier North-Holland Biomedical Press, Amsterdam, 1981 pp 27–47.
7. Krabbe K H. Bidrag til kundsgaben om corpus pineale hos pattedyrene. Kgl Dan Vidensk Selsk Biol Nedd 2:1–126, 1919.
8. Vollrath L. Comparative morphology of the vertebrate complex. *In* The Pineal of Vertebrates including Man, ed J Ariëns Kappers, P Pévet. Prog Brain Res 52, Elsevier, Amsterdam, 1979, pp 25–38.
9. Vollrath L. The Pineal Organ. Handbuch der mikroskopischen Anatomie des Menschen, vol. 7. Springer Verlag, Berlin, 1981.
10. Vollrath L, Boeckmann D. Comparative anatomy of the rodent pineal complex. Gen Comp Endocrinol 34:Abstr 39, 1978.
11. Ariëns Kappers, J The development of topographical relations and innervations of the epiphysis cerebri in albino rat. Z Zellforsch 52:163–215, 1960.
12. Sheridan M N, Reiter R J. Observations in the pineal system in the hamster. II. Fine structure of the deep pineal. J Morphol 131:163–171, 1970.
13. Boeckmann D. Morphological investigation of the deep pineal of the rat. Cell Tiss Res 210:283–294, 1980.
14. Hülsemann M. Vergleichende histologische Untersuchungen über das Vorkommen von Gliafasern in der Epiphysis cerebri von Säugetieren. Acta Anat (Basel) 66:249–278, 1967.
15. Moore R Y. Indoleamine metabolism in the intact and denervated pineal, pineal stalk and habenula. Neuroendocrinology 19:323–330, 1975.
16. Pévet P, Balemans M G M, Legerstee W C, Vivien-Roels B. Circadian rhythmicity in the activity of hydroxyindole-O-methyltransferase (HIOMT) in the formation of melatonin and 5-methoxytryptophol in the pineal, retina and Harderian gland of the golden hamster. J Neural Transm 49:229–245, 1980.
17. Reiter R J, Vaughan M K, Blask D E. Possible role of cerebrospinal fluid in the transport of pineal hormones in mammals. *In* Brain-Endocrine Interaction. The Ventricular System in Neuroendocrine Mechanisms, vol 2, ed K M Knigge, D E Scott, H Kobayashi. Karger, Basel, 1975, pp 337–354.
18. Ariëns Kappers. J The pineal, an introduction. *In* The Pineal Gland, ed G E W Wolstenholme, J Knight. Churchill, Livingstone, London & Edinburgh, 1971, pp 3–34.
19. Hewing M. A liquor contacting area in the pineal recess of the golden hamster *(Mesocricetus auratus)*. Anat Embryol 153:295–304, 1978.

20. Hewing M. Cerebrospinal fluid-contacting area in the pineal recess of the vole *(Microtus agrestis)*, guinea pig *(Cavia cobaya)* and rhesus monkey *(Macaca mulatta)*. Cell Tiss Res 209:473–484, 1980.

21. Fleischhauer K. Fluorescenzmikroskopische Untersuchungen über den Stofftransport zwischen Ventrikkelliquor und Gehirn. Z Zellforsch 62:639–654, 1964.

22. Pavel S. Arginine vasotocin as a pineal hormone. J Neural Transm Suppl 13:135–155, 1978.

23. Pavel S. The mechanism of action of vasotocin in the mammalian brain. *In* The Pineal Gland of Vertebrates including Man, eds J Ariëns Kappers, P Pévet, Prog Brain Res 52, Elsevier, Amsterdam, 1979, pp 445–458.

24. Legait H, Legait E, Contet-Audonneau J L, Mur J M, Roux M, Richoux J P, Sirjean D, Dussart G. Etude des corrélations liant les volumes de l'hypophyse, de l'épiphyse et de l'OSH au poids somatiques et au volume de l'hypothalamus chez les Rongeurs. Bull Ass Anat (Nancy) 59(164):185–201, 1975.

25. Legait H, Bauchot R, Stephan H, Contet-Audonneau J L. Etude des corrélations liant le volume de l'épiphyse aux poids somatique et physiologique chez les rongeurs, les insectivores, les chiroptères, les prosimiens et les simiens. Mammalia 40:327–337, 1976.

26. Legait H, Bauchot R, Contet-Audonneau J L. Etude des corrélations liant les volumes des lobes hypophysaires et de l'épiphyse au poids somatique et au poids encéphalique chez les Chiroptères. Bull Ass Anat (Nancy) 60(168):175–188, 1976.

27. Quay W B. Greater pineal volume at higher latitudes in Rodentia: exponential relationship and its biological interpretation. Gen Comp Endocrinol 41:340–348, 1980.

28. Quay W B. Volumetric and cytologic variation in the pineal body of *Peromyscus leucopus* (Rodentia) with respect to sex, captivity and day-length. J Morphol 98:471–495, 1956.

29. Quay W B. Quantitative morphology and environmental response of the pineal gland in the collared lemming *(Dicrostonyx groenlandicus)*. Am J Anat 153:545–562, 1978.

30. Legait H, Roux M, Dussart G, Richoux J P, Contet-Audonneau J L. Données morphométriques sur la glande pinéale du Loir *(Glis glis)* et du Lérot *(Eliomys quercinus)* au cours du cycle annuel. C R Soc Biol (Paris) 169:132–136, 1975.

31. Reiter R J. Pineal control of a seasonally reproductive rhythm in male golden hamsters exposed to natural daylight and temperature. Endocrinology 92(2):423–430, 1973.

32. Reiter R J. Interaction of photoperiod, pineal and seasonal reproduction as exemplified by findings in the hamster. Prog Reprod Biol 169–190, 1978.

33. Hoffman K. Photoperiod, pineal, melatonin and reproduction in hamsters. *In* The Pineal Gland of Vertebrates including Man, ed. J Ariëns Kappers, P Pévet. Prog Brain Res 52, Elsevier North-Holland, Amsterdam, 1979, pp 397–415.

34. Pévet P. Secretory processes in the mammalian pinealocyte under natural and experimental conditions. *In* The Pineal Gland of Vertebrates including Man, ed J Ariëns Kappers, P Pévet. Prog Brain Res 52. Elsevier North-Holland, Amsterdam, 1979, pp 149–194.

35. Pévet P. Ultrastructure of the mammalian pinealocytes. *In* The Pineal, Anatomy and Biochemistry, ed R J Reiter. CRC Press, Boca Raton, Florida, 1981, pp 121–154.

36. Pévet P, Haldar-Misra C, Öcal T. The independency of an intact pineal gland of the inhibition by 5-methoxytryptamine of the reproductive organs in the male hamster. J Neural Transm 1981 52:95–106, 1981.

37. Vivien-Roels B. Activité sexuelle et glande pinéale. La Recherche 113:833–835, 1980.

38. Vivien-Roels B. Pineal control of reproduction in non mammalian vertebrates. *In* The Pineal Organ. Photobiology-Biochronometry-Endocrinology, ed A Oksche, P Pévet. Elsevier North-Holland Biomedical Press, Amsterdam, 1981, pp 315–334.

39. Tilney F, Warren L F. The morphology and evolutional significance of the pineal body. The American Anatomical Memoirs, No. 9, The Wistar Institute, Philadelphia, 1919.

40. Elden C A, Keyes M C, Marshall C E. Pineal body of the northern fur seal *(Callorhinus ursinus)*. A model for studying the probable function of the mammalian pineal body. Am J Vet Res 32:639–647, 1971.

41. Cuello A C, Tramezzani J H. The epiphysis cerebri of the Weddell seal: its remarkable size and glandular pattern. Gen Comp Endocrinol 12:153–164, 1969.

42. Ralph C L. The pineal gland and geographical distribution of animals. Int J Biometeorol 19:289–303, 1975.

43. Quay W B. Histological structure and cytology of the pineal organ in birds and mammals. In *Structure and Function of the Episphysis cerebri*, ed J Ariëns Kappers, J P Schadé. Prog Brain Res 10. Elsevier/North-Holland, Amsterdam, 1965, pp. 49–86.

44. Hill W C O. Notes on the dissection of two dugongs. J Mammal 26:153–175, 1945.

45. DeLany M J, Happolid, D C D. Ecology of African Mammals. Longman, London, 1979.

46. Bertler Å, Falck B, Owman C. Cellular localization of 5-hydroxytryptamine in the rat pineal gland. Kgl Fysiogr Sällsk Lund, Förhdl. 33:13–16, 1963.

47. Owman C. On the presence of 5-hydroxytryptamine in pineal nerves. Biochem Pharmacol 12:Suppl 112, 1963.

48. Owman C. Sympathetic nerves probably storing two types of monoamines in the rat pineal gland. Int J Neuropharmacol 3:105–112, 1964.

49. Neff N H, Barrett R E, Costa E. Kinetic and fluorescent histochemical analysis of serotonin compartments in rat pineal gland. Eur J Pharmacol 5:348–356, 1969.

50. Taxi J, Droz B. Etude de l'incorporation de noradrénaline-^{3}H(NA-^{3}H) et de 5-hydroxytryptophane-^{3}H(5-HTP-^{3}H) dans l'épiphyse et le ganglion cervical supérieur. CR Acad Sci (Paris) D 263:1326–1329, 1966.

51. Romijn H J. Structure and innervation of the pineal gland of the rabbit, *Oryctolagus cuniculus* (L.) with some functional considerations. A light and electronmicroscopic investigation. Thesis, Free University of Amsterdam, 1972.

52. Nielsen J T, Møller M. Innervation of the pineal gland in the Mongolian gerbil *(Meriones unguiculatus)*. A fluorescence microscopical study. Cell Tiss Res 187:235–250, 1978.

53. Matsushima S, Reiter R J. Fine structural features of adrenergic nerve fibres and endings in the pineal gland of the rat, ground squirrel and chinchilla. Am J Anat 148:463–478, 1977.

54. Ueck M. Innervation of the vertebrate pineal. In The Pineal Gland of Vertebrates including Man, ed J Ariëns Kappers, P Pévet. Prog Brain Res 52, Elsevier/North-Holland, Amsterdam, 1979, pp 45–88.

55. Owman C. Localization of neuronal and parenchymal monoamines under normal and experimental conditions in the mammalian pineal gland. In Structure and Function of the Epiphysis Cerebri eds J. Ariëns Kappers and J. P. Schadé, Prog Brain Res 10:423–453, Elsevier/North-Holland, Amsterdam, 1965.

56. Björklund A, Owman C, West K A. Peripheral sympathetic innervation and serotonin cells in the habenular region of the rat brain. Z Zellforsch 127:570–579, 1972.

57. Reiter R J, Hedlund L. Peripheral sympathetic innervation of the deep pineal of the golden hamster. Experientia (Basel) 22:1071–1072, 1976.

58. Matsushima S, Ito T. Diurnal changes in sympathetic nerve endings in the mouse pineal: semi-quantitative electron microscopic observations. J Neural Transm 33:275–288, 1972.

59. Pellegrino de Iraldi A, De Robertis, E. Action of reserpine, iproniazid and pyrogallol on nerve endings of the pineal gland. Int J Neuropharmacol 2:231–239, 1963.

60. Rodin A E, Turner R A. The relationship of intravesicular granules to the innervation of the pineal gland. Lab Invest 14:1644–1652, 1965.

61. Romijn H J. Structure and innervation of the pineal gland of the rabbit, *Oryctolagus cuniculus* (L.) III. An electron microscopic investigation of the innervation. Cell Tiss Res 157:25–51, 1975.

62. Machado A B M. Straight OsO_4 versus glutaraldehyde-OsO_4 in sequence as fixatives for the granular vesicles in sympathetic axons of the rat pineal body. Stain Technol 42:293–300, 1967.

63. Jaim-Etcheverry G, Zieher L M. Cytochemistry of 5-hydroxytryptamine at the electron microscope level. II. Localization of the autonomic nerves of the rat pineal gland. Z Zellfosch 86:393–400, 1968.

64. Ariëns Kappers. J The mammalian pineal organ. J Neurovisc Relat Suppl. 9:140–184, 1969.

65. Kenny G C T. The "nervi conarii" of the monkey. (An experimental study). J Neuropathol Exp Neurol 20:563–570, 1961.

66. Romijn H J. Structure and innervation of the pineal gland of the rabbit, *Oryctolagus cuniculus* (L.). I. A light microscopic investigation. Z Zellforsch 139:473–485, 1973.

67. Romijn H J. Parasympathetic innervation of the rabbit pineal gland. Brain Res 55:431–436, 1973.

68. Schrier B K, Klein D C. Absence of choline acetyltransferase in rat and rabbit pineal gland. Brain Res 79:347–351, 1974.

69. Eränkö O, Rechard L, Eränkö L, Cunningham A. Light and electron microscopic histochemical observations on cholinesterase-containing sympathetic nerve fibres in the pineal body of the rat. Histochem J 2:479–489, 1970.

70. Trueman T, Herbert J. Monoamines and acetylcholinesterase in the pineal gland and habenula of the ferret. Z Zellforsch 109:83–100, 1970.

71. David G F X, Anand Kumar T C. Histochemical localization of cholinesterase in neural tissue of pineal in rhesus monkey. Experientia (Basel) 34:1067–1068, 1978.

72. Romijn H J. The influence of some sympatholytic, parasympatholytic and serotonin synthesis inhibiting agents on the ultrastructure of the rabbit pineal organ. Cell Tiss Res 167:167–177, 1976.

73. Le Gros Clark W E. The nervous and vascular relations of the pineal gland. J. Anat (Lond) 74:471–492, 1939/40.

74. Bargmann W. Die Epiphysis Cerebri. *In* Handbuch der mikroskopischen Anatomie des Menschen, vol. 6, no. 4, ed W v Möllendorff. Springer Verlag, Berlin, 1943, p 309.

75. Kenny G C T. The innervation of the mammalian pineal body (a comparative study). Proc Aust Assoc Neurol 3:133–140, 1965.

76. Matsushima S, Reiter R J. Electron microscopic observations on neuron-like cells in the ground squirrel pineal gland. J Neural Transm 42:223–237, 1978.

77. David G F X, Herbert J. Experimental evidence for a synaptic connection between habenula and pineal ganglion in the ferret. Brain Res 64:327–343, 1973.

78. David G F X, Herbert J, Wright G D S. The ultrastructure of the pineal ganglion in the ferret. J Anat (Lond) 115:79–97, 1973.

79. Hartmann F. Uber die Innervation der Epiphysis cerebri einiger Säugetiere. Z Zellforsch 46:416–429, 1957.

80. Nielsen J T, Møller M. Nervous connections between the brain and the pineal gland in the cat (Felis catus) and the monkey *(Cercopethicus aethiops)*. Cell Tiss Res 161:293–301, 1975.

81. Pévet P. Correlations between pineal gland and sexual cycle. An electron microscopic and histochemical investigation on the pineal gland of the hedgehog, mole, mole-rat and white rat. Thesis, University of Amsterdam, 1976.

82. Korf H W, Wagner U. Evidence for a nervous connection between the brain and the pineal organ in the guinea pig. Cell Tiss Res 209:505–510, 1980.

83. Ariëns Kappers J. Short history of pineal discovery and research. *In* The Pineal Gland of Vertebrates including Man, ed J Ariëns Kappers, P Pévet. Prog Brain Res 52, Elsevier, North-Holland Biomedical Press, Amsterdam, 1979, pp 3–22.

84. Hülsemann M. Development of the innervation in the human pineal organ. Light and electron microscopic investigations. Z Zellforsch 115:396–415, 1971.

85. Møllgaard K, Møller M. On the innervation of the human fetal pineal gland. Brain Res 52:428–432, 1973.

86. Møller M. The ultrastructure of the human fetal pineal gland. 1) Cell types and blood vessels. Cell Tiss Res 152:13–30, 1974.

87. Møller M. Presence of a pineal nerve (nervus pinealis) in the human fetus. A light and electron microscopic study of the innervation of the pineal gland. Brain Res 154:1–12, 1978.

88. Møller M, Møllgaard K, Kimble J E. Presence of a pineal nerve in sheep and rabbit fetuses. Cell Tiss Res 158:451–459, 1975.

89. Schapiro S, Salas M. Effects of age, light and sympathetic innervation on electrical activity of the rat pineal gland. Brain Res 28:47–55, 1971.

90. Dafny N, McClung R. Pineal body: neural recording. Experientia (Basel) 31:321–322, 1975.

91. McClung R, Dafny N. Neurophysiological properties of the pineal body. II. Single unit recording. Life Sci 16:621–628, 1975.

92. Rønnekleiv O K, Kelly M J, Møller M, Wuttke W. Electrophysiological and morphological evidence of direct central innervation of the pineal gland, Pflügers Arch Supp 373:Abstr 187, 1978.

93. Dafny N, McClung R, Strada S J. Neurophysiological properties of the pineal body. I. Field potentials. Life Sci 16:611–620, 1975.

94. Dafny N. Electrophysiological evidence of photic, acoustic, and central input to the pineal body and hypothalamus. Exp Neurol 55:449–457, 1977.

95. Pévet P, Buijs R M, Dogterom J, Vivien-Roels B, Holder F C, Guerné J M, Reinharz A, Swaab D F, Ebels I, Neacsu C. Peptides in the mammalian pineal gland. In Pineal Function, eds L D Matthews, R F Seamark, Elsevier/North-Holland, Amsterdam, 1981, pp 173–184.

96. Pévet P, Pineal peptides in the fetus and in young and adult mammals. In Melatonin Rhythm, eds D K Klein, S Karger, 1982 (in press).

97. Pévet P. Peptides in the pineal gland of vertebrates. Ultrastructural, histochemical, immunocytochemical and radioimmunological aspects. In The Pineal Organ. Photobiology-Biochronometry-Endocrinology, eds A Oksche, P Pévet, Elsevier/North-Holland, Amsterdam, 1981, pp 211–235.

98. Buijs R M, Swaab D F. Immunoelectron microscopical demonstration of vasopressin and oxytocin synapses in the limbic system of the rat. Cell Tiss Res 204:355–365, 1979.

99. Buijs R M. Vasopressin and oxytocin innervation of the rat brain. Thesis, University of Amsterdam, 1980.

100. Barry J. Les voies extra-hypophysaires de la neurosécrétion diencephalique. Ass Anatomistes 89:264–276, 1956.

101. Bargmann W. Neurosekretion und hypothalamisch-hypophysäres System. Verh Anat Ges 51:30–45, 1954.

102. Suomalainen P. Stress and neurosecretion in the hibernating hedgehog. Dall Museum Comp Zool Harvard Coll 124:271–283, 1960.

103. Lukaszyk A, Reiter R J. Neurosecretion in the pineal gland of Macaca rhesus. Experientia (Basel) 30:654–655.

104. Lukaszyk A, Reiter R J. Histophysiological evidence for the secretion of polypeptides by the pineal gland. Am J Anat 143:451–464, 1975.

105. Japha J L, Eder T J, Goldsmith E D. A histochemical study of aldehyde fuchsin-positive material and "high-esterase cells" in the pineal gland of the mongolian gerbil. Am J Anat 149:23–38, 1977.

106. Reinharz A C, Czernichow P, Valloton M B. Neurophysin-like protein in bovine pineal gland. J Endocrinol 62:35–44, 1974.

107. Reinharz A C, Valloton M B. Presence of two neurophysins in human pineal gland. Endocrinology 100:994–1001, 1977.

108. Legros J J, Louis F, Demoulin A, Franchimont P. Immunoreactive neurophysins and vasotocin in human foetal pineal glands. J Endocrinol 69:289–290, 1976.

109. Buijs R M, Pévet P. Vasopressin and oxytocin containing fibres in the pineal gland and subcommissural organ of the rat. Cell Tiss Res 205:11–17, 1980.

110. Pévet P. Unpublished data.

111. Dogterom J, Snijdewint F G M, Pévet P, Swaab D F. Studies on the presence of vasopressin, oxytocin and vasotocin in the pineal gland, subcommissural organ and foetal pituitary gland: failure to demonstrate vasotocin in mammals. J Endocrinol 84:115–123, 1980.

112. Negro-Villar A, Sanchez-Franco F, Kwiatkowski M, Samson W K. Failure to demonstrate radioimmunoassayable arginine vasotocin in mammalian pineals. Brain Res Bull 4:789–792, 1980.

113. Pévet P, Reinharz A C, Dogterom J. Neurophysins, vasopressin and oxytocin in the bovine pineal gland. Neurosci Lett 16:301–306, 1980.

114. Barry J. Immunofluorescence study of the preoptico-terminal LRH tract in the female squirrel monkey during the estrous cycle. Cell Tiss Res 198:1–13, 1979.

115. Uddman R, Alumets J, Haakanson R, Loren I, Sundler F. Vasoactive intestinal peptide (VIP) occurs in nerves of the pineal gland. Experientia 36:1119–1120, 1980.

116. Møller M, Fahrenkrug J, Ottesen B. The presence of vasoactive intestinal peptide (VIP) in nerve fibres connecting the brain and the pineal gland of the cat. EPSG Newsletter Suppl. 3, p 45, 1981.

117. Pévet P. On the presence of different populations of pinealocytes in the mammalian pineal gland. J Neural Transm 40:289–304, 1977.

118. Karasek M. Ultrastructure of the pineal body in white rats in normal conditions and after pituitary gland extraction. Endokrynol Pol 22:15, 1971.

119. Clabough J W. Cytological aspects of pineal development in rats and hamsters. Am J Anat 137:215–230, 1973.

120. Zimmerman B L, Tso M O M. Morphological evidence of photoreceptor differentiation of pinealocytes in the neonatal rat. J Cell Biol 66:60–75, 1975.

121. Pévet P, Collin J P. Les pinealocytes de mammifère: diversité, homologies origine. Etude chez la Taupe adulte (*Talpa europaea*, L.). J Ultrastruct Res 57:22–31, 1976.

122. Pévet P, Ariëns Kappers J, Voûte A M. Morphologic evidence for differentiation of pinealocytes from photoreceptor cells in the adult noctule bat (*Nyctalus noctula*, Schreber). Cell Tiss Res 182:99–109, 1977.

123. Wolfe D E. The epiphyseal cell: an electron microscopic study of its intercellular relationship and intracellular morphology in the pineal body of the albino rat. Prog Brain Res 10:332–376, 1965.

124. Pévet P, Ariëns Kappers J, Nevo E. The pineal gland of the mole-rat (*Spalax ehrenbergi*, Nehring). I. The fine structure of pinealocytes. Cell Tiss Res 174:1–24, 1976.

125. Pévet P, Ariëns Kappers J, Voûte M. The pineal gland of nocturnal mammals. I. The pinealocytes of the bat *Nyctalus noctula*, Schreber. J Neural Transm 40:47–68, 1977.

126. Pévet P, Racey P A. The pineal gland of nocturnal mammals. II. The ultrastructure of the pineal gland in the pipistrelle bat (*Pipistrellus pipistrellus*, L.), Presence of two populations of pinealocytes. Cell Tiss Res 216:253–271, 1981.

127. Arstila A U. Electron microscopic studies on the structure and histochemistry of the pineal gland of the rat. Neuroendocrinology 2, Suppl 6:1–101, 1967.

128. Gusek W. Die Feinstruktur der Rattenzirbel und ihr Verhalten unter Einflusz von Antiandrogenen und nach Kastration. Endokrinologie 67:129–151, 1976.

129. Welsh M G. Effects of superior cervical ganlionectomy, constant light and blinding on the gerbil pineal gland: an ultrastructural analysis. Anat Rec 190:580–589, 1978.

130. Matsushima S, Reiter R J. Comparative ultrastructural studies of the pineal gland of rodents. *In* Electron Microscopic Concepts of Secretion: Ultrastructure of Endocrine and Reproductive Organs, ed M Hess. Wiley, New York, 1975, pp 335–336.

131. Sheridan M N, Reiter R J. The fine structure of the pineal gland in the Pocket Gopher (*Geomys bursarius*, L.). Am J Anat 36:363–382, 1973.

132. Wartenberg H. The mammalian pineal organ: electron microscopic studies on the fine structure of pinealocytes, glial cells and on the perivascular compartment. Z Zellforsch 86:74–97, 1968.

133. Lues G. Die Feinstruktur der Zirbeldrüse normaler, trächtiger und experimentell beeinfluszter Meerschweinchen. Z Zellforsch 114:38–60, 1971.

134. Bererni A, Abbas-Terki M. Structure fine de l'epiphyse du Magot d'Algerie (*Macacus sylvanus*, L.). Bull Ass Anat 148:285–294, 1970.

135. Upson R H, Benson B, Satterfield V. Quantification of ultrastructural changes in the mouse pineal in response to continuous illumination. Anat Rec 184:311–324, 1976.

136. Romijn H T, Mud M T, Wolters P S. Electron microscopic evidence of glycogen storage in the dark pinealocytes of the rabbit pineal gland. J Neural Transm 38:231–237, 1977.

137. Flight W F G. On the pineal body of the urodele, *Diemictylus viridescens viridescens*. Thesis, University of Utrecht, 1975.

138. Meiniel A. Detection and localization of biogenic amines in the pineal complex of *Lampetra planeri* (Petromyzontidae). *In* The Pineal Gland in Vertebrates including Man, ed J Ariëns Kappers, P Pévet. Prog Brain Res 52, Elsevier/North-Holland, Amsterdam, 1979, pp 303–307.

139. Vivien-Roels B, Meiniel A. Preliminary ultrastructural and autoradiographic observations on the pineal organ of the rockling (Fish, *teleostei*) (abstract). XIth Conference European Society Comparative Endocrinology, Jerusalem, August 10–15, 1981.

140. Meiniel A, Hartwig H G. Indoleamines in the pineal complex of *Lampetra planeri* (Petromyzontidae). A fluorescence and microspectrofluorimetric study. J Neural Transm 48:65–84, 1980.

141. Petit A. Contribution à l'étude de l'épiphyse des reptiles: le complexe épiphysaire des lacertiliens et l'epiphyse des Ophidiens. Etude embryologique, structurale, ultrastructurale; analyse qualitative et quantitative de la sérotonin dans les conditions normales et expérimentales. Thesis, University of Strasbourg, 1976.

142. McNulty J A. The pineal of the troglophilic fish, Chlorogaster agassizi: an ultrastructural study. J Neural Transm 43, 47–71, 1978.

143. McNulty J A. A light and electron microscopic study of the pineal in the blind goby, *Typhlogobius californiensis* (Pisces: Gobiidae). J Comp Neurol 181, 197–212, 1978.

144. McNulty J A. Fine structure of the pineal organ in the troglobytic fish. *Typhlichtyes subterraneous* (Pisces: Amblyopsidae). Cell Tiss Res 195:535–545, 1978.

145. Pévet P, Kuyper M A. The ultrastructure of pinealocytes in the golden mole (*Amblysomus hottentotus*) with special reference to the granular vesicles. Cell Tiss Res 191:39–56, 1978.

146. Falck B, Hillarp NA, Thieme G, Torp A. Fluorescence of catecholamines and related compounds condensed with formaldehyde. J Histochem Cytochem 10:348–354, 1962.

147. Collin J P. Recent advances in pineal cytochemistry. Evidence of the production of indoleamines and proteinaceous substances by rudimentary photoreceptor cells and pinealocytes of Amniota. *In* The Pineal Gland of Vertebrates including Man, ed J Ariëns Kappers, P Pévet. Prog Brain Res 52, Elsevier/North-Holland, Amsterdam, 1979, pp 271–296.

148. Hori S, Kuroda Y, Saito K, Ohotani S. Subcellular localization of tryptophan-5-monooxygenase in bovine pineal glands and raphe nuclei. J Neurochem 27:911–914, 1976.

149. Romijn J H, Mud M T, Wolters P S. A pharmacological and autoradiographic study on the ultrastructural localization of indoleamine synthesis in the rabbit pineal gland. Cell Tiss Res 185:199–214, 1977.

150. Collin J P, Meiniel A. Métabolisme des indolamines dans l'organe pinéal de Lacerta (reptiles, lacertiliens). I. Intégration sélective de 5-HTP-^{3}H(5-hydroxytryptophane-^{3}H) et rétention de ses dérivés dans les photorecepteurs rudimentaires sécrétoires. Z Zellforsch 142:549–570, 1973.

151. Meiniel A. Activités 5-hydroxytryptophane decarboxylasique (5-HTPDT) et monoamine oxydasique (MAO) dans l'organe pineal embryonnaire de Lacerta vivipara J. Etude qualitative et quantitative de l'incorporation du 5-HTP-^{3}H dans les conditions expérimentales et histoenzymologie des monoamine oxydases. J Neural Trans 41:175–208, 1977.

152. Juillard M T, Collin J P. L'organe pinéal aviaire: étude ultracytochimique et pharmacologique d'un "pool" granulaire de 5-hydroxytryptamine chez la perruche (*Melopsittacus undulatus*, Shaw). J Microsc Biol Cell 26:133–138, 1976.

153. Hakanson R, Owman C, Sporrong B, Sundler F. Electron microscopic classification of amine-producing endocrine cells by selective staining of ultrathin sections. Histochemie 27:226–242, 1971.

154. Meiniel A, Collin J P, Hartwig H G. Pinéale et troisième oeil de *Lacerta vivipara* (J) au cours de la vie embryonnaire et postnatale. Etude cytophysiologique des monoamines en microscopie de fluorescence et microspectrofluorimetrie. Z Zellforsch 144:89–115, 1973.

155. Juillard M T, Collin J P. Pools of serotonin in the pineal gland of the mouse. The mammalian pinealocyte as a component of the diffuse neuroendocrine system. Cell Tiss Res 213:273–291, 1980.

156. Sheridan M N, Sladek Jr J R. Histofluorescence and ultrastructural analysis of hamster and monkey pineal. Cell Tiss Res 614:145–152, 1975.

157. Sheridan M N, Keppel J F. The effect of p-chlorophenylalanine (pCPA) and 6-hydroxydopamine (6-HD) on ultrastructure features of hamster pineal parenchyma. Anat Rec 169:427–435, 1971.

158. Karasek M. Ultrastructure of rat pineal gland in organ culture; influence of norepinephrine, dibutyryl cyclic adenosine 3-5-monophosphate and adenohypophysis. Endokrinologie 64(1):106–114, 1974.

159. Lin H S, Hwang B H, Tseng C Y. Fine structural changes in the hamster pineal gland after blinding and superior cervical ganglionectomy. Cell Tiss Res 158:285–299, 1975.

160. Romijn H J. The ultrastructure of the rabbit pineal gland after sympathectomy, parasympathectomy, continuous illumination, and continuous darkness. J Neural Transm 36:183–194, 1975.

161. Freund D, Arendt J, Vollrath L. Tentative immunohistochemical demonstration of melatonin in the rat pineal gland. Cell Tiss Res 181:239–244, 1977.

162. Bubenik G A, Brown G M, Uhir I, Grota L J. Immunohistological localization of N-acetylindolealkylamines in pineal gland, retina and cerebellum. Brain Res 81:233–242, 1974.

163. Vivien-Roels B, Pévet P, Dubois M P, Arendt J, Brown G M. Immunohistochemical evidence for the presence of melatonin in the pineal gland, the retina and the Harderian gland. Cell Tiss Res 217:105–115, 1981.

164. Smith A R. Conditions influencing the serotonin and tryptophan metabolism in the epiphysis cerebri of the rabbit. A fluorescence histochemical, microscopic and electrophoretic study. Thesis, University of Amsterdam, 1972.

165. Smith A R, Jongkind J F, J Ariëns Kappers. Distribution of quantification of serotonin-containing and autofluorescent cells in the rabbit pineal organ. Gen Comp Endocrinol 18(2):364–371, 1972.

166. Smith A R, Ariëns Kappers J, Jongkind J F. Alterations in the distribution of yellow fluorescing rabbit pinealocytes produced by p-chlorophenylalanine and different conditions of illumination. J Neural Transm 33:91–113, 1972.

167. Pévet P, Juillard M T, Smith A R, Ariëns Kappers J. The pineal gland of the mole (*Talpa europaea* L.). III. A fluorescence histochemical study. Cell Tiss Res 165:297–306, 1976.

168. Pévet P. The pineal gland of the mole (*Talpa europaea* L.). 1) The fine structure of the pinealocytes. Cell Tiss Res 153:277–292, 1974.

169. Karasek M, Marek K. Influence of gonadotropic hormones on the ultrastructure of rat pinealocytes. Cell Tiss Res 188:133–141, 1978.

170. Karasek M, Pawlikowski M, Ariëns Kappers J, Stepien H. Influence of castration followed by administration of LH-RH on the ultrastructure of rat pinealocytes. Cell Tiss Res 167:325–339, 1976.

171. Karasek M, Pawlikowski M, Pévet P, Stepien H. Ultrastructural and fluorescence histochemical studies of the rat pineal gland after castration. Ann Med Sect Pol Acad Sci 21:57–58, 1976.

172. Pévet P, Smith A R, Van de Kar L, Van Bronswijk H. Effect of castration on the rat

pineal gland: a fluorescence histochemical and biochemical study. Experientia 31:1237–1238, 1975.

173. Smith A R, Pévet P, Van de Kar L, Van Oostrom R. Effect of gonadotropic hormones on the rat pineal gland. A fluorescence histochemical and biochemical study. J Neural Transm 36:217–226, 1975.

174. Bowie E P, Herbert D C. Immunocytochemical evidence for the presence of arginine vasotocin in the rat pineal gland. Nature (Lond) 261:66, 1976.

175. Pévet P, Swaab D F. Immunocytochemical evidence for the presence of an α-MSH-like compound in the rat pineal. J Physiol (Paris) 75:75–77, 1979.

176. Pévet P, Ebels I, Swaab D F, Mud M, Arimura A. Presence of AVT-, α-MSH-, LHRH- and somatostatin-like compounds in the rat pineal gland and their relationship with the UMO5R pineal fraction: An immunocytochemical study. Cell Tiss Res 200:341–353, 1980.

177. Swaab D F, Fisser B. Immunocytochemical localization of α-melanocyte stimulating hormone (α-MSH)-like compounds in the rat nervous system. Neurosci Lett 7:313–317, 1977.

178. Bowie E P, Eng L F. A comparative study of astrocytes and AVT cells in the rat pineal. Anat Rec 192(1):121, 1978.

179. Juillard M T. The proteinaceous content and possible physiological significance of dense-cored vesicles in hamster and mouse pinealocytes. Ann Biol Anim Biophys 19:413–428, 1979.

180. Pévet P, Yadav M. The pineal gland of equatorial mammals. I. The pinealocytes of the Malaysian rat (Rattus sabanus). Cell Tiss Res 210:417–433, 1980.

181. Karasek M. Some functional aspects of the ultrastructure of rat pinealocytes. Endocrinol Exp (Bratisl) 15:17–25, 1981.

182. Renold A. Insulin biosynthesis and secretion. A still unsettled topic. N Engl J Med 282:173–282, 1970.

183. Haldar-Misra C, Pévet P. Unpublished data.

184. Romijn H J, Gelsema A J. Electron microscopy of the rabbit pineal organ in vitro. Evidence of norepinephrine-stimulated secretory activity of the Golgi apparatus. Cell Tiss Res 172:365–377, 1976.

185. Aguado, L I, Benelbaz G A, Gutierez L S, Rodriguez E M. Ultrastructure of the rat pineal gland grafted under the kidney capsule. Cell Tiss Res 176:131–142, 1977.

186. Sheridan M N. Pineal gland fine structure. In Brain Endocrine Interactions. II. The Ventricular System, 2nd Int Symp, Shizuoka, Japan, 1974, pp 324–336.

187. Haldar-Misra C, Pévet P. Influence of noradrenaline on the pineal peptide/protein synthesis. An ultrastructural study in the mouse pineal in vitro. EPSG Newsletter Suppl. 3, 32, 1981.

188. Clabough J W. Ultrastructural features of the pineal gland in normal and light de-prived golden hamsters. Z Zellforsch 114:151–164, 1971.

189. Pévet P, Jarvis C. Unpublished data.

190. Matsushima S, Kachi T, Mukai S, Morisawa Y. Functional relationship between sympathetic nerves and pinealocytes in the mouse pineal: quantitative electron microscopic observations. Arch Histol Jap 40:279–291.

191. Karasek M, Marek K, Kunert-Radek J. Ultrastructure of rat pinealocytes in vitro: influence of gonadotropic hormones and LH-RH. Cell Tiss Res 195:547–556, 1978.

192. Upson R H, Benson B. Effects of blinding on the ultrastructure of mouse pinealocytes with particular emphasis on the dense-cored vesicles. Cell Tiss Res 183:491–498, 1977.

193. Gittes R F, Chu E W. Reversal of the effect of pinealectomy in female rats by multiple isogenic transplants. Endocrinology 77:1061–1067, 1965.

194. Roux M, Richoux J P, Cordonnier J L. Influence de la photoperiode sur l'ultrastructure de l'épiphyse avant et pendant la phase génitale saisonnière chez la femelle du Lérot (Eliomys quercinus). J Neural Transm 41:209–223, 1977.

195. Matsushima S, Morisawa Y, Petterborg L S, Zeagler J W, Reiter R J. Ultrastructure of pinealocytes of the cotton rat, *Sigmodon hospidus.* Cell Tiss Res 204:407–416, 1979.

196. Pévet P. The pineal gland of the mole (*Talpa europaea* L.). IV. Effect of pronase on material present in cisternae of the granular endoplasmic reticulum of pinealocytes. Cell Tiss Res 182:215–219, 1977.

197. Pévet P. The pineal gland of the mole. VI. Fine structure of fetal pinealocytes. Cell Tiss Res 206:417–430, 1980.

198. Pévet P, Smith A R. The pineal gland of the mole (*Talpa europaea,* L.). II. Ultrastructural variations observed in the pinealocytes during different parts of the sexual cycle. J Neural Transm 36:227–248, 1975.

199. Roux M, Richoux J P. Effets de l'énucléation oculaire bilatérale sur l'ultrastructure de l'épiphyse chez la femelle du Lérot (*Eliomys quercinus* L.) Corrélations avec l'axe hypothalamo-hypophyso-ovarien. Reprod Nutr Develop 21:47–57, 1981.

200. Pévet P. Etude ultrastructurale de l'épiphyse du Hérisson mâle. Evolution et fonction du cycle sexuel. Thèse III cycle. University of Poitiers, 1972.

201. Pévet P, Soboureau M. L'épiphyse du Hérisson (*Erinaceus europaeus,* L.) mâle. 1. Les pinéalocytes et leurs variations ultrastructurales considérées au cours du cycle sexuel. Z Zellforsch 143:367–385, 1973.

202. Pévet P, Saboureau M. Effect of serotonin administration on the ultrastructure of pinealocytes during the period of maximal sexual activity of the male hedgehog (*Erinaceus europaeus,* L.). Experientia 30:1069–1070, 1974.

203. Pévet P. Cytological aspects of indoleamine secretion in the pineal gland. *In Melatonin—Current Status and Perspectives,* ed N Burna, W Schloot. Pergamon, Oxford, 1981, pp 23–34.

204. Pévet P, Balemans M G M, Barry F A M, Noordegraff E M. The pineal gland of the mole (*Talpa europaea,* L.). V. Activity of hydroxyindole-O-methyltransferase (HIOMT) in the formation of melatonin/5-hydroxytryptophol in the eyes and the pineal gland. Ann Biol Anim Biochem Biophys 18:259–284, 1978.

205. Balemans M G M, Pévet P, Legerstee W C, Nevo E. Preliminary investigations on melatonin and 5-methoxytryptophol synthesis in the pineal, retina and Harderian gland of the mole rat and in the pineal of the mouse "eyeless." J Neural Transm 49:247–255, 1980.

206. Pévet P, Balemans M G M, De Reuver G F. The pineal gland of the mole (*Talpa europaea,* L.). VII. Activity of hydroxyindole-O-methyltransferase (HIOMT) in the formation of 5-methoxytryptophan, 5-methoxytryptamine, 5-methoxyindole-3-acetic acid, 5-methoxytryptophol and melatonin in the eyes and the pineal. J Neural Transm 51:271–282, 1981.

207. Barratt G F, Nadakavukaren M J, Frehn J L. Effect of melatonin implants on gonadal weights and pineal gland fine structure of the Golden hamster. Tissue Cell 9:335–345, 1977.

208. Benson B, Krasovich M. Circadian rhythm in the number of granulated vesicles in the pinealocytes of mice. Effect of sympathectomy and melatonin treatment. Cell Tiss Res 184:499–506, 1977.

209. Freire F, Cardinali D P. Effects of melatonin treatment and environmental lighting on the ultrastructural appearance, melatonin synthesis, norepinephrine turnover and microtubule protein content of the rat pineal gland. J Neural Transm 37:237–257, 1975.

210. Lu K S, Lin H S. Cytochemical studies on cytoplasmic granular elements in the hamster pineal gland. Histochemistry 61:177–187, 1979.

211. Matthews C D, Leong A Y S. A possible role for the pineal gland and melatonin in the diffuse neuroendocrine system (DNES). *In Melatonin—Current Status and Perspectives,* ed N Birau, W Schlott, Pergamon, Oxford, 1981, pp 77–82.

212. Öcal T, Pévet P. Unpublished data.

213. Povtliege P. L'influence des oestrogènes sur l'ultrastructure de greffons hypophysaires chez la ratte. J Microscopie 4:485–496, 1965.

214. Bjersing L. On the ultrastructure of granulosa lutein cells in porcine corpus luteum. Z Zellforsch 82:187–211.

215. King J C, Williams T H, Gerall A A. Transformations of hypothalamic arcuate neurons. I. Changes associated with stages of the estrous cycle. Cell Tiss Res 153:497–515, 1975.

216. McNeill M E. Membranous structures in pinealocytes of the infertile diabetic mutant mouse (C57BL/Ks-db/db). J Neural Transm 42:207–221, 1978.

217. Roux M, Richoux J P, Dussart G. Etude ultrastructurale de l'épiphyse du Lérot (Eliomys quercinus, L.). Bull Ass Anat 58(163):1–12, 1974.

218. Hoffman R A, Reiter R J. Pineal gland. Influence on gonads of male hamster. Science 148:1609–1611, 1965.

219. Reiter R J. The pineal and its hormones in the control of reproduction in mammals. Endocrinol Rev 1:109–131, 1980.

220. Clabough J W, Norvell J E. Effects of castration, blinding, and the pineal gland on the Harderian glands of the male golden hamster. Neuroendocrinology 12:344–353, 1973.

221. Quay W B. Pineal Chemistry in Cellular and Physiological Mechanisms. Charles C Thomas, Springfield, Ill, 1974.

222. Kachi T, Matsushima S, Ito T. Diurnal changes in glycogen content in the pineal cells of the male mouse: a quantitative histochemical study. Z Zellforsch 118:310–314, 1971.

223. Kachi T, Matsushima S, Ito T. Diurnal variations in pineal glycogen content during the oestrous cycle in female mice. Arch Histol Jap 35:153–159, 1973.

224. Kachi S, Ito T. Effect of continuous darkness on diurnal rhythm in glycogen content in pineal cells of the mouse: a semi-quantitative histochemical study. Anat Rec 179:405–410, 1974.

225. Kachi T, Matsushima S, Ito T. Effects of continuous lighting on glycogen in the pineal cells of the mouse: a quantitative histochemical study. Z Zellforsch 118:214–220, 1971.

226. Gregorek J C. The ultrastructure of the pineal gland of normal and enucleated gerbils. Anat Rec 175:133, 1973.

227. Quay W B. Cytologic and metabolic parameters of pineal inhibition by continuous light in the rat (Rattus norvegicus). Z Zellforsch 60:479–490, 1963.

228. Kachi T, Ito T. Neural control of glycogen content and its diurnal rhythm in mouse pineal cell. Am J Physiol 232:E584–E589, 1977.

229. Pévet P. Vacuolated pinealocytes in hedgehog (Erinaceus europaeus L.). Cell Tiss Res 159:303–309, 1975.

230. Welsh M G, Reiter R J. The pineal gland of the gerbil, Meriones unguiculatus. I. An ultrastructural study. Cell Tiss Res 193:323–336, 1978.

231. Clementi F, Muller E, Zanoboni A. Pineal function and modifications of its ultrastructural aspects. In Proceedings of the 2nd International Congress on Endocrinology. London, Excerpta Medica, International Congress Series no. 83, 1964, pp 364–366.

232. Povlishock J T, Kriebel R M, Siebel H R. A light and electron microscopic study of the pineal gland of the ground squirrel Citellus tridecemlineatus. Am J Anat 143:465–484, 1975.

233. Quay W B. Reduction of mammalian pineal weight and lipid during continuous light. Gen Comp Endocrinol 1:211–217, 1961.

234. Zweens J. Influence of the oestrous cycle and ovariectomy on the phospholipid content of the pineal gland in the rat. Nature 197:1114–1115, 1963.

235. Zweens J. Alterations of the pineal lipid content in the rat under hormonal influences. Prog Brain Res 10:540–551, 1965.

236. Perrelet A, Orci L, Rouiller C. Clarification of the osmiophilic granules of the rat pinealocytes by p-chlorophenylalanine. Experientia (Basel) 24:1047–1049, 1968.

237. De Martino C, De Luca F, Paluello F M, Tonietti G, Orci L. The osmiophilic granules of the pineal body in rats. Experientia (Basel) 19:639–641, 1963.

238. Richoux J P, Roux M, Legait H. Etude de l'appareil génital femelle et de l'épiphyse du lérot dans diverses conditions au cours de la période hivernale. J Physiol (Paris) 70:21B, 1975.

239. Roux M, Richoux J P. Liposome variations in the pinealocytes of an hibernator. EPSG Newsletter Suppl 3:51, 1981.

240. Cordonnier J L, Roux M. Etude en histofluorescence des monoamines épiphysaires chez le Lérot (*Eliomys quercinus* L.) dans diverses conditions expérimentales au cours de la période hivernale. Ann Endocrinol (Paris) 39:403–410, 1978.

241. Gusek W, Santoro A. Zur Ultrastruktur der Epiphysis cerebri der Ratte. Endokrinologie 41:105–129, 1961.

242. Vollrath L, Huss H. The synaptic ribbons of the guinea pig pineal gland under normal and experimental conditions. Z Zellforsch 139:417–429, 1973.

243. Vollrath L. Synaptic ribbons of a mammalian pineal gland—circadian changes. Z Zellforsch 145:171–183, 1973.

244. Theron J J, Biagio R, Meyer A C, Boekkooi S. Microfilaments, the smooth endoplasmic reticulum and synaptic ribbons fields in the pinealocytes of the baboon *(Papio ursinus)*. Am J Anat 154:151–162, 1979.

245. Kurumado K, Wataru M. A morphological study of the circadian cycle of the pineal gland of the rat. Cell Tiss Res 182:565–568, 1977.

246. Kurumado K, Mori W. Synaptic ribbon in the human pinealocyte. Acta Pathol Jap 26:381–384, 1976.

247. Karasek M, Vollrath L. "Synaptic" ribbons of the rat pineal gland: circadian rhythmicity in vitro? EPSG Newsletter Suppl 3:38, 1981.

248. Vollrath L, Kantarjian A, Howe C. Mammalian pineal gland: 7-day rhythmic activity? Experientia (Basel) 31:458–460, 1975.

249. Wurtman R J, Axelrod J, Kelly D E. The Pineal. Academic, New York, 1968.

250. Mori W, Kurumado K. Circadian change in number of synaptic ribbons in pinealocytes of normal and blinded rats. J Neural Transm Suppl 13:383, 1978.

251. Karasek M. Quantitative changes in number of "synaptic" ribbons in rat pinealocytes after orchidectomy and in organ culture. J Neural Transm 38:149–157, 1976.

252. Arstila A U, Kalimo H O, Hyppää M. Secretory organelles of the rat pineal gland: electron microscopic and histochemical studies in vitro and in vivo. *In* The Pineal Gland, A CIBA Symposium. eds G E W Wolstenholm, J Knight, Churchill, Livingstone, London and Edinburgh, 1971, pp 147–164.

253. McNeill M E, Whitehead D S. The synaptic ribbons of the guinea pig pineal gland in sterile, pregnant and fertile but non-pregnant females and in reproductively active males. J Neural Transm 45:149–164, 1979.

254. Miline R, Krstric R, Devecerski V. Sur le comportement de la glande pinéale dans des conditions de stress. Acta Anat (Basel) 71:352–402, 1968.

255. Krštić R. Influence du froid sur la morphodynamique de la glande pinéale du rat. Acta Anat (Basel) 86:320–321, 1973.

256. Hopsu V K, Arstila A U. An apparent somato-somatic synaptic structure in the pineal gland of the rat. Exp Cell Res 37:484–487.

257. Vivien-Roels B. L'épiphyse des Chéloniens. Etude embryologique, structurale, ultrastructurale; analyse qualitative et quantitative de la sérotonine dans des conditions normales et expérimentales. Thesis, University of Strasbourg, 1976.

258. Krštić R. Ultracytochemistry of the synaptic ribbons in the rat pineal organ. Cell Tiss Res 166:135–143, 1976.

259. Knyihar E, Laszlo I, Csillik B. Thiamime pyrophosphatase activity in neurotubuli and synaptic vesicles. Neurobiology 3:327–334, 1973.

260. Japha J L, Eder T J, Goldsmith E D. Calcified inclusions in the superficial pineal gland of the Mongolian gerbil, *Meriones unguiculatus*. Acta Anat (Basel) 94:533–544, 1976.

261. Reiter R J, Lukaszyk A J, Vaughan M K, Blask D E. New horizons of pineal research. Am Zoologist 16:93–101, 1976.

262. Diehl B J M. Occurrence and regional distribution of calcareous concretions in the rat pineal gland. Cell Tiss Res 195:359, 1978.
263. Milofsky A. The fine structure of the pineal in the rat, with special reference to parenchyma. Anat Rec 127:435–436, 1957.
264. Møller M, Ingild A, Bock E. Immunohistochemical demonstration of S-100 protein and GFA protein in interstitial cells of rat pineal gland. Brain Res 140:1–13, 1978.
265. Bowie E P. Immunocytochemical evidence for the presence of an albuminlike substance in the rat pineal gland. Histochemistry 66:83–87, 1980.
266. Krštić R. A combined scanning and transmission electron microscopic study and electron probe analysis of human pineal acervuli. Cell Tiss Res 174:129–137, 1976.

ALFRED J. LEWY, M.D., Ph.D.

BIOCHEMISTRY AND REGULATION OF MAMMALIAN MELATONIN PRODUCTION

INTRODUCTION

This chapter focuses on the biochemistry and regulation of the synthesis of melatonin. Other texts (1) can provide a comprehensive review of other aspects of pineal biochemistry. Because of some apparent species differences (particularly between phyla), emphasis will be on data from the laboratory rat. Regulation of melatonin secretion in humans will also be discussed.

A thorough understanding of the biochemistry of melatonin synthesis is essential in understanding how secretion of this hormone is regulated. Although measurement of melatonin has become increasingly important (particularly in humans), measurement of intermediate substances has been, and will continue to be, useful in assessing regulation of melatonin secretion in nonhuman species. The principal intermediates are norepinephrine, serotonin, adenyl cyclase, cyclic AMP, hydroxyindole-O-methyltransferase (HIOMT), and serotonin N-acetyltransferase—the rate-limiting step in the synthesis of melatonin (2). The regulation of

From the Sleep and Mood Disorders Laboratory, Department of Psychiatry, and Department of Pharmacology, Oregon Health Sciences University, Portland, Oregon 97201.

melatonin secretion by the endogenous circadian pacemaker and by the environmental light/dark cycle will also be covered in some detail, since this area has apparently not received adequate attention in previous reviews.

History

From antiquity to the Renaissance, the early pinealologists were fascinated by the human pineal's location in the center of the brain, positioned behind the third ventricle and midway between the lateral ventricles. It was therefore thought to be directing flow of the "vital fluids" (3,4). In the latter part of the last century and the beginning of the present one, anatomists discovered photosensorylike cells in pineal tissue of some submammalian species (5–7), thus suggesting another function for the pineal. Other scientists were struck by the changes in size in this organ associated with disorders of puberty (8,9), imparting on the pineal the distinction of perhaps being a gland. Within the past 25 years, the modern era of research was initiated by Lerner and his associates who proposed the molecular structure of the active skin-lightening principle in the pineal to be N-acetyl-5-methoxytryptamine, or melatonin (10). Soon after, Ariëns Kappers identified the innervation of the pineal (or epiphysis cerebri) as primarily, if not exclusively, postganglionic sympathetic neurons (11).

Embryology and Histology

Embryologically, the human pineal derives from the neural crest, forming part of the diencephalic roof situated between the habenular commissure rostrally and the posterior commissure caudally; it is therefore part of the epithalamus (12). In some submammalian pineal glands, pinealocytes are photosensitive; for many of these species, the pineal is located superficially and is known as a parietal "eye" capable of photoreception but not vision (13). In mammals, the pineal remains in contact with the environmental light/dark cycle through a neuroanatomical pathway (see the later section on Circadian Anatomy).

The pinealocyte is an unusual type of cell, having some characteristics of endocrine cells and some characteristics of neurons. Some scientists consider the pineal to be a "paraneuron," because (1) the pinealocyte produces substances related to neurotransmitters; (2) the pinealocyte contains synaptic vesicles; (3) the pineal secretes substances in response to stimuli mediated by a receptor in the cell membrane; and (4) the pinealocyte has its origin in the neuroectoderm (14). The pinealocyte has also been thought to be part of the APUD (amine uptake precursor and decarboxylase cell) system (15).

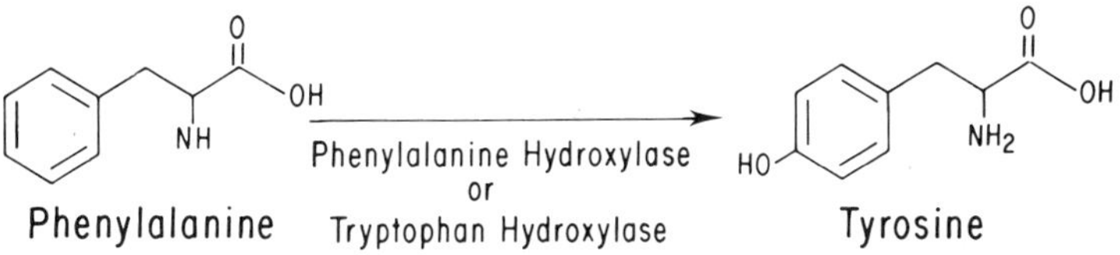

FIGURE 1. Synthesis of tyrosine.

BIOCHEMISTRY

Presynaptic Biochemistry

To emphasize the regulatory functions of the various constituents of the pineal, this section begins with the synthesis of norepinephrine.

NOREPINEPHRINE SYNTHESIS

With the onset of nighttime darkness, sympathetic neurons increase their firing rate (16). There is a modest rise in norepinephrine levels (17) and a significant increase in norepinephrine turnover (18). Enucleation or optic nerve transection causes a loss in the nighttime increase in norepinephrine activity; levels remain intermediate between those of day and night (19). Superior cervical ganglionectomy decreases norepinephrine levels (20); decentralization (accomplished by sectioning the preganglionic neurons of the superior cervical ganglia) reduces norepinephrine levels, but to a lesser extent.

Norepinephrine ultimately derives from tyrosine, which, in the pineal, derives primarily from dietary phenylalanine. Phenylalanine uptake is significant in the pineal, whereas tyrosine uptake is minimal (21). Tyrosine is synthesized from phenylalanine by an enzyme in the pineal thought to be tryptophan hydroxylase, not phenylalanine hydroxylase (21–23). Pineal tryptophan hydroxylase may not be the same enzyme as brain tryptophan hydroxylase (21–23). The synthesis of tyrosine from phenylalanine is shown in Figure 1.

The next step is the conversion of tyrosine to DOPA (dihydroxyphenylalanine) by tyrosine hydroxylase (17), the rate-limiting step in norepinephrine synthesis (Figure 2). Tyrosine hydroxylase, which in-

FIGURE 2. Synthesis of l-DOPA (dihydroxyphenylalanine).

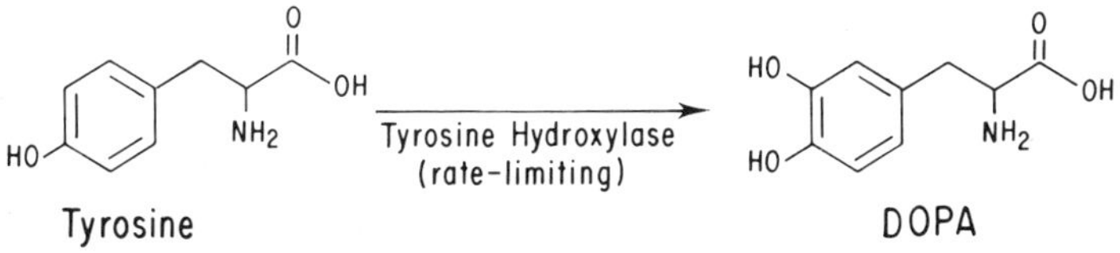

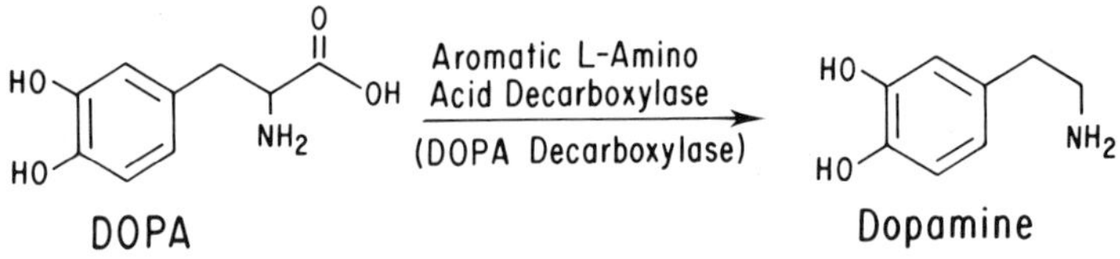

FIGURE 3. Synthesis of dopamine.

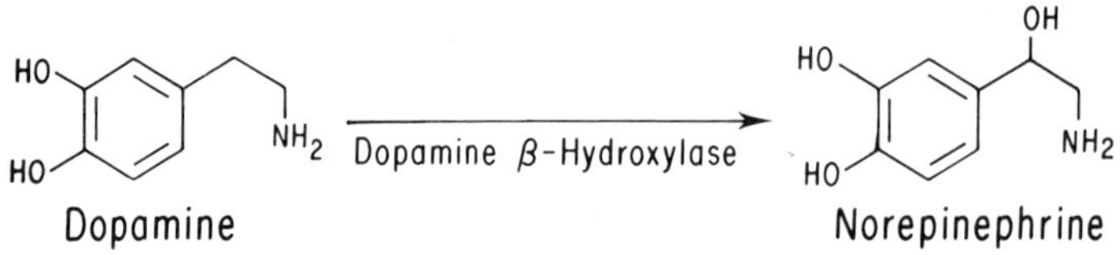

FIGURE 4. Synthesis of norepinephrine.

creases by more than 50% at night, is highly concentrated in pineal tissue (24).

DOPA is converted to dopamine (Figure 3) by the enzyme DOPA decarboxylase (or aromatic l-amino acid decarboxylase, as it is more commonly known, since this enzyme is reputed to have many substrates) (25,26). This enzyme requires pyridoxal phosphate as a cofactor; its concentration in the pineal gland is the highest in the body (27). Although the significance is not clear, denervation increases the concentration of DOPA decarboxylase (20,28) in the pineal.

Norepinephrine is synthesized from dopamine by the enzyme dopamine beta-hydroxylase (Figure 4). This enzyme also has other substrates (28). It requires ascorbic acid for activity and contains copper, which explains why it is susceptible to inhibition by drugs that bind copper, such as disulfiram (tetraethylthiuram) (29,30).

INACTIVATION OF NOREPINEPHRINE

On release into the synaptic cleft, norepinephrine can interact with the pineal's beta-adrenergic receptors postsynaptically (Figure 5). Norepinephrine is then deactivated by four types of mechanisms. One mechanism is diffusion away from the synapse. Another deactivating mechanism is reuptake into the presynaptic neuron. The presynaptic neurons are very efficient at removing norepinephrine from the synaptic cleft and serve an important function in protecting the postsynaptic receptors from circulating catecholamines (released by other sympathetic nerves or by the adrenal medulla) (31,32), because there is apparently no "blood-brain barrier" for biogenic amines in the pineal (33). An uptake blocker is usually necessary to facilitate stimulation of the pineal's beta-adrenergic receptors by circulating catecholamines released in response to stress (34,35).

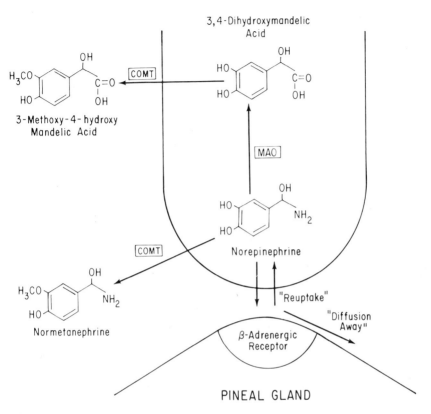

FIGURE 5. Inactivation of norepinephrine by diffusion away, reuptake, MAO (mono-amine oxidase), and COMT (catechol-0-methyltransferase).

Other deactivating mechanisms are related to enzymatic degradation to nonactive metabolites. Monoamine oxidase (MAO), primarily of the A type, is located in the presynaptic nerve. The B type is located mainly in the pinealocyte (26,36). With denervation, there is a loss of MAO_A, but not MAO_B, activity. There is no circadian rhythm in MAO activity, but there is a rhythm in the activity of the other deactivating enzyme, catechol-O-methyltransferase (COMT) (37), (more activity during the day than at night). That the rhythm of this extraneuronal enzyme's activity is inverse to the rhythm of pineal norepinephrine synthesis (but corresponds to the circadian rhythm of circulating catecholamines) may indicate that COMT is another way in which the pineal's beta-adrenergic receptors are protected from circulating agonists, particularly during the day. The pineal's beta-adrenergic receptors are stimulated exclusively by norepinephrine released by the pineal's sympathetic neurons. Metabolites of norepinephrine are shown in Figure 5.

Postsynaptic Biochemistry

BETA-ADRENERGIC RECEPTOR

Postsynaptically, norepinephrine stimulates a beta-l-adrenergic receptor (38,39). Although norepinephrine is thought to have more alpha-adrenergic than beta-adrenergic activity, the postsynaptic receptor in the pineal is a beta-adrenergic receptor. Consequently, norepinephrine is blocked by propranolol but not by alpha-adrenergic antagonists such as phenoxybenzamine (40). Isoproterenol is a particularly potent beta-adrenergic agonist (41), because it is not taken up into the presynaptic neurons.

During each 24-hour period, the pineal's beta-adrenergic receptors undergo a marked change in number, which is a function of the degree of previous stimulation. The binding of labeled alprenolol (a beta-adrenergic drug) is twice as great at the end of the light period as it is at the beginning of the light period (39,42), reflecting a change in Bmax or number of receptors. Through continued stimulation by norepinephrine, perhaps more receptor sites are occupied at night; by the end of the day, more receptors are made available. Isoproterenol stimulates the synthesis of melatonin six times greater in the evening than in the morning, suggesting that other postsynaptic factors in addition to receptor number are responsible for the diurnal rhythm of responsivity (43).

N-ACETYLTRANSFERASE

Stimulation of the pineal's beta-adrenergic receptors by norepinephrine initiates a sequence of events (Figure 6) that culminate in the induction of N-acetyltransferase (44), the rate-limiting step in the synthesis of melatonin. N-acetyltransferase synthesizes N-acetylserotonin from serotonin, using acetyl CoA as a cofactor (Figure 7).

N-acetyltransferase activity accurately reflects melatonin synthesis, although there may be species variability (45,46). N-acetyltransferase activity increases at least twentyfold (2,47,48) during the night. The increase in activity can be blocked by reserpine, which depletes stores of norepinephrine, and by propranolol, a beta-adrenergic blocker (49). Isoproterenol stimulation of N-acetyltransferase activity is also blocked by propranolol (41).

Induction of N-acetyltransferase activity involves an increase in both mRNA and protein synthesis; consequently, cyclohexamide, an inhibitor of protein synthesis, can block stimulatory effects of isoproterenol on N-acetyltransferase activity and can block the nighttime rise in N-acetyltransferase due to norepinephrine stimulation (49,50). Cyclohexamide causes a slow decline in N-acetyltransferase activity with a half-life of about 1 hour. Induction also involves mRNA synthesis, since N-acetyltransferase can be inhibited by actinomycin D (51).

However, light (47) and propranolol (41), which block norepinephrine stimulation immediately, cause a rapid decrease in N-acetyltransferase activity (or N-acetylserotonin levels) with a half-life of about 10 minutes.

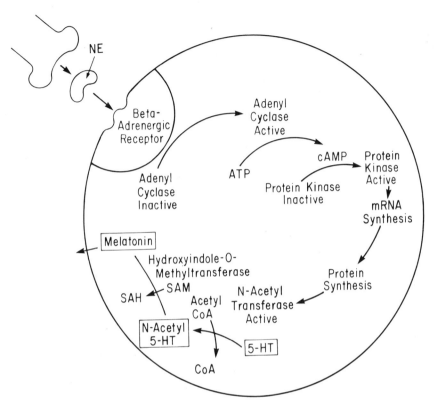

FIGURE 6. Sequence of biochemical events in the synthesis of melatonin after adrenergic stimulation of the pineal gland. (**NE** = norepinephrine, **ATP** = adenosine triphosphate, **cAMP** = cyclic AMP, **CoA** = coenzyme A, **SAH** = S-adenosylhomocysteine; see text and Figure 8 for definition of other abbreviations).

Reinduction of N-acetyltransferase activity can be blocked by cyclohexamide but not by actinomycin D (51). Furthermore, isoproterenol cannot stimulate N-acetyltransferase synthesis immediately, but only after a delay of 1–2 hours, typical of the usual lag time following lights-out (38). These data suggest that (1) the lag time at the beginning of the night is due to induction of N-acetyltransferase (requiring mRNA and protein synthesis); (2) the need for mRNA synthesis decreases after the lag period, and (3) there is an additional function for norepinephrine stimulation, namely, the maintenance of N-acetyltransferase activity. Although it is probable that synthesis of de novo protein is required for N-acetyltransferase activity, the specific protein has not yet been identified.

The additional function of norepinephrine stimulation of the beta-adrenergic receptor is maintenance of N-acetyltransferase in an active

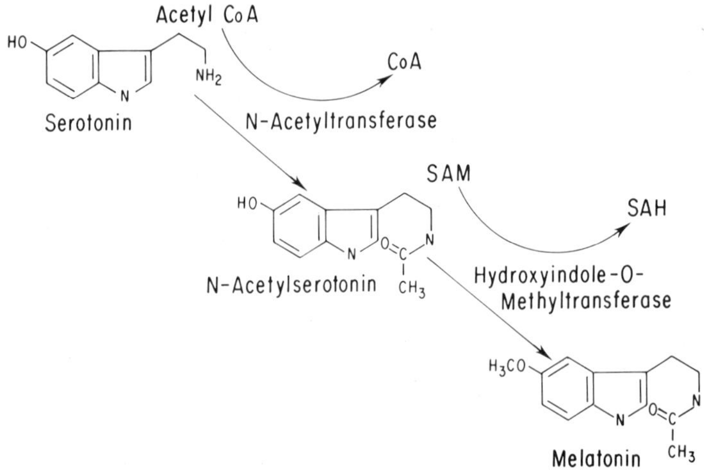

FIGURE 7. Synthesis of N-acetylserotonin and melatonin (see text and Figure 6 for definition of abbreviations).

form. Both protein synthesis and maintenance of N-acetyltransferase in the active form appear to be mediated by an increase in adenyl cyclase activity and cyclic AMP production.

Cyclic AMP is derived from ATP through the action of adenyl cyclase, which requires a divalent cation such as magnesium for activity (52). The first evidence identifying a beta-adrenergic receptor in the pineal came from work by Weiss and Costa (53), which showed that beta-adrenergic stimulation increased adenyl cyclase activity. Cyclic AMP is more highly concentrated in the pineal than in any other brain region (54).

At first, it was reported that the circadian rhythm in cyclic AMP levels was 180° out of phase with norepinephrine turnover and N-acetyltransferase activity. However, with improved methodology, it has been recently shown that cyclic AMP levels are greatest during the night (55). The activity of phosphodiesterase (which was discovered in the pineal by Weiss and Costa, 56) is also greatest at night and least during the day (57). Much of the work concerning the role of cyclic AMP has been through the use of dibutyryl cyclic AMP, which is not metabolized by phosphodiesterase and which mimics the effects of norepinephrine in the pineal (58,59).

Presumedly, cyclic AMP acts through a cyclic AMP-dependent protein kinase (60). The concentration of protein kinase is greater in the pineal than in any brain region (60). However, the protein kinase specifically involved in the synthesis or activation of N-acetyltransferase has not yet been identified.

HYDROXYINDOLE-O-METHYLTRANSFERASE

Melatonin is synthesized from N-acetylserotonin by the enzyme hydroxyindole-O-methyltransferase (HIOMT) (see Figure 7); S-adenosylmethionine (SAM) is a cofactor (44). HIOMT was at one time considered to be rate-limiting, but it at most has a twofold increase at night (61). Constant light over several days decreases HIOMT activity (61,62); some workers, however, have not found a rhythm in HIOMT activity (63,64). It is not clear if norepinephrine is involved in the stimulation of HIOMT activity (65). HIOMT, once believed to be exclusively found in the pineal, is apparently also found in the retina and the Harderian gland (66,67), but the Harderian gland enzyme may be of a different type (66). The postmortem decline in HIOMT is slow (even at room temperature) (68); therefore, measurement of postmortem levels of pineal HIOMT may be informative, including in humans (69–71).

SAM is formed from ATP by methionine-forming enzyme (72). The pineal gland contains high levels of methionine, much higher than in the brain (73,74). Levels of SAM can be increased by addition of dietary methionine (75).

The effects of various treatments on HIOMT activity are not clear. Hypothesized cholinergic control (76) is in dispute, since choline acetyltransferase appears not to be present in the rat pineal (77). Similarly, reports of parasympathetic innervation of the rabbit pineal (78) are confounded by the fact that choline acetyltransferase is also not present in the rabbit pineal (77). Acetyl cholinesterase has apparently been measured in the sympathetic fibers innervating the pineal, which is apparently diminished by 6-hydroxydopamine and ganglionectomy (27,83,84), but again this work must be evaluated in the light that there may be no choline acetyltransferase in the pineal (77).

SEROTONIN SYNTHESIS

The circadian rhythm in serotonin (5-HT) was the first circadian rhythm discovered in the pineal (85,86). The concentration of 5-HT in the pineal (0.5 mM) is higher than any region in the brain—more than 250-fold (87) and perhaps higher than in any organ in the body (87,88). Serotonin has a circadian rhythm in pineal levels of 10–20 µg/g at night and 60–90 µg/g during the day (89,90). There is also a high turnover of serotonin (87,88). Sympathetic control of the circadian rhythm in serotonin levels was discovered by Fiske (91) and Snyder et al. (92). Isoproterenol stimulates the reduction in serotonin levels (93). Some scientists feel that the decline in serotonin levels during the night may be mainly due to its metabolism to N-acetylserotonin and to melatonin (2,93,94), since alpha-methyl-para-tyrosine (an inhibitor of tyrosine hydroxylase) increases serotonin concentrations in the pineal (95,96).

Uptake of dietary tryptophan from the circulation is the first step in increasing the concentration of serotonin in the pineal. Serotonin is stored both in sympathetic nerves and in the pinealocytes (97,98). In the rabbit pineal gland, uptake of tryptophan is as high as 0.5–0.6 μg/g (99). The concentration of tryptophan is greatest in the pineal at the end of the light period and declines abruptly after the onset of darkness (100) (which is 180° out of phase with the rhythm of plasma tryptophan, implying that the uptake of tryptophan is not rate-limiting in the synthesis of serotonin and that pineal tryptophan is used mainly at night).

Tryptophan hydroxylase, the rate-limiting step (101,102) in the synthesis of serotonin (Figure 8), converts tryptophan to 5-hydroxytryptophan (5-HTP). It is found in higher concentrations in the pineal than in any other tissue in the body and requires a reduced pteridine cofactor, oxygen, and ferrous iron for its activity (101,103). Tryptophan hydroxylase in the pineal is also higher than in any other part of the brain (101). It appears to have a circadian rhythm in its activity, which was not originally noted (104,105). Its activity is greatest at night, suggesting that its "role" in the pineal is to supply serotonin for nighttime use. Exposure to continuous light reduces its activity and abolishes its circadian increase (105). Unlike for the brain enzyme, levels of tryptophan do not appear to saturate the pineal enzyme (21). It was first reported that tryptophan hydroxylation was stimulated by norepinephrine (106); however, a more recent study has shown that norepinephrine does not appear to stimulate tryptophan hydroxylase activity (21). This remains a confusing area, since propranolol can apparently inhibit tryptophan hydroxylase activity in vivo (104).

Serotonin is formed by decarboxylation of 5-HTP by 5-HTP decarboxylase (also known as aromatic l-amino acid decarboxylase) (Figure 8). This enzyme requires pyridoxal phosphate (107). It has greater activity than does tryptophan hydroxylase; consequently, 5-HTP is rapidly converted to serotonin. 5-HTP does not exist in high concentrations in the

FIGURE 8. Synthesis of 5-hydroxytryptophan and serotonin.

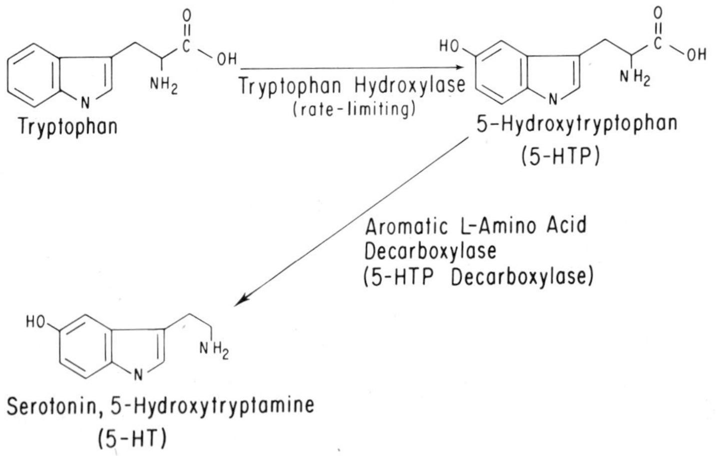

Tryptophan

Tryptophan Hydroxylase
(rate-limiting)

5-Hydroxytryptophan
(5-HTP)

Aromatic L-Amino Acid
Decarboxylase
(5-HTP Decarboxylase)

Serotonin, 5-Hydroxytryptamine
(5-HT)

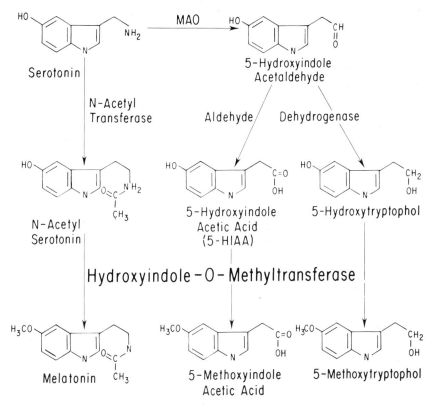

FIGURE 9. Metabolism of serotonin.

pineal; accordingly, 5-HTP decarboxylase is not considered to be rate-limiting. There is also no 24-hour rhythm in this enzyme's activity (108).

Serotonin can be metabolized by MAO to form 5-hydroxyindole acetaldehyde (109,110). This compound then is rapidly oxidized by aldehyde dehydrogenase to 5-hydroxyindole acetic acid (5-HIAA) (111,112). These compounds are shown in Figure 9. In the rabbit, approximately one-third of pineal tryptophan is converted directly to kynurenine (113).

MELATONIN

Melatonin, or N-acetyl-5-methoxytryptamine, was identified by Lerner as the most active substance in the pineal capable of blanching amphibian melanocytes (10,114–121), a biological effect that forms the basis for the bioassay (121–129). The potency of melatonin is more than 10,000 times greater than the potency of any other compound. The concentration of melatonin in rat pineal gland is 0.4–4.0 μg/g during the day and 2.0–7.0 μg/g at night (130,131).

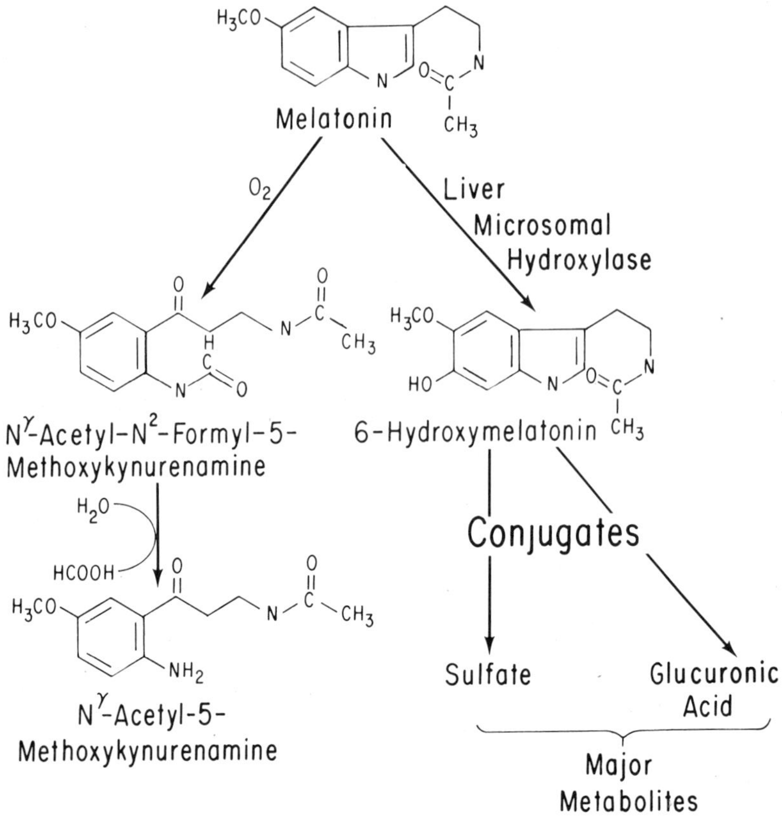

FIGURE 10. Metabolism of melatonin.

Melatonin has a melting point of 117°C. It does not go into aqueous solution easily. This can be facilitated, however, by dissolving it in a small amount of ethanol, methanol, or chloroform (10,118,119).

Melatonin has a half-life of between 10 and 40 minutes (132–134). In rats, more than 90% is cleared in a single pass through the liver (135). In mice, 70–80% is converted in the liver microsomal system to 6-hydroxymelatonin, which is subsequently conjugated as a sulfate (70%) or as a glucuronide (6%) (132). In humans (136), perhaps the glucuronide fraction is slightly higher. Less than 1% is excreted unchanged. It is possible that as much as 12% is excreted as N-acetyl-5-methoxykynurenamine (132,137) (see Figure 10). Chlorpromazine inhibits 6-hydroxylation of melatonin (138–140).

OTHER COMPOUNDS

This chapter will not discuss other compounds in the pineal, although the enzymes just discussed synthesize many other indoles, such as 5-

methoxytryptophol and 5-hydroxytryptophol (see Figure 9). It is too soon to tell how important these or other pineal indoles are (141); this topic should be the subject of a future text. Pineal peptides are discussed in other chapters of this book (see the chapters by Pévet, Reiter, Relkin).

IMPLICATIONS OF ADRENERGIC INNERVATION

The pineal is unique in its sympathetic innervation. Most *endocrine* glands are regulated by blood-born substances usually of pituitary origin. (Some *exocrine* glands are innervated by peripheral postganglionic neurons.) The adrenal medulla (which is considered by some to be a homologous variant of a postganglionic sympathetic neuron since it synthesizes and secretes catecholamines) is innervated by *preganglionic* fibers (from splanchic nerves); however, the pineal is innervated by *postganglionic* neurons from the superior cervical ganglia. What is also remarkable (and has important implications) is that these neurons do not respond to stress (34,35). The "fight or flight" response typical of the sympathetic nervous system as a whole does not include the sympathetic nerves of the pineal (which are discretely regulated by an endogenous circadian pacemaker).

The pineal is also unusual in that melatonin production is not regulated by parasympathetic nerves (see the earlier section on Hydroxyindole-O-Methyltransferase). A few studies, however, suggest in at least some species the existence of efferent innervation to the pineal whose function is not as yet known (142–145). New evidence may come to light, but at this time it seems safe to assume that neuroregulation of melatonin production is exclusively sympathetic (11–13). The pineal apparently also has presynaptic alpha-2 autoadrenoceptors (146). [Postsynaptic pineal alpha-adrenergic receptors appear to regulate phosopholipid metabolism in the pineal (147).] It is too soon to know the role of prostaglandins (148) or cyclic GMP (149,150) in the pineal.

The Pineal as a Model of Adrenergic Function

Because the pineal is innervated by peripheral postganglionic sympathetic neurons that appear to be exclusively involved in the regulation of melatonin production, this gland has advantages as an experimental model for evaluation of adrenergic function. It is particularly useful since synthesis of melatonin normally does not exceed basal levels during the day and since stress (which increases the levels of circulating catecholamines) does not influence melatonin production due to highly active uptake mechanisms (34,35). (Since melatonin production is not affected by stress, measurement of melatonin is not a "marker" for stress.) It is also important to remember that the pineal is a peripheral, not a central, organ (its beta-adrenergic receptors are outside of the blood-brain barrier).

In animal experimentation, the pineal gland facilitates several ways in which to evaluate adrenergic function. Because the nerves of the pineal are quiescent during the day (and firing rate can be suppressed at any time by light), neuronal firing can be manipulated without the use of drugs. During the day, postsynaptic function can be selectively evaluated (since the presynaptic nerves are quiescent) by administration of an agonist, such as isoproterenol (see Figure 11, top). Because uptake mechanisms function day and night, these mechanisms can be evaluated by comparing responses to isoproterenol (which is not taken up presynaptically) and to norepinephrine (which is). During the night, the sympathetic nerves are active. Nighttime measurement of melatonin secretion is a measure of both pre- and postsynaptic function (see Figure 11, bottom).

FIGURE 11. Stimulation of melatonin production during the day by exogenous administration of isoproterenol, a beta-adrenergic agonist that is not taken up into the presynaptic neuron (top); nighttime production of melatonin by endogenously released norepinephrine **(NE)** from the pineal's adrenergic neurons (bottom).

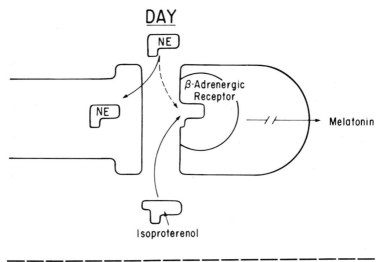

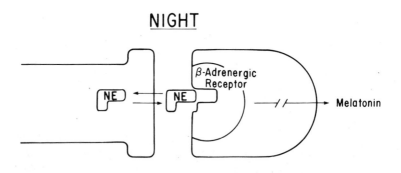

A hypothetical experiment would be as follows. Suppose a drug caused a 50% reduction of melatonin reduction at night and a 50% decrease in melatonin levels in response to isoproterenol during the day. This would indicate that the drug had primarily postsynaptic activity and relatively little presynaptic activity. On the other hand, suppose the drug caused only 10% reduction in response to isoproterenol during the day but a 50% reduction at night. Then it would be reasonable to conclude that the drug had primarily a presynaptic effect.

Human Adrenergic Studies

As is the case for melatonin in all mammals studied to date, human melatonin appears to be under adrenergic control. Patients with transection of the cervical spinal cord have disturbed melatonin secretory patterns (151). Patients with Shy-Drager syndrome (multiple system atrophy) and idiopathic orthostatic hypotension, diseases that are manifested by central and peripheral sympathetic lesions, have reduced levels of plasma melatonin (152) and urinary 6-hydroxymelatonin (153). These data suggest that the human pineal is regulated by sympathetic adrenergic neurons. Vaughan originally demonstrated in one healthy subject that propranolol blocks nighttime melatonin secretion (154). This was later confirmed in a psychiatric patient (155) and in several human subjects (author's unpublished data).

Doses of 120–140 mg administered orally at night can completely reduce melatonin secretion to daytime levels or below (author's unpublished data). Propranolol may therefore be used to help evaluate adrenergic function of the human pineal in vivo. The amount of propranolol that causes 50% reduction of melatonin levels may be related to pineal beta-adrenergic receptor function. Propranolol may also have a use in the treatment of hypersecretion of melatonin. Administration of propranolol also affords the opportunity to understand the relationship between melatonin secretion and secretion of other endocrine substances. After reducing melatonin secretion with propranolol, changes in the levels of other hormones could be assessed. Administration of the same dose of propranolol on a subsequent night in addition to an infusion of physiologic levels of melatonin would control for any beta-adrenergic and/or nonspecific effects of propranolol; thus hormonal changes due to the reduction of melatonin levels can be specifically determined.

CLONIDINE

Human melatonin secretion is also reduced by clonidine. (156). This alpha-adrenergic agonist is primarily selective for presynaptic alpha-2 adrenergic autoreceptors but stimulates postsynaptic alpha-1 and alpha-2 adrenergic receptors as well.

Clonidine, which passes through the blood-brain barrier, has been used to evaluate alpha-adrenergic receptors in a variety of disorders, including affective disorders (157). Clonidine's effects have been evaluated by measuring growth hormone or blood pressure. However, these physiological variables may be regulated by more than one neurotransmitter. Also, compensatory autonomic mechanisms can confound the cardiovascular effects of clonidine. Consequently, measurement of melatonin secretion in response to clonidine may provide a more specific index of alpha-2-adrenoceptor function; however, the location of these receptors remains to be demonstrated.

One hour after intravenous administration of clonidine, melatonin levels are reduced; there is a linear dose-response relationship (156). Oral clonidine is also effective; this may be a more practical route of administration. After oral administration, there is a lag time and a longer duration of action. It may also be possible to measure urinary 6-hydroxymelatonin sulfate in an overnight collection in order to quantify melatonin excretion.

MANIC-DEPRESSIVE PATIENTS

Naturalistic measurement of melatonin remains the simplest way of evaluating adrenergic activity. In a preliminary study, plasma melatonin secretion was measured in five manic-depressive patients, in both manic and depressed states (158). Problems of age, sex, drug regimen, or time of year that might confound the results were avoided, since patients also were on the same drug regimen in both phases of the illness and were studied at the same time of year in each mood state. Melatonin levels were increased in mania compared to depression, which is compatible with increased adrenergic activity in mania compared to depression.

Wetterberg et al. also found that unipolar patients have decreased melatonin levels when depressed, compared to when they are not depressed (159). Jimerson et al. studied bipolar depressed patients and found no difference in urinary immunoreactive melatonin (160); however, they compared patients to healthy subjects. Since it is not known if phase of the menstrual cycle, age, sex, and time of year affect melatonin secretion, it is recommended that these variables be controlled for as much as possible. Either the "area under the curve" of plasma melatonin levels or an overnight (or 24-hour) urinary 6-hydroxymelatonin sulfate level is the optimal method of measuring adrenergic function.

HUMAN BETA-ADRENERGIC AGONIST STUDIES

Although the human pineal is probably regulated by sympathetic adrenergic neurons, stimulation of these beta-adrenergic receptors during the day in humans is difficult, since the dose of these drugs that would be necessary to stimulate melatonin secretion would cause untoward cardiovascular effects. At least 1 hour of continuous stimulation is necessary to provide sufficient time for the induction of N-acetyltransferase. This problem may have been avoided in a recent investigation by studying volunteers who exercised for a length of time on an exercycle, which produced a twofold increase in melatonin levels (161). This increase is considerably less than the response seen in experimental animals with isoproterenol, but assay specificity may have contributed to this apparent difference in response. Using the gas chromatography-negative chemical ionization mass spectrometric (neg CI GCMS) assay (162), doses of isoproterenol, tyramine, l-DOPA, and dopamine (which caused a 50% increase in heart rate for 1 hour) were insufficient to raise melatonin levels significantly (author's unpublished data). Negative results in attempting to stimulate melatonin production during the day in some species (such as man) is possibly a dosage problem.

HUMAN PLASMA MELATONIN ASSAY

Assays for melatonin are the subject of another chapter in this book (see Lynch). However, some discussion of GCMS assays is warranted here. There seems to be a growing consensus that the neg CI GCMS assay is the most accurate of the human plasma melatonin assays (163). However, GCMS assays require expensive instrumentation that is difficult to maintain. Therefore, a principal use for this assay is validation of other assays.

As with all assays, the lower the values, the more specific the assay. To compare an assay to the neg CI GCMS assay, plasma levels of melatonin should be low during the day (ideally 2–10 pg/ml) and in the range of 25–100 pg/ml at night. The dynamic range is perhaps more important: with the mass spectral assay, there is a ten- to fiftyfold increase from day to night. Values that are similar to those of the GCMS assay at night but higher than the GCMS values during the day probably indicate the presence of a consistent level of a contaminant that appears to be relatively greater during the day than at night. Ideally, values should be corrected for recovery, since artifactually lower results could occur due to low or variable recovery. (The values of the neg CI GCMS assay are corrected for recovery.) There is a broad range of specifities among the various assays; however, absolute specificity is not necessary for many types of studies. Nonetheless, it is important to interpret data from a particular assay according to its specificity and the requirements for each experiment.

GCMS is considered to be highly specific, since compounds are identified (by molecular weight as well as by retention time) as they are quantified. However, not all GCMS assays are optimally specific. It is important that a deuterated internal standard be used. The deuterated internal standard is chemically similar to endogenous melatonin and melatonin of the external standard curve except that it has a slightly higher molecular weight. When added to the plasma at the initiation of the assay, the deuterated internal standard coextracts, coderivatizes, cochromatographs, and cofragments with the nondeuterated (endogenous) melatonin. Measurement of two fragment ions at a characteristic intensity ratio is the mass spectral "fingerprint" for the parent molecule.

Retention times are known exactly for each injection; the retention time of plasma melatonin is the same as that of the internal standard. Interfering substances (should they occur) can be visually noted since they are characterized by "shoulders" preceding or following the melatonin peak. A recovery is calculated for each sample; thus each point of the external standard curve and each plasma sample is corrected for any losses that might occur during the assay.

Adequate sensitivity has been a problem for GCMS. The neg CI GCMS assay (162) has the requisite sensitivity for measuring plasma melatonin (minimal detectable concentration < 1 pg/ml) and is among the most sensitive of the human plasma melatonin assays (164). Since it uses a deuterated internal standard, this assay also has a high degree of specificity and precision.

Urinary 6-Hydroxymelatonin

Measurement of 6-hydroxymelatonin sulfate in the urine has been performed with mass spectral assays using deuterated internal standards (165,166). The day/night dynamic range in the concentration of this urinary metabolite is similar to plasma melatonin (as measured by the neg CI GCMS assay). Only low levels of 6-hydroxymelatonin are excreted during the day, implying that marked daytime pulsatile secretion of melatonin does not occur (again, this is in agreement with the plasma melatonin data as measured by the neg CI GCMS assay, since it is rare that plasma levels above 10 pg/ml are found in sighted healthy humans during the day).

The urinary 6-hydroxymelatonin assay is the method of choice for measuring amplitude of secretion; the plasma melatonin assay is the method of choice for evaluating timing of secretion. Urine is difficult to collect in shorter than 6-hour intervals; consequently, only a gross estimate of the day/night rhythm can be obtained. Measurement of plasma melatonin, however, requires many time points, not only for determination of onset, maximum, or offset of secretion, but also for description of a curve of values under which an area can be calculated. Measurement of urinary excretion of 6-hydroxymelatonin usually involves fewer data points per subject.

The Question of Extrapineal Melatonin

After pinealectomy, rats have very little plasma melatonin during the day or night or after administration of isoproterenol as measured by the neg CI GCMS assay (minimal detectable concentration < 1 pg/ml) (167) (see Figure 12). Pelham reported similar results in the chicken using a bioassay (168,169). Arendt found that only after complete pinealectomy could sheep plasma melatonin be abolished (170). It is not known as yet exactly how low are the "true" levels of melatonin and 6-hydroxymelatonin after pinealectomy, because these levels approach the minimal detectable concentration of the most sensitive assays. Measurement of

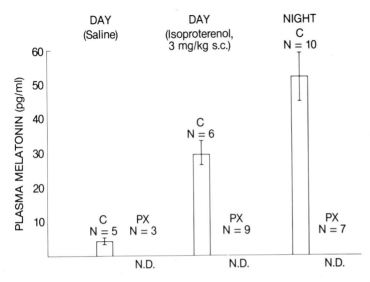

FIGURE 12. Pinealectomized **(PX)** rats have nondetectable (N.D.) plasma melatonin (minimal detectable concentration < 1 pg/ml using the negative chemical ionization mass spectral assay), whereas sham-operated controls **(C)** have low, but measurable concentrations during the day and higher concentrations during the night or after daytime administration of a beta-adrenergic agonist (isoproterenol). *From Lewy et al. (167).*

substantial amounts of melatonin in the circulation after pinealectomy most likely indicates an assay specificity problem. Reduction of melatonin at night in humans after administering propranolol (154,155, author's unpublished data) suggests that most of human plasma melatonin is derived from the pineal gland, since it is unlikely that other sources of melatonin would be under beta-adrenergic regulation.

The existence of extrapineal sources of melatonin remains controversial. The presence of melatonin in other organs needs to be demonstrated in pinealectomized animals to rule out the pineal as a source for melatonin. Identification of melatonin by immunohistological techniques using antibodies whose specificity has not been absolutely assured leaves unanswered the question of the true identity of "immunoreactive melatonin" in extrapineal tissue. Demonstration of melatonin production in a tissue culture after adding serotonin is not adequate proof of extrapineal synthesis in vivo; identification of extrapineal N-acetyltransferase and HIOMT activity should also include evidence of serotonin in those organs at adequate concentrations. If extrapineal sources of melatonin exist, it is unlikely that they make a significant contribution to plasma or urine levels.

Abolition of plasma melatonin after pinealectomy provides validation for using circulating levels to estimate pineal secretion of this hormone and provides the basis for further work with plasma levels as a marker for adrenergic activity as well as for the circadian system.

REGULATION: THE CIRCADIAN SYSTEM

One of the reasons that plasma melatonin and urinary 6-hydroxyme-latonin are useful markers for adrenergic function is that melatonin secretion can be manipulated nonpharmacologically by light exposure, thus increasing versatility of experimental design. Melatonin secretion is also a highly useful marker for the circadian system and may be unique for assessing the effects of environmental light.

Circadian Anatomy

For more than 50 years, it has been known that the endogenous circadian pacemaker is located in the brain (171,172). In many species of animals, the pacemaker is thought to be located in the suprachiasmatic nucleus (SCN) of the hypothalamus (173–176). There may be more than one functional pacemaker and more than one anatomical pacemaker. However, with regard to melatonin production by the pineal gland, there is increasing agreement that there is one pacemaker and that it is located in the SCN.

Lesioning of the SCN results in a decrease of N-acetyltransferase activity (65,177). For this reason, it was thought that the SCN "turns on" the sympathetic stimulation of the pineal. In other words, when the SCN is "on," the pineal is "on." Recent studies may have challenged this view, since stimulation of some SCN neurons causes a decrease in sympathetic activity (178). Also, both inhibitory and excitatory responses have been recorded in response to light (178,179). However, these neurophysiological studies are difficult to interpret and do not necessarily rule out that SCN activity results in an "on" signal. (Should the SCN prove to be "off" at night, then there must be a center of "on" activity caudal to the SCN, which is inhibited by the SCN during the day.) Studies of uptake of 2-deoxy-D-(C^{14}) glucose show increased uptake during the day compared to night (180,181). However, the greatest uptake in these studies occurs during exposure to light at night, which suggests that this assay might be measuring synaptic activity at the interface of the SCN, as well as activity within the SCN itself. Future studies are necessary to determine with certainty whether the SCN is "on" or "off" at night with respect to sympathetic stimulation of the pineal.

The effects of light on the SCN are mediated by the retinohypothalamic tract (RHT) (182). The RHT extends from the retina (or the optic nerve) to the contralateral (70%) and ipsilateral (30%) SCN (183). For several years, it was thought that the inferior accessory optic tract mediated effects of light on the SCN-pineal system (177); however, the effects of light on this system appear to be mediated by the RHT (65). Circadian

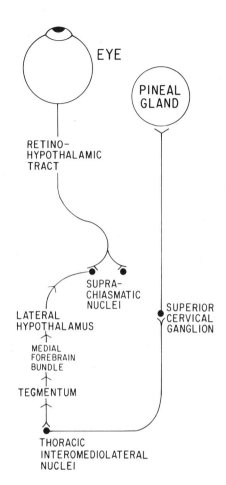

EYE

PINEAL
GLAND

RETINO-
HYPOTHALAMIC
TRACT

SUPRA-
CHIASMATIC
NUCLEI

LATERAL
HYPOTHALAMUS

SUPERIOR
CERVICAL
GANGLION

MEDIAL
FOREBRAIN
BUNDLE

TEGMENTUM

THORACIC
INTEROMEDIOLATERAL
NUCLEI

FIGURE 13. Schematic diagram of the neuroanatomical connections from the retina to the pineal gland.

anatomy is schematically represented in Figure 13. Other inputs to the SCN may come from the ventral nucleus of the lateral geniculate body (184,185) and midbrain raphe nuclei (186), but they are probably not important for entrainment of the SCN by the light/dark cycle (187–189).

The neural pathway from the SCN to the sympathetic outflow is not entirely known. A multisynaptic pathway of an unknown number of synapses connects the SCN to the interomediolateral nuclei of the upper thoracic segments in the spinal cord where the preganglionic sympathetic fibers originate (12). This pathway traverses the tuberal and lateral hypothalamus, the medial forebrain bundle, and the rostral part of the mesencephalic tegmentum. Preganglionic sympathetic fibers synapse with postganglionic sympathetic fibers in the superior cervical ganglion (SCG). Postganglionic fibers course back up into the brain as the nervi conarii (11).

Effects of Light in Animals

Light has three effects on melatonin production: (1) the light/dark cycle entrains the endogenous pacemaker that drives the melatonin production rhythm; (2) light suppresses melatonin production; (3) the changing lengths of daylight and darkness regulate the annual (seasonal) patterns of melatonin production.

ENTRAINMENT BY THE LIGHT/DARK CYCLE

The effect of the light/dark cycle on the circadian rhythm of melatonin production is so profound that at first it was thought that the light/dark cycle directly regulated melatonin production, i.e., that melatonin production passively followed environmental conditions of light and dark. Later, it was discovered that the rhythm persisted in blinded animals or animals kept in constant darkness (2,190,191). Identification of the neuroanatomical innervation of the SCN and its function led scientists to conclude that the light/dark cycle regulates melatonin production through its effects on an endogenous hypothalamic circadian pacemaker (the SCN).

Circadian means "about a day" or about 24 hours (192). When an animal is not entrained to the light/dark cycle, it displays a circadian rhythm of approximately, but not precisely, 24 hours; this is termed "free-running." In constant darkness, the melatonin production rhythm free-runs with the activity/rest cycle (melatonin production still occurs at "night," that is, during the activity phase of nocturnal animals or during the rest phase of diurnal animals) (191,193,194). The activity rhythm and the melatonin production rhythm are "hands of the clock" not the "clock" itself, which is presumedly the SCN.

The period (τ, or tau) of the free-running endogenous pacemaker is a characteristic of an individual animal and usually of a particular species. Some animals have endogenous periods that are longer than 24 hours ($\tau>24$), some shorter than 24 hours ($\tau<24$) (195,196). In general, the former is more common in diurnal animals, the latter in nocturnal animals (195,196). Why is the endogenous free-running period (τ) of the biological clock not precisely 24 hours? Perhaps because a biological clock can never be as precise as a physical clock. Perhaps being slightly different than 24 hours permits greater flexibility for accommodation to the changes in the times of dawn and dusk throughout the year. Pittendrigh has reasoned that internal phase relationships would be unstable if the period of the endogenous pacemaker were to be exactly 24 hours (197).

When endogenous rhythms are synchronized by an environmental time cue, such as the 24-hour light/dark cycle, they are "entrained." The period of the environmental cycle must be close to the endogenous period (τ) for entrainment to occur. The "range of entrainment" is the range in the periods of the environmental cycle that are capable of synchronizing the endogenous pacemaker.

PHASE RESPONSE CURVE

The interaction of light as a zeitgeber (literally, time giver) with the endogenous pacemaker can be described and predicted by a phase response curve (PRC). This topic has not been dealt with in previous pineal texts, so it deserves a detailed discussion here. The PRC was first discovered by exposing an animal free-running in constant darkness to a

FIGURE 14. Schematic diagrams of hypothesized phase response curves for animals with endogenous circadian periods equal to (top), greater than (middle), or less than (bottom) 24 hours.

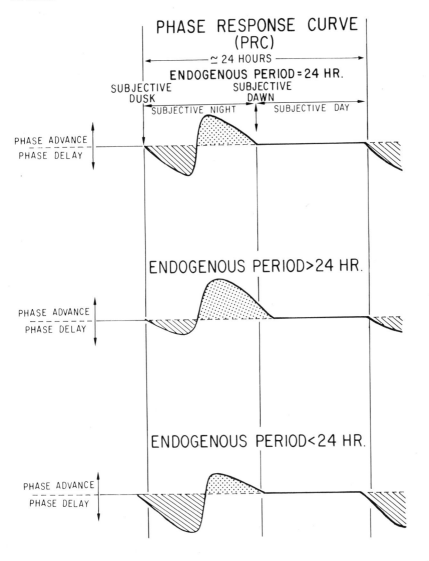

short (15-minute) pulse of light. The animal responded with an advance in phase or a delay in phase, depending on the phase at which the light pulse occurred (197). Phase refers to a specific time within a circadian cycle. Because the animal is in constant darkness, the term "subjective day" refers to that part of the animal's time spent in behavior typical during the day (rest for nocturnal animals, activity for diurnal animals). Subjective night refers to that part of the animal's time spent typically during the night (rest for diurnal animals, activity for nocturnal animals). Subjective dawn and dusk refer to the transitions between activity and rest.

If the light pulse occurs during the animal's subjective night, the animal will respond with either an advance or a delay; if the light pulse occurs during the animal's subjective day, the animal will not respond with much of a phase shift. This is true for both diurnal and nocturnal animals. During subjective night, the closer the pulse occurs to subjective dawn, the more likely the animal will respond with an advance in phase; the closer to dusk, the more likely there will be a delay in phase. In the middle of the night, there is an inflection point where an advance is separated from a delay by only a few minutes. An anthropomorphic explanation might be that, if the light pulse occurs during the first half of night, the animal "thinks" of it as "dusk;" if in the second half of night, as "dawn." In general, the closer the pulse is to the middle of the night, the greater the magnitude of the response (in either direction). Thus, the middle of the night is a time where the maximum phase advance is separated from the maximum phase delay by only a few minutes (Figure 14). Since the animal is in constant darkness, it continues to free-run throughout this procedure, relative to the transient phase shift due to the light pulse. A PRC has recently been described measuring chicken N-acetyltransferase activity (198), although the full effect was not determined because the animals were sacrificed the day after the light pulse: several circadian cycles are needed to realize the full response to a light pulse. In the rat, a light pulse as short as 1 minute can shift the phase of the N-acetyltransferase activity rhythm (199).

SKELETON PHOTOPERIOD

What happens under entrained conditions? Another experimental paradigm for evaluating the PRC is the skeleton photoperiod. This is accomplished by two 15-minute pulses of light several hours apart. The pulse that occurs near the phase-advance portion of the PRC will function as "dawn"; the pulse that occurs close to the phase delay part of the PRC functions as "dusk." The relative magnitude of the phase advance compared to the phase delay produces a net effect.

Consider an animal with a free-running period longer than 24 hours, for example, 25 hours. For stable steady-state entrainment to 24 hours, each day the light/dark cycle must advance the endogenous pacemaker 1 hour. The net effect must also include a phase advance to compensate for any phase delay that might result each day from the action of light on the phase-delay portion of the PRC. If $\tau > 24$ hours, then the animal must advance more than delay each day for entrainment to a 24-hour period. A major factor in determining the shape of the PRC is whether an animal's endogenous period is greater than or less than 24 hours (see Figure 14).

NATURAL CONDITIONS

In nature, animals are exposed to a photoperiod that is several hours in duration. It is not simple to generalize from the skeleton photoperiod to the natural photoperiod. However, the margins of the natural photoperiod seem to be most important for entrainment, because of the typical shapes of the PRCs. That portion of the PRC with the greatest area under it would be most significant in determining the daily net change in phase. As can be seen in Figure 14, if $\tau > 24$ hours, the animal will have a greater area under the advance part of its PRC, and if $\tau < 24$ hours, it will have a greater area under the delay part of the PRC. The greater the difference between τ and 24 hours, the more asymmetric the PRC. In nature, there may be significant species variation. For example, in Drosophila, in every photoperiod of 12 or more hours of continuous light, the endogenous pacemaker is stopped at midcycle (197). It is not clear if this phenomenon occurs in mammals.

It is also not clear what happens to the phase of circadian rhythms during the changing seasons. On the one hand, one might expect phases of circadian rhythms to be constant throughout the year, since dawn and dusk change symmetrically. However, it is possible that some circadian rhythms might change their phases during the year (especially in animals with very asymmetrical PRCs), since the PRC must shift its phase (at least transiently and particularly during times of increased rate of change in the photoperiod) to maintain stable 24-hour steady-state entrainment. This will be discussed under Photoperiodism.

SUPPRESSANT EFFECT OF LIGHT

The suppressant effect of light appears to be unique to melatonin production by the pineal gland. It is thought that the retinohypothalamic tract mediates both the entrainment effect of light and the suppressant effect of light (65). For this reason, the suppressant effect may be a way of assessing the properties of light important for the entrainment effect.

In experimental animals, very dim light is sufficient to suppress melatonin production. As little as 1–2 lux will suppress N-acetyltransferase activity by 50% in the rat (200). Less than 500 lux will completely suppress N-acetyltransferase activity in the sheep and the monkey (201,202). Suppression occurs immediately, with the decline in melatonin levels corresponding to its half-life in plasma or CSF (134). On return to darkness, N-acetyltransferase and melatonin levels resume their pretreatment values within a few minutes. However, in the rat, melatonin production resumes slowly, and only if the light pulse occurs during the first half of the night (49,203). One minute of light is sufficient for suppression of melatonin production in the rat or the hamster (203,204). The effects of light on hydroxyindole-O-methyltransferase have been discussed earlier. They do not appear to be as dramatic as the effects of light on N-acetyltransferase, but apparently they are mediated by the same neural pathways (65).

There is one study of the wavelengths important for light suppression of melatonin production. The action spectrum has a peak in the blue-green range, which corresponds to the middle of the visual spectrum and to the action spectrum for rhodopsin (205).

"CLOCK-GATE" MODEL

It is useful at this point to propose a model (which may be modified in the future) relating the entrainment and suppressant effects of light. Because of the suppressant effect of light, darkness acts as a "gate" that must be open in order for melatonin production to be expressed, providing that it coincides with the proper circadian phase (as set by the endogenous "clock" or pacemaker, the SCN). Light also entrains the endogenous pacemaker in a relationship described by a PRC. In other words, light entrains the clock (the endogenous pacemaker for melatonin production), but light can also suppress the "hand of the clock" (melatonin production per se).

In this model, the signal to initiate melatonin production begins only after *both* the clock is "on" and the gate is open (i.e., between dusk and dawn). It is assumed in this model, perhaps arbitrarily, that the "clock on" phase and the "clock off" phase of the endogenous pacemaker are each 12 hours in duration when entrained to a 24-hour light/dark cycle and are approximately 12 hours long during free-running conditions. The width of the gate, however, varies according to the length of the scotoperiod (dark period): the gate is open wider in the winter than in the summer. Therefore, in the summer, gating effects are most profound. In the winter, there may be little or no gating.

As discussed previously (under N-Acetyltransferase), there is a lag period between the signal to initiate melatonin production and the increase in N-acetyltransferase activity. The lag period is present primarily in the first part of the night. Presumably, once mRNA necessary for N-acetyltransferase activity is synthesized initially, it does not need to be synthesized for the remainder of the night.

A significant feature of the clock-gate model is that when the clock is on *before* dusk (that is, the gate is not yet open), the clock can be on and yet the signal to initiate melatonin production can be off; that is, the later dusk occurs, the later melatonin production begins (Figure 15, top, middle). However, when "clock on" begins *after* dusk (Figure 15, bottom), the onset of melatonin production is related not to the time of dusk but to the time of "clock on." Thus, in the winter, melatonin production may occur late in relation to dusk, not only because dusk is occurring earlier but also because "clock on" is occurring after dusk.

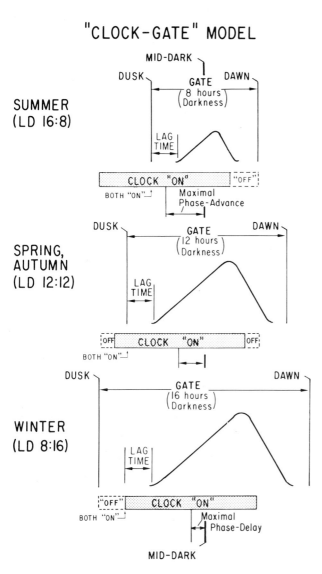

FIGURE 15. "Clock-gate" model proposed to explain how the light/dark cycle **(LD)** entrains the "clock" (the endogenous pacemaker) for melatonin production and how darkness gates the expression of melatonin production.

Furthermore, "clock on" may actually be changing its phase in relation to real (solar) time. This annual shift in phase has been indicated relative to middark in Figure 15.

The essence of the clock-gate model is that the hand of the clock is not necessarily providing accurate information about the clock itself. To use melatonin secretion as a meaningful marker for the endogenous pacemaker, the gate must be maximally open. This means that *on the day of the experiment only*, darkness must occur before the expected "clock on" and continue until after the expected "clock off."

An implication of the clock-gate model is that whereas entrainment to a new light/dark cycle is best seen several days after a shift, gating effects are best observed on the first day of the shift. This principle is illustrated in a recent paper by Illnerová and Vaněček (206). (The reader may find the following discussion more meaningful after examining Figure 1 of their paper.) The day after lengthening the scotoperiod from 12 to 16 hours, the onset of melatonin production occurred *earlier*, but there was no change in the offset. However, after several days, both the onset and the offset shifted *later*. According to the clock-gate model, the interpretation of these data would be that the earlier timing of the onset on the day after the shift represented the actual time of "clock on" on the previous 12:12 light/dark cycle (which had appeared to be later on the 12:12 schedule because of the gating effect of that schedule). The later timing of both onset and offset after several days on the new light/dark cycle suggests that the endogenous pacemaker shifted to a delayed phase position relative to where it was on the previous 12:12 light/dark cycle (see Figure 15, middle and bottom, for a schematic representation of the difference between entrainment to a 12:12 light/dark cycle and entrainment to an 8:16 light/dark cycle).

In the same study (206), when rats were switched from a 12:12 light/dark cycle to a 16:8 schedule, gating effects were also, as predicted by the clock-gate model, most notable on the day after the shift: the onset of melatonin production shifted *later* (due to gating by the later-occurring dusk) and the offset of melatonin production occurred *earlier* (suppressed by the earlier-occurring dawn). After several days on the 16:8 schedule, offset shifted to an even more phase-advanced position. indicating the time of "clock off" before dawn (see Figure 15, middle and top, for a schematic representation of the difference between entrainment to a 12:12 light/dark cycle and entrainment to an 16:8 light/dark cycle).

The clock-gate model explains Illnerová and Vaneček's data (206) by assuming that dawn is more important than dusk in entraining the endogenous pacemaker for melatonin production. As discussed earlier (under Phase Response Curve), in an animal with $\tau > 24$ hours, dawn is expected to be more effective than dusk, since the phase-advance portion of the curve is more pronounced (see Figure 14, middle). Whether dawn is more, less, or equally as important as dusk for entraining the endogenous pacemaker in an animal with $\tau < 24$ hours can only be answered with experimental data in such species. It is possible that this model may have to be modified to include the possibility that in another species dusk may be more important than dawn for entrainment or that both are equally important. However, data from the rat (206–208) and the Djungarian hamster (209), as interpreted by the clock-gate model, indicate that dawn is more important. Although for entrainment dawn appears to be more important than dusk, dusk appears to be more important than dawn for the gating effect under most light/dark schedules [acutely increasing the scotoperiod symmetrically affects the onset of melatonin production more than the offset (206,210)].

Because light acutely suppresses melatonin production, it is tempting to link suppression of melatonin production with the entrainment effect of light. Indeed, they both appear to be mediated by the retinohypothalamic tract and perhaps by the same neurotransmitters (65,211,212). Operationally, however, these two effects of light appear to be different, and it is still possible that the pathways mediating the suppressant and the entrainment effects of light may not be the same. During steady-state entrainment to most light/dark cycles, melatonin production in the Djungarian hamster, Syrian hamster and the rat decreases before lights on (206,209,210). (In other species, however, melatonin production may not begin to decline until at or after lights on.) Under natural conditions, this matter becomes even more complicated.

One endogenous pacemaker was assumed for the clock-gate model. However, there may be two pacemakers involved in the timing of melatonin production, one for onset and one for offset. (These alternative possibilities can be tested experimentally.) Also, at the present time it is not known whether or not the maximum amplitude of production changes as a function of the length of night. (In Figure 15, it was arbitrarily assumed that the longer the duration of melatonin production, the greater its maximum amplitude.) Another unanswered question is whether or not there is a shift in the phase of the endogenous pacemaker throughout the year. In the rat, there appears to be a phase delay in the winter relative to a phase advance in the summer (206). Although a seasonal change in the phase of the endogenous pacemaker can be explained by the clock-gate model (see Figure 15), this is a modifiable part of the model and may vary from species to species. A phase change dependent on time of year (or length of photoperiod) will be discussed in more detail under Photoperiodism.

In summary, the clock-gate model is proposed in order to relate the gating of melatonin production (that is due to the suppressant effect of light) to the timing of the melatonin production rhythm by an endogenous pacemaker (that is entrained by the light/dark cycle). In the rat (206–208) and the Djungarian hamster (209), it appears that dawn may be more important than dusk for entrainment (in these animals, $\tau > 24$ hours) whereas dusk appears to be more important than dawn for gating. (Gating is best demonstrated immediately after changing the light/dark cycle whereas several days must pass before the full effects of entrainment can be known.) Onset of melatonin secretion, because of its abrupt increase from low daytime levels and of the absence of beta-adrenergic subsensitivity at this time of day (39,42,43), is probably the most accurate marker for the phase of the endogenous pacemaker—providing that dusk does not occur before "clock on." Therefore, on the experimental day, dusk should be advanced before the suspected time of "clock on."

Several assumptions were made for the clock-gate model—some of which are not as yet proved, some of which may be erroneous. This model will probably undergo several modifications. Its purpose is to aid in the construction of specific, testable hypotheses.

PATTERNS OF MELATONIN SECRETION

The greatest *amplitude* of melatonin secretion during the night may be related to the degree of pineal adrenergic activity. It is not known, as yet, if there is significant change in the maximum amplitude reached at different times of the year (206,207), if natural conditions are different from artificial ones, or if there is a difference between species.

It is clear, however, that in most species studied the *duration* of melatonin production increases during the long nights of winter and decreases during the short nights of summer. This seems to be true in rats (206), Syrian hamsters (210), Djungarian hamsters (209), Siberian hamsters (213), mice (214), sheep (215,216), and elephant seals (217). Although duration of melatonin production appears to be proportional to the length of night, this relationship may not be apparent if the lengths of the scotoperiods are not sufficiently different (45). The relationship between duration of melatonin production and length of the scotoperiod is best understood by the gating effect of darkness. Is there a change in the *timing* of the endogenous pacemaker for melatonin secretion as well?

In order to characterize *timing*, the components of the pattern of melatonin production must be distinguished: onset, maximum, and offset. The timing of the maximum (and to some extent, the offset) is confounded by increasing beta-adrenergic subsensitivity during the night (39,42,43). But, in using onset and offset as markers for timing, one encounters a paradox. In the summer, there appears to be a phase delay in the onset but a phase advance in the offset of melatonin production (the opposite occurs in the winter). Assuming one pacemaker drives the melatonin production rhythm, should onset or should offset be used to indicate the phase of the endogenous pacemaker? According to the clock-gate model (Figure 15), there appears to be a phase delay of the pacemaker in the winter and a phase advance in the summer (in animals with $\tau > 24$ hours). The model suggests that the apparent (but opposite) changes in the time of onset of melatonin production (phase delay in the summer and phase advance in the winter) are "artifacts" due to gating. This is why the use of onset of melatonin production as an accurate marker for the phase of the endogenous pacemaker requires that the time of lights off be advanced before the suspected time of onset on the day of the experiment.

PHOTOPERIODISM

There are two basic models for photoperiodism. One is termed the external coincidence model (218,219) and the other, the internal coincidence model (220). In the external coincidence model, a photoperiodic event, such as reproduction, occurs when light illuminates a critical interval of the circadian cycle. Because the duration of melatonin production appears to be a function of the length of the scotoperiod, it is possible that melatonin secretion participates in photoperiodic events as explained by an external coincidence model. In the internal coincidence model, it is hypothesized that the phase angle between two circadian rhythms changes according to the length of the photoperiod. In Figure 15, the phase of the endogenous pacemaker for the melatonin production rhythm appears to be a function of the length of the photoperiod (phase advance in the summer relative to a phase delay in the winter). (A change in an internal phase angle could also result from a change in the duration of the scotoperiod, if separate pacemakers regulate the time of onset and the time of offset of melatonin production.) Consequently, whether the melatonin production rhythm is driven by one or two pacemakers, it may be involved in the timing of photoperiodic events according to an internal coincidence model. Thus, melatonin production could be related to photoperiodic phenomena according to either the internal or the external coincidence model. Reproductive effects attributed to photoperiodism and the pineal are discussed in detail in other chapters in this book (see Reiter).

Certain aspects of natural environmental light have not been discussed in detail but are worth identifying. What is the role of twilight (its duration and spectral characteristics) in entrainment of circadian rhythms and in photoperiodism? Twilight is longest in the summer, shortest at the equinoxes, and at a midpoint in the winter (221). There is also a "shift toward the red" during twilight (222,223). The length of the natural photoperiod is constantly changing, with its greatest rate of change at the equinoxes (221). If the phase response curve undergoes a seasonal phase-angle change, the greatest rate of change may be during the equinoxes. These are potential areas for further research.

Effects of Light in Humans

SUPPRESSANT EFFECT OF LIGHT IN HUMANS

Previous investigators have had difficulty in attempting to demonstrate effects of light in humans, leading many to speculate that humans are different in their response to light (154,224–231) compared to all other warm-blooded species tested, including nonhuman primates (231). Recently, however, it has been shown that light suppresses human melatonin secretion (232); humans apparently require bright artificial light or sunlight for suppression of melatonin secretion that is accomplished with low intensities of light in other species.

First, sunlight was tested (232).[1] The sleep/wake cycles of two healthy volunteer subjects were phase-delayed in the laboratory; that is, they

---

[1]The idea that sunlight might be effective in suppressing human melatonin secretion (though ordinary room light was ineffective) came from an instance of self-experimentation (AJL): shortly after returning to Washington, D.C., from a two-week stay in Sydney, Australia, the author's 9 A.M. plasma melatonin level was quite low. (It should have been at a higher level, based on the phase of the author's endogenous pacemaker.)

slept between 3 and 11 A.M. for several days. After 7 days, melatonin secretion was maximal during the late morning (between 9 and 10 A.M.). On the eighth day of the study, the volunteers were awakened at 7 A.M. and exposed to sunlight. Melatonin concentrations declined precipitously. It appeared that sunlight was indeed capable of suppressing melatonin secretion in humans.

Why was sunlight (and not ordinary artificial light) effective? Since sunlight is more intense than ordinary room light (at all wavelengths), intensity was the next variable selected to be studied. The intensity of sunlight on a sunny afternoon is 100,000 lux; ordinary room light is rarely more than 500 lux and is usually 200-300 lux (223). By increasing intensity from 500 lux to 2500 lux, the intensity at practically each wavelength was increased, despite a change in light spectra.

Six volunteers were studied under different light intensities during an interruption of sleep between 2 and 4 A.M. Five hundred lux fluorescent light had little or no effect in reducing melatonin concentrations, but 2500 lux incandescent light[2] profoundly reduced melatonin secretion (Figure 16). Moreover, two of these subjects who were also exposed to 1500 lux appeared to have a 50% reduction of melatonin secretion at this intensity, thus suggesting a dose-response relationship between light intensity and suppression of melatonin secretion (Figure 17). This relationship has been previously shown in the rat with respect to N-acetyltransferase activity (200).

These findings have several implications. First, the human pineal appears to be regulated in the same way as is the pineal in other species. [The SCN has been identified in humans as well as in other primates (233,234).] These results also suggest that the human pineal may function in a similar way as in other mammals.

The second implication is that, perhaps on the basis of intensity, humans have adapted to ordinary room light, yet may still remain sensitive to the natural (brighter) sunlight/dark cycle. Thus, the changing length of the natural photoperiod might affect humans in ways similar to the effects in other animal species. It is hoped that these results will stimulate more studies of seasonal rhythms in humans.

The third implication of these findings is that a "bright light/dim light" paradigm may be a useful research strategy for investigating the effects of light in humans. Most previous studies of the effects of light in humans have resulted in negative or ambiguous findings (235), with very few exceptions. For example, Sharp has shown a change in urine volume by prolonging darkness and holding constant the activity/rest cycle in humans (236). Among the most dramatic findings is the effect of light on human eosinophylls (237). The brighter the light, the greater the decrease in eosinophyll count. But this effect might have been due to increased cortisol secretion caused by stress as a result of exposure to

---

[2]Fluorescent light (Vita-Lite) of this intensity is similarly effective, produces less glare and heat, and is currently being used in these studies.

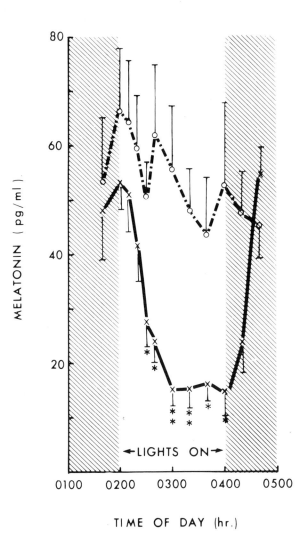

FIGURE 16. Effect of 500 lux (O) and 2500 lux (X) on human plasma melatonin levels (*n* = 6). Each point represents the mean ± SEM for six subjects. A paired *t*-test, a two-way analysis of variance with repeated measures, and the Newman-Keuls statistic for the comparison of means showed significant differences between 2:30 and 4 A.M. (*, $p < 0.05$; **, $p < 0.01$). *From Lewy et al. (232).* ©1980 by the Am Assoc Adv Sci.

bright light, since cortisol is known to reduce the peripheral eosinophyll count (235). Previous studies that used insufficiently intense light should be repeated with bright artificial light or sunlight.

Why do humans require brighter light? Is it evolutionary? This is unlikely, since the discovery of fire was not a long time ago by evolutionary standards. A more likely explanation is that short-term adap-

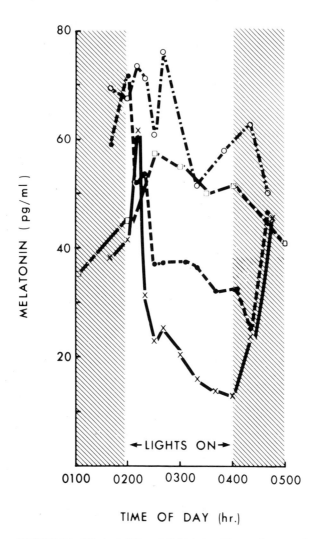

FIGURE 17. Effect of different light intensities on human plasma melatonin levels (□, dark; O, 500 lux; ●, 1500 lux; X, 2500 lux). The averaged values for two subjects are shown. *From Lewy et al. (232).* ©1980 by the Am Assoc Adv Sci.

tation occurs in the retina, retinohypothalamic tract, or SCN. Recent preliminary evidence suggests that there may be an annual rhythm in light sensitivity (author's unpublished data): if a person is exposed to 100,000 lux during a bright, sunny summer day and is tested that night with 500 lux, he will have a response relatively subsensitive compared to that after having been exposed to 20,000 lux during a winter day. This type of short-term adaptation may be responsible for the apparent species differences. To confirm this, laboratory animals that have been reared in the wild should be tested. Either a toxic effect of light or a form of short-term adaptation has recently been demonstrated in the rat: dim light permitted melatonin production, when it was alternated with bright light (238,239). Other possible explanations for apparent species differences may relate to whether or not an animal is diurnal or nocturnal, or is albino.

HUMAN ENTRAINMENT BY LIGHT

To evaluate the entrainment effects of light in humans, blind subjects were studied. Previous work on blind subjects has produced suggestive, but not conclusive, experimental data. This might have resulted because studies were in general not done longitudinally. For example, in an initial study of melatonin patterns in 10 blind subjects, subjects were studied for only 1 day (240). "Phase dispersion" was found in this group. Melatonin onset occurred in these blind subjects at all times of the evening or early morning. (In sighted subjects, melatonin secretion begins regularly between 10 P.M. and 1 A.M.)

More informative data were obtained, however, by longitudinally studying two of these subjects once a week for 4 weeks. Studied in this way, these two subjects displayed markedly unusual circadian melatonin secretory rhythms (240). One subject appeared to be entrained to a 24-hour period but was more than 120° phase-delayed from normal. The other subject was "free-running," with a period of approximately 24.7 hours.

Although only two subjects were studied, these data suggest that light is important in the entrainment of the circadian melatonin secretory rhythm. Many researchers have thought that, unlike the case in other animals, light has little or no effect in the entrainment of human circadian rhythms. Are past negative results due to the use of insufficiently intense light? These studies should be repeated using bright artificial light or sunlight.

Some additional data suggest that sunlight has different effects than does artificial light, particularly with regard to entrainment of human circadian rhythms. Sunlight deprivation may increase the number of days necessary for reentrainment of circadian rhythms after flight across several time zones (241). Field studies, compared to laboratory simulation, of air travel across time zones have been noted to produce different results (242). Perhaps these differences are due to the fact that the laboratory simulations were conducted with ordinary room light. In a few subjects studied under isolated conditions, the light/dark cycle has been shown to be able to entrain the temperature rhythm, whereas the activity/rest rhythm continued to free-run (243). The range of entrainment of the human temperature rhythm appears to be greater under the natural light of the summer Arctic (244) than under ordinary room light (243). Finally, the light/dark cycle appears to be capable of entraining at least part of the circadian cortisol secretory rhythm (245).

Light may have two separate effects on circadian rhythms: (1) light (of any intensity) is a social (or behavioral) cue and is somewhat effective for synchronizing the activity/rest cycle; (2) light of higher intensity may also act as a direct zeitgeber on the endogenous pacemaker for the melatonin secretory rhythm (and perhaps on the endogenous pacemaker for the body temperature rhythm and other circadian rhythms as well). It is important to note that the activity/rest cycle may modify the structure of the light/dark cycle (by the opening and closing of the eyes). It is reasonable, then, to hypothesize a "closed-loop" system in which (1) the temperature (and melatonin) endogenous pacemaker is particularly sensitive to entrainment by light (of sufficient intensity); (2) the activity/ rest rhythm (or its pacemaker) is affected by the core body temperature rhythm (or its pacemaker) (246,247); and (3) the activity/rest cycle su- perimposes a structure on the light/dark cycle, thus closing the loop. Such a closed-loop system might provide for stable steady-state entrain- ment.

HUMAN PHOTOPERIODISM

There are a few epidemiological studies of seasonal rhythms in human physiology and disease (248). Human seasonal rhythms have generally not been attributed to changes in the photoperiod, probably since data on effects of light in humans have been so unimpressive. It is hoped that melatonin research related to effects of sunlight and bright artificial light will stimulate more seasonal studies in humans as well as the testing of possible photoperiodic responses. Again, the bright light/dim light paradigm may be useful here.

In a highly preliminary study of one individual, photoperiodic effects of light were evaluated (249). A manic-depressive patient with a 13-year history of winter depressions and springtime remissions was exposed to bright artificial light between 6 and 9 A.M. and between 4 and 7 P.M. during the first week of December 1980. After 4 days of exposure to these "long" days, using bright, full spectrum light (Vita-Lite), he "switched" out of his typical winter depression (which normally happens in the spring). More patients were studied in December 1981 using the bright light/dim light paradigm.

"MARKERS" FOR THE ENDOGENOUS PACEMAKER
AND THE PROBLEM OF "MASKING"

The peaks and troughs of the circadian rhythms of cortisol and thyroid- stimulating hormone secretion and core body temperature straddle the dawn and dusk transitions (250). Melatonin secretion is unique in that its active phase is confined to night, completely confined between dawn and dusk. Melatonin secretion is also unique among circadian rhythms in that its active phase occurs at night in all species of animals, whether they are diurnal or nocturnal. Other circadian rhythms have a 180° phase- angle difference when diurnal animals are compared to nocturnal animals (250). For these reasons, melatonin has been thought to be a highly useful marker for the phase and period of its endogenous pacemaker, and perhaps it functions as part of the endogenous biological clock as well.

One of the major methodological problems facing circadian rhythm research has been that of masking. Activity causes an increase in core body temperature; inactivity and sleep decrease temperature (251). Stress increases cortisol secretion (252). Melatonin secretion appears to be free from these types of masking effects. Acute changes in the activity/rest cycle do not seem to affect the rhythm of melatonin secretion (224,225); that is, sleep deprivation has no effect (224,229). It is also likely that diet does not affect the rhythm of melatonin secretion (216,253) nor does stress (34,35,152,254–256), nor is melatonin secretion related to the stages of sleep (257,258; author's unpublished data). Aside from specific drugs that can affect the amplitude of melatonin secretion, melatonin secretion is masked only by light. By reducing light intensity below threshold (which in the case of human research permits a fairly high intensity), this masking effect can be avoided.

EXAMPLES OF MELATONIN SECRETION AS A MARKER

The study of manic-depressive patients provides an opportunity to examine "abnormal" conditions of melatonin secretion. In a previous section of this chapter (on Manic-Depressive Patients), abnormalities in the amplitude of secretion were described that might be a function of pineal adrenergic activity. Many of these patients are also thought to have phase-advanced circadian rhythms in cortisol secretion, core body temperature, and many other physiological variables (259). Melatonin secretion appears to be consistent with the "phase-advance hypothesis" (259) in that melatonin secretion seems to have an earlier timing in mania compared to depression and in depression compared to healthy subjects (158).

Recently, the response to light was studied in a group of manic-depressive patients compared to a group of controls matched for age but not sex (260). Patients were more sensitive to light than the control subjects; that is, melatonin secretion was suppressed to twice the extent in the patient group compared to the control group when exposed to 500 or 1500 lux. A group of euthymic (i.e., neither manic nor depressed) patients also appeared to be supersensitive to light, suggesting that this finding might possibly be a "trait marker" and might possibly explain the phase-advanced circadian rhythms observed in these patients (256).

SPECULATION ON THE FUNCTION OF MELATONIN

As a marker, melatonin secretion appears to be extremely useful. But is this "hand of the clock" also part of the "clock" itself? In another chapter of this book (see Reiter), evidence is presented for the functional role of melatonin in the timing of seasonal reproductive rhythms in certain species of animals. Does melatonin function as a part of the biological clock in humans as well? The fact that light suppresses human melatonin secretion and may be important for the entrainment of the timing of melatonin secretion in humans suggests that melatonin serves some function involving the circadian system of humans.

What *specific* function might that be? Melatonin could be a chemical messenger communicating circadian time as well as the season of the year. Melatonin could act directly on the SCN, perhaps modulating the phase or period of the endogenous pacemaker (261–266). (Administration of melatonin has different effects depending on the time of day of administration and the experimental light/dark cycle (267–269).)

More specifically, it seems possible that the function of melatonin is related to the effects of light, since melatonin is produced only at night and in some species it blanches skin (114–129), thus permitting more light radiation to penetrate. In the trout (270,271) and guinea pig retina (272), melatonin also causes pigment aggregation, thus permitting more light radiation to stimulate retinal photoreceptors. In fact, melatonin appears to increase the retinotoxic effects of high-intensity light (273,274). Therefore, a possible role for melatonin might be that it modulates the organism's circadian and circannual responses to light. A specific testable "circadian system-light sensitization" hypothesis might be that melatonin secretion by the pineal gland makes the retina, retinohypothalamic tract, and/or SCN more responsive to light. Gern has discussed a similar hypothesis with regard to the retina (275). Perhaps melatonin's skin-lightening effect in phylogenetically primitive animals has been extended to sensitize the circadian system to light in more evolutionarily advanced animals, such as humans.

CONCLUSIONS

1. In mammals, melatonin production appears to be regulated by beta-adrenergic receptors that undergo changes in Bmax related to previous stimulation. An alpha-2-adrenoceptor may also be involved in melatonin production.
2. Afferent innervation of the pineal that regulates melatonin production appears to be exclusively sympathetic.
3. Under most circumstances, N-acetyltransferase is the rate-limiting step in melatonin production, although there may be species variability.
4. Adenyl cyclase, mRNA, and protein synthesis are necessary for the initial nighttime activation of N-acetyltransferase, although the specific protein for activation has not yet been identified and the specific protein kinase that presumably mediates the action of cyclic AMP has not yet been identified.
5. Stimulation of the beta-adrenergic receptor and the concomitant increase in cyclic AMP also appear to maintain N-acetyltransferase in the active form throughout the night (and may involve continued protein synthesis).

6. Most of the rhythms of constituent substances necessary for melatonin synthesis are in phase with the rhythm of melatonin secretion.
7. Research on prostaglandins and cyclic GMP is too new for comment
at the present time.
8. Although this topic is still controversial, the contribution to circulating levels of melatonin by extrapineal production (if it does occur)
appears to be extremely low, if not entirely absent.
9. The suprachiasmatic nucleus (SCN) appears to be the locus of the
"clock" (or endogenous circadian pacemaker) for regulating melatonin production. Whether or not it is the only clock for melatonin
production or if it is the clock for other circadian rhythms as well,
remains to be determined. It is not known whether it is actually
"on" or "off" during the nighttime sympathetic stimulation of the
pineal.
10. The retinohypothalamic tract (and not the inferior accessory optic
tract as once believed) mediates the effects of light on the SCN.
Other innervation of the SCN does not seem to be related to melatonin production.
11. There are two, possibly three, distinct effects of light on pineal production of melatonin: (a) acute suppression, (b) entrainment of the
circadian rhythm, and (c) photoperiodic changes in the pattern and
timing.
12. The duration of melatonin production appears to be greater during
the long nights of winter compared to the short nights of summer.
It is not known whether or not there is a difference in amplitude at
different times of the year (or under different photoperiods) nor is
it known whether or not there is a seasonal phase-angle change in
the endogenous pacemaker that regulates the timing of melatonin
production.
13. The human pineal appears to be regulated in much the same way
as is the pineal in other mammalian species, except that humans
apparently require bright artificial light or sunlight. This may be due
to previous history of light exposure.
14. In order to assess the phase of the endogenous pacemaker for melatonin production, it is recommended that on the night of the study,
dusk be advanced (and dawn delayed). In order to measure amplitude of secretion accurately, ambient lighting during the night should
be reduced below threshold levels. Gating is best evaluated immediately after an acute change in the light/dark cycle; entrainment
effects of the light/dark cycle are best evaluated after several days.
15. A "clock-gate" model is described in this chapter for the purpose of
formulating specific testable hypotheses for understanding how the
light/dark cycle entrains the endogenous pacemaker (the "clock")
for melatonin production and how darkness gates (that is, light
suppresses) the expression of melatonin production (the "hand of
the clock").
16. The strategy for testing light can be related to intensity. Bright light
should have biological effects that dim light lacks. Therefore, a "bright

light/dim light" paradigm is suggested as a method for evaluating biological effects of light, particularly in humans.

17. Humans may be sensitive to seasonal changes in the length of the natural photoperiod unconfounded by indoor lighting, perhaps because of adaptation to the lower intensity of indoor lighting.

18. In addition to the clock-gate model, two other specific testable hypotheses are suggested in this chapter: (a) the "closed-loop" hypothesis for understanding the interaction between the light/dark cycle and the circadian system; and (b) the "circadian system-light sensitization" hypothesis for melatonin function. These and other hypotheses will, it is hoped, lead to the generation of increasingly meaningful and interpretable data.

(See page 128 for Note Added in Proof.)

REFERENCES

1. Quay W B. Pineal Chemistry in Cellular and Physiological Mechanisms. Charles C Thomas, Publisher, Springfield, Ill. 1974.

2. Klein D C, Weller J. Indole metabolism in the pineal gland: a circadian rhythm in N-acetyltransferase. Science 169:1093–1095, 1970.

3. Descartes R. De Homine, Figuris et Latinitate Donatus a Schuyl, F., Lugduni Batavorum, 1662.

4. Descartes R. Description du corps humain et Passions de l'Ame. In Oeuvres, vol XI, ed C Adam, P Tannery. Paris, 1909.

5. Ahlborn F. Über die Bedeutung der Zirbeldrüse (Glandula pinealis, Commissur, Epiphysis cerebri). Z Zool 40:331–337, 1884.

6. Rabl-Rüeckhardt H. Zur Deutung der Zirbeldrüse (Epiphyse). Zool Anz 9:536–547, 1886.

7. Studnicka K K. Die Parietalorgane. In Lehrbuch der vergleichenden mikroskopischen Anatomie, vol 5, ed A Oppel. Springer, Jena, 1905.

8. Huebner O. Tumor der Glandula pinealis. Dtsch Med Wschr 24:214, 1898.

9. Kitay J I, Altschule M D. The Pineal Gland, A Review of the Physiologic Literature. Harvard University Press, Cambridge, Mass. 1954.

10. Lerner A B, Case J D, Heinzelman R V. Structure of melatonin. J Am Chem Soc 81:6084–6085, 1959.

11. Ariëns Kappers J. The development, topographical relations and innervation of the epiphysis cerebri in the albino rat. Z Zellforsch Mikrosk Anat 52:163–215, 1960.

12. Ariëns Kappers J, Smith A R, DeVries R A C. The mammalian pineal gland and its control of hypothalamic activity. In The Pineal Gland of Vertebrates Including Man—Progress in Brain Research, vol 52, ed J Ariëns Kappers, P Pévet. Elsevier/North-Holland, Amsterdam 1979, pp 149–174.

13. Ariëns Kappers J. Short history of pineal discovery and research. In The Pineal Gland of Vertebrates Including Man—Progress in Brain Research, vol 52, ed J Ariëns Kappers, P Pévet. Elsevier/North-Holland, Amsterdam, 1979, pp 3–22.

14. Ueck M, Wake K. The pinealocyte—a paraneuron. In The Pineal Gland of Vertebrates Including Man—Progress in Brain Research, vol 52, ed J Ariëns Kappers, P Pévet. Elsevier/North-Holland, Amsterdam, 1979, pp 141–147.

15. Pearse A G E. The cytochemistry and ultrastructure of polypeptide hormone producing cells of the APUD series and the embryology, physiology, and pathologic implications of the concept. J Histochem Cytochem 17:303–313, 1969.

16. Taylor A N, Wilson R W, Electrophysiological evidence for the action of light on the pineal gland in the rat. Experientia 26:267–269, 1970.

17. Levitt M, Spector S, Sjoerdsma A, Udenfriend S. Elucidation of the rate-limiting step in norpinephrine biosynthesis in the perfused guinea pig heart. J Pharmacol Exp Ther 148:1–8, 1965.

18. Brownstein M J, Axelrod J. Pineal gland: a 24-hour rhythm in norepinephrine turnover. Science 184:163–165, 1974.

19. Moore R Y, Heller A, Bhatnager R K, Wurtman R J, Axelrod J. Central control of the pineal gland: visual pathways. Arch Neurol 18:208–218, 1968.

20. Pellegrino de Iraldi A, Zieher L M. Noradrenaline and dopamine content of normal, decentralized and denervated pineal gland of the rat. Life Sci 5:149–154, 1966.

21. Bagchi S P, Zarycki E P. The effect of p-chlorophenylalanine on the hydroxylation of phenylalanine in the pineal gland and brainstem. Fed Proc 30:381, 1971.

22. Bensinger R E, Klein D C, Weller J L, Lovenberg W. Radiometric assay of total tryptophan hydroxylation by intact cultured pineal glands. J Neurochem 23:111–117, 1974.

23. Jequier E, Robinson D S, Lovenberg W, Sjoerdsma A. Further studies on tryptophan hydroxylase in rat brainstem and beef pineal. Biochem Pharmacol 18:1071–1081, 1969.

24. McGeer E G, McGeer P L. Circadian rhythm in pineal tyrosine hydroxylase. Science 153:73–74, 1966.

25. Lovenberg W, Weissbach H, Udenfriend S. Aromatic l-amino acid decarboxylase. J Biol Chem 237:89–93, 1962.

26. Snyder S H, Axelrod J. A sensitive assay for 5-hydroxytryptophan decarboxylase. Biochem Pharmacol 13:805–806, 1964.

27. Snyder S H, Axelrod J, Wurtman R J, Fischer J E. Control of 5-hydroxytryptophan decarboxylase activity in the rat pineal gland by sympathetic nerves. J Pharmacol Exp Ther 147:371–375, 1965.

28. Laduron P, Belpaire F. Transport of noradrenaline and dopamine-beta-hydroxylase in sympathetic nerves. Life Sci 7:1–7, 1968.

29. Goldstein M, Lauber E, McKereghan M R. The inhibition of dopamine-beta-hydroxylase by tropolone and other chelating agents. Biochem Pharmacol 13:1103–1105, 1964.

30. Musacchio J, Kopin I J, Snyder S. Effects of disulfiram on tissue norepinephrine content and subcellular distribution of dopamine, tyramine, and their beta-hydroxylated metabolites. Life Sci 3:769–775, 1964.

31. Gfeller E, Green A, Snyder S H, Regional differences in (³H) noradrenaline accumulation in monkey brain (Macacairus). Brain Res 11:263–267, 1968.

32. Steinman A M, Smerin S E, Barchas J D. Epinephrine metabolism in mammalian brain after intravenous and intraventricular administration. Science 165:616–617, 1969.

33. Axelrod J. The pineal gland: a neurochemical transducer. Science 184:1341–1348, 1974.

34. Klein D C, Parfitt A. A protective role of nerve endings in stress-stimulated increase in pineal N-acetyltransferase activity. In Catecholamines and Stress, eds E. Usdin, R. Kvetnanasky, I. J. Kopin. Pergamon Press, New York, 1976, pp 119–128.

35. Parfitt A, Klein D C. Increase caused by desmethylimipramine in the production of (³H) melatonin by isolated pineal glands. Biochem Pharmacol 26:904–905, 1977.

36. Vacas M I, Cardinali D P. Effects of castration and reproductive hormones on pineal serotonin metabolism in rats. Neuroendocrinology 28:187–195, 1979.

37. Bäckström M, Wetterberg L. Catechol-0-methyltransferase, histamine-N-methyltransferase and methanol forming enzyme in the rat pineal gland. Life Sci 11:293–299, 1972.

38. Parfitt A, Weller JL, Klein DC. Beta adrenergic-blockers decrease adrenergically stimulated N-acetyltransferase activity in pineal glands in organ culture. Neuropharmacology 15:353–358, 1976.

39. Zatz M, Kebabian J W, Romero J A, Lefkowitz R J, Axelrod J. Pineal adrenergic receptor: correlation of binding of ³H-alprenolol with stimulation of adenylate cyclase. J Pharmacol Exp Ther 196:714–722, 1976.

40. Wurtman R J, Shein H M, Larin F. Mediation by beta-adrenergic receptors of effect of norepinephrine on pineal synthesis of ¹⁴(C) serotonin and ¹⁴(C) melatonin. J Neurochem 18:1683–1687, 1971.

41. Deguchi T, Axelrod J. Induction and superinduction of serotonin N-acetyltransferase by adrenergic drugs and denervation in rat pineal organ. Proc Natl Acad Sci USA 69:2208–2211, 1972.

42. Kebabian J W, Zatz M, Romero J A, Axelrod J. Rapid changes in rat pineal beta-adrenergic receptor. Alterations in 1-(³H) alprenolol binding and adenylate cyclase. Proc Natl Acad Sci USA 72:3735–3739, 1975.

43. Romero J A, Axelrod J. Regulation of sensitivity to beta-adrenergic stimulation in induction of pineal N-acetyltransferase. Proc Natl Acad Sci USA 72:1661–1665, 1975.

44. Axelrod J, Weissbach, H. Purification and properties of hydroxyindole-O-methyltransferase. J Biol Chem 236:211–213, 1961.

45. Tamarkin L, Reppert S M, Klein D C. Regulation of pineal melatonin in the Syrian hamster. Endocrinology 104:385–389, 1979.

46. Panke E S, Rollag M D, Reiter R J. Pineal melatonin concentrations in the Syrian hamster. Endocrinology 104:194–197, 1979.

47. Klein D C, Weller J. Rapid light-induced decrease in pineal serotonin N-acetyltransferase activity. Science 177:532–533, 1972.

48. Ellison N, Weller J L, Klein D C. Development of a circadian rhythm in the activity of pineal serotonin N-acetyltransferase. J Neurochem 19:1335–1341, 1972.

49. Deguchi T, Axelrod J. Control of circadian change of serotonin N-acetyltransferase in the pineal organ by the beta-adrenergic receptor. Proc Natl Acad Sci USA 69:2547–2550, 1972.

50. Brownstein M, Saavedra J M, Axelrod J. Control of pineal N-acetylserotonin by a beta-adrenergic receptor. Mol Pharmacol 9:605–611, 1973.

51. Romero J A, Zatz M, Axelrod J. Beta-adrenergic stimulation of pineal N-acetyltransferase: adenosine 3′,5′-cyclic monophosphate stimulates both RNA and protein synthesis. Proc Natl Acad Sci USA 72:2107–2111, 1975.

52. Robison G A, Schmidt M J, Sutherland E W. On the development and properties of the brain adenyl cyclase system. In Role of Cyclic AMP in Cell Function, ed P Greengard, E Costa. Raven Press, New York, 1970, pp 11–30.

53. Weiss B, Costa E. Adenyl cyclase activity in rat pineal gland: effects of chronic denervation and norepinephrine. Science 156:1750–1752, 1967.

54. Ebadi M S, Weiss B, Costa E. Distribution of cyclic adenosine monophosphate in rat brain. Arch Neurol 24:353–357, 1971.

55. Mikuni M, Saito Y, Koyama T, Yamashita I. Circadian variation of cyclic AMP in the rat pineal gland. J Neurochem 36:1295–1297, 1981.

56. Weiss B, Costa E. Selective stimulation of adenyl cyclase activity in rat pineal by pharmacologically active catecholamines. J Pharmacol Exp Ther 161:310–319, 1968.

57. Minneman K P, Iversen L L. Diurnal rhythm in rat pineal cyclic nucleotide phosphodiesterase activity. Nature 260:59–61, 1976.

58. Berg G R, Klein D C. Pineal gland melatonin production: site of action of norepinephrine and dibutyryl cyclic adenosine monophosphate. Fed Proc 29:615, 1970.

59. Shein H M, Wurtman R J. Cyclic adenosine monophosphate stimulation of melatonin and serotonin synthesis in cultured rat pineals. Science 166:519–520, 1969.

60. Fontana J A, Lovenberg W. A cyclic AMP-dependent protein kinase of the bovine pineal gland. Proc Natl Acad Sci USA 68:2787–2790, 1971.

61. Axelrod J, Wurtman R J, Snyder S. Control of hydroxyindole-O-methyltransferase activity in the rat pineal gland by environmental lighting. J Biol Chem 240:949–954, 1965.

62. Wurtman R J, Axelrod J, Phillips L S. Melatonin synthesis in the pineal gland: control by light. Science 142:1071–1073, 1963.

63. Quay W B. Lack of rhythm and effect of darkness in rat pineal content of N-acetyl-serotonin-O-methyltransferase. Physiologist 10:286, 1967.

64. Lynch H J, Ralph C L. Diurnal variation in pineal melatonin and its nonrelationship to HIOMT activity. Am Zool 10:300, 1970.

65. Klein D C, Moore R Y. Pineal N-acetyltransferase and hydroxyindole-O-methyl transferase: control by the retinohypothalamic tract and the suprachiasmatic nucleus. Brain Res 174:245–262, 1979.

66. Cardinali D P, Wurtman R J. Hydroxyindole-O-methyl transferase in rat pineal, retina and harderian gland. Endocrinology 91:247–252, 1972.

67. Nagle C A, Cardinali D P, Rosner J M. Light regulation of rat retinal hydroxyindole-O-methyl transferase (HIOMT) activity. Endocrinology 91:423–426, 1972.

68. Quay W B, Smart L I. Substrate specificity and post-mortem effects in mammalian pineal acetylserotonin methyltransferase activity. Arch Int Physiol Biochim 75:197–210, 1967.

69. Wurtman R J, Axelrod J, Barchas J D. Age and enzyme activity in the human pineal. J Clin Endocrinol Metab 24:299–301, 1964.

70. Otani T, Györkey F, Farrell G. Enzymes of the human pineal body. J Clin Endocrinol Metab 28:349–354, 1968.

71. Smith J A, Mee T J X, Padwick D J, Spokes E G. Human post-mortem pineal enzyme activity. J Clin Endocrinol Metab 14:75–81, 1981.

72. Guchhait R B, Grau J E. Biosynthesis of S-adenosyl-1-methionine in the rat pineal gland. J Neurochem 31:921–925, 1978.

73. Baldessarini R J, Kopin I J. Assay of tissue levels of S-adenosylmethionine. Anal Biochem 6:289–292, 1963.

74. Baldessarini R J, Kopin I J. S-adenosylmethionine in brain and other tissues. J Neurochem 13:769–777, 1966.

75. Baldessarini R J. Factors influencing S-adenosylmethionine levels in mammalian tissues. In Amines and Schizophrenia, eds H E Himwich, S S Kety, J R Smythies. Pergamon Press, Oxford, 1967, p 199.

76. Wartman S A, Branch B J, George R, Taylor A N. Evidence for a cholinergic influence on pineal hydroxyindole-O-methyltransferase activity with changes in environmental lighting. Life Sci 8:1263–1270, 1969.

77. Schrier B K, Klein D C. Absence of choline acetyltransferase in rat and rabbit pineal gland. Brain Res 79:347–351, 1974.

78. Romijn H J. Parasympathetic innervation of the rabbit pineal gland. Brain Res 55:431–436, 1973.

79. Eränkö O, Rechardt L, Eränkö L, Cunningham A. Acetylcholinesterase (AChE) activity in the sympathetic nerve fibres of the pineal body (PB) of the rat. Scand J Clin Lab Invest 25(Suppl 113):82, 1970.

80. Eränkö O, Rechardt L, Eränkö L, Cunningham A. Light and electron microscopic histochemical observations on cholinesterase-containing sympathetic nerve fibers in the pineal body of the rat. Histochem J 2:479–489, 1970.

81. Manocha S L. Histochemical distribution of acetylcholinesterase and simple esterases in the brain of squirrel monkey (Saimiri sciureus). Histochemie 21:236–248, 1970.

82. Trueman T, Herbert J. The distribution of monoamines and acetylcholinesterase in the pineal gland and habenula of the ferret. J Anat 106:406, 1970.

83. Machado A B M, Lemos V P J. Histochemical evidence for a cholinergic sympathetic innervation of the rat pineal body. J Neurovisc Relat 32:104–111, 1971.

84. Turkervitsch N. Eigentümlichkeiten der embryologischen Entwicklung des Epiphysengebiets des Schafes (Ovis Aries L). Morphol Jahrb 79:305–330, 1937.

85. Quay W B. Circadian rhythm in rat pineal serotonin and its modifications by estrous cycle and photoperiod. Gen Comp Endocrinol 3:473–479, 1963.

86. Quay W B. Effect of dietary phenylalanine and tryptophan on pineal and hypothalamic serotonin levels. Proc Soc Exp Biol Med 114:718–721, 1963.

87. Neff N H, Barrett R E, Costa E. Kinetic and fluorescent histochemical analysis of the serotonin compartments in rat pineal gland. Eur J Pharmacol 5:384–390, 1969.

88. Neff N H, Lin R C, Ngai S H, Costa E. Turnover rate measurements of brain serotonin in unanesthetized rats. Adv Biochem Psychopharmacol 1:91–109, 1969.

89. Roth W D. Metabolic and morphologic studies on the rat pineal organ during puberty. In Structure and Function of the Epiphysis Cerebri, Progress in Brain Research, vol 10, ed J Ariëns Kappers, J P Schade. Elsevier, Amsterdam, 1965, pp 552–563.

90. Lovenberg W, Jequier E, Sjoerdsma A. Tryptophan hydroxylation in mammalian systems. Adv Pharmacol 6A:21–36, 1968.

91. Fiske V M. Serotonin rhythm in the pineal organ: control by the sympathetic nervous system. Science 146:253–254, 1964.

92. Snyder S H, Zweig M. Axelrod J, Fischer J E. Control of circadian rhythm in serotonin content of the rat pineal gland. Proc Natl Acad Sci USA 53:301–305, 1965.

93. Brownstein M, Holz R, Axelrod J. The regulation of pineal serotonin by a beta-adrenergic receptor. J Pharmacol Exp Ther 186:109–113, 1973.

94. Klein D C. The pineal gland: a model of neuroendocrine regulation. In The Hypothalamus, vol 56, eds S Reichlin, R J Baldessarini, J B Martin. Raven Press, New York, 1978, pp 303–327.

95. Klein D C, Berg G R. Pineal gland: stimulation of melatonin production by norepinephrine involves cyclic AMP-mediated stimulation of N-acetyltransferase. In Role of Cyclic AMP in Cell Function, Advances in Biochemical Psychopharmacology, vol 3, ed P Greengard, E Costa. Raven Press, New York, 1970, pp 241–263.

96. Zweig M, Axelrod J. Relationship between catecholamines and serotonin in sympathetic nerves of the rat pineal gland. J Neurobiol 1:87–97, 1969.

97. Bertler À, Falck B, Owman C. Cellular localization of 5-hydroxytryptamine in the rat pineal gland. Kungl Fysiografiska Sällskapets i Lund Forhandlingar 33:13, 1963.

98. Bertler À, Falck B, Owman C. Studies on 5-hydroxytryptamine stores in pineal gland of rat. Acta Physiol Scand 63(Suppl 239):1–18, 1964.

99. Smith A R. Conditions influencing serotonin and tryptophan metabolism in the epiphysis cerebri of the rabbit; a fluorescence histochemical, microchemical and electrophoretic study. Thesis, Purmerend, The Netherlands, Nooy's Drukkerij, 1972.

100. Sugden D. Circadian change in rat pineal tryptophan content: lack of correlation with serum tryptophan. J Neurochem 33:811–813, 1979.

101. Lovenberg W, Jequier E, Sjoerdsma A. Tryptophan hydroxylation: measurements in pineal gland, brain stem, and carcinoid tumor. Science 155:217–218, 1967.

102. Studnitz W V. Tryptophanhydroxylase im Corpus pineale beim Menschen. Experientia 23:711, 1967.

103. Ichiyama A, Nakamura S, Nishizuka Y, Hayaishi O. Tryptophan-5-hydroxylase in mammalian brain. Adv Pharmacol 6A:5–17, 1968.

104. Shibuya H, Toru M, Watanabe S. A circadian rhythm of tryptophan hydroxylase in rat pineals. Brain Res 138:364–368, 1978.

105. Sitaram B R, Lees G J. Diurnal rhythm and turnover of tryptophan hydroxylase in the pineal gland of the rat. J Neurochem 31:1021–1026, 1978.

106. Shein H M, Wurtman R J, Axelrod J. Synthesis of serotonin by pineal glands of the rat in organ culture. Nature 213:730–731, 1967.

107. Lovenberg W, Weissbach H, Udenfriend S. Aromatic 1-amino acid decarboxylase. J Biol Chem 237:89–93, 1962.

108. Snyder S H, Axelrod J, Zweig M, Circadian rhythm in the serotonin content of the rat pineal gland: regulating factors. J Pharmacol Exp Ther 158:206–213, 1967.

109. Udenfriend S, Titus E, Weissbach H, Peterson R E. Biogenesis and metabolism of 5-hydroxyindole compounds. J Biol Chem 219:335–344, 1956.

110. Weissbach H, Redfield B G, Udenfriend S. Soluble monoamine oxidase: its properties and actions on serotonin. J Biol Chem 229:953–963, 1957.

111. Keglevic D, Kveder S, Iskric S. Indolealdehydes-intermediates in indolealkylamine metabolism. Adv Pharmacol 6A:79–89, 1968.

112. Feldstein A, Williamson O. Serotonin metabolism in pineal homogenates. Adv Pharmacol 6A:91–96, 1968.

113. Fujiwara M, Shibata M, Watanabe Y, Nukiwa T, Hirata F, Mizuno N, Hayaishi O. Indoleamine 2,3-dioxygenase: formation of 1-kynurenine from 1-tryptophan in cultured rabbit pineal gland. J Biol Chem 253:6081–6085, 1978.

114. Gianferrari L. Influenza dell'alimentazione con capsule surrenali, ipofisi ed epifisi su la pigmentazione cutanea ed il ritmo respiratorio di Salmo fario. Arch Sci Biol (Bologna) 3:39, 1922.

115. Huxley J S, Hogben L T. Experiments on amphibian metamorphosis and pigment responses in relation to internal secretions. Proc R Soc Lond (Biol) 93:36–53, 1922.

116. McCord C P, Allen F P. Evidence associating pineal gland function with alterations in pigmentation. J Exp Zool 23:207–224, 1917.

117. Lerner A B, Case J D. Pigment cell regulatory factors. J Invest Dermatol 32:211–221, 1959.

118. Lerner A B, Case J D, Takahashi Y. Isolation of melatonin and 5-methoxyindole-3-acetic acid from bovine pineal glands. J Biol Chem 235:1992–1997, 1960.

119. Lerner A B, Case J D, Takahashi Y, Lee T H, Mori W. Isolation of melatonin, the pineal gland factor that lightens melanocytes. J Am Chem Soc 80:2587, 1958.

120. Lazo-Wasem E A, Graham C E. Quantitative in vivo assay of pineal melanophore contracting principle (melatonin). Fed Proc 19:150, 1960.

121. Lerner A B, Wright M R. In vitro frog skin assay for agents that darken and lighten melanocytes. Methods Biochem Anal 8:294–307, 1960.

122. Mori W, Lerner A B. A microscopic bioassay for melatonin. Endocrinology 67:443–450, 1960.

123. Tomatis M E, Orias R. Changes in melatonin concentration in pineal gland in rats exposed to continuous light or darkness. Acta Physiol Lat Am 17:227–233, 1967.

124. Kastin A J, Schally A V. In vivo assay for melanocyte lightening substances. Experientia 22:389, 1966.

125. Ralph C L, Lynch H J. A quantitative melatonin bioassay. Gen Comp Endocrinol 15:334–338, 1970.

126. Bagnara J T. The pineal and the body lightening reaction of larval amphibians. Gen Comp Endocrinol 3:86–100, 1963.

127. Quay W B, Bagnara J T. Relative potencies of indolic and related compounds in the body-lightening reaction of larval Xenopus. Arch Int Pharmacodyn Ther 150:137–143, 1964.

128. Van de Veerdonk F C G. Separation method for melatonin in pineal extracts. Nature 208:1324–1325, 1965.

129. Barchas J D, Lerner A B. Localization of melatonin in the nervous system. J Neurochem 11:489–491, 1964.

130. Quay W B. Circadian and estrous rhythms in pineal melatonin and 5-OH indole-3-acetic acid. Proc Soc Exp Biol Med 115:710–713, 1964.

131. Lynch H J. Diurnal oscillations in pineal melatonin content. Life Sci 10:791–795, 1971.

132. Kopin I J, Pare M B, Axelrod J, Weissbach H. The fate of melatonin in animals. J Biol Chem 236:3072–3075, 1961.

133. Kveder S, McIsaac W M. The metabolism of melatonin (N-acetyl-5-methoxytryptamine) and 5-methoxytryptamine. J Biol Chem 236:3214–3220, 1961.

134. Reppert S M, Perlow M J, Tamarkin L, Klein D C. A diurnal melatonin rhythm in primate cerebrospinal fluid. Endocrinology 104:295–301, 1979.

135. Pardridge W M, Mietus L J. Transport of albumin-bound melatonin through the blood-brain barrier. J Neurochem 34:1761–1763, 1980.

136. Jones R L, McGee P L, Greiner A C. Metabolism of exogenous melatonin in schizophrenic and non-schizophrenic volunteers. Clin Chim Acta 26:281–285, 1969.

137. Hirata F, Hayaishi O, Tokuyama T, Senoh S. In vitro and in vivo formation of two new metabolites of melatonin. J Biol Chem 249:1311–1313, 1974.

138. Wurtman R J, Axelrod J, Anton-Tay F. Inhibition of the metabolism of ^{3}H-melatonin by phenothiazines. J Pharmacol Exp Ther 161:367–372, 1968.

139. Ozaki Y, Lynch H J, Wurtman R J. Melatonin in rat pineal, plasma and urine: 24-hour rhythmicity and effect of chlorpromazine. Endocrinology 98:1418–1424, 1976.

140. Smith J H, Mee T J X, Barnes J D. Decreased serum melatonin levels in chlorpromazine-treated psychiatric patients. J Neural Transm Suppl 13:397, 1978.

141. Silman R E, Hooper R J L, Leone R M, Edwards R, Grudzinskas J G, Gordon Y D, Chard T, Savage M, Smith I, Mullen P E. 5-methoxytryptophan and pituitary function in man. In The Pineal Gland of Vertebrates Including Man, Progress in Brain Research, vol 52, ed J Ariëns Kappers, P Pévet. Elsevier North-Holland, New York, 1978, pp 507–511.

142. David G F X, Herbert J. Experimental evidence for a synaptic connection between habenula and pineal ganglion in the ferret. Brain Res 64:327–343, 1973.

143. Nielsen J T, Møller M. Nervous connections between the brain and the pineal gland in the cat (Felis catus) and the monkey (Cercopithecus aethiops). Cell Tiss Res 161:293–301, 1975.

144. Møller M. Presence of a pineal nerve (nervus pinealis) in the human fetus; a light and electron microscopical study of the innervation of the pineal gland. Brain Res 154:1–12, 1978.

145. Rønnekleiv O K, Kelly M J, Wuttke W. Single unit recordings in the rat pineal gland: evidence for habenulo-pineal neural connections. Exp Brain Res 39:187–192, 1980.

146. Pelayo F, Dubocovich M L, Langer S Z. Regulation of noradrenaline release in the rat pineal through a negative feedback mechanism mediated by presynaptic alpha-adrenoceptors. Eur J Pharmacol 45:317–318, 1977.

147. Nijjar M S, Smith T L, Hauser G. Evidence against dopaminergic and further support for beta-adrenergic receptor involvement in the pineal phosphatidylinositol effect. J Neurochem 34:813–821, 1980.

148. Cardinali D P, Ritta M N, Speziale N S, Gimeno M F. Release and specific binding of prostaglandins in bovine pineal gland. Prostaglandins 18:577–589, 1979.

149. O'Dea R F, Gagnon C, Zatz M. Regulation of cyclic GMP in the rat pineal and posterior pituitary glands. J Neurochem 31:733–738, 1978.

150. Klein D C, Auerbach D A, Weller J L. Seesaw signal processing in pineal cells: homologous sensitization of adrenergic stimulation of cyclic GMP accompanies homologous desensitization of beta-adrenergic stimulation of cyclic AMP. Proc Natl Acad Sci USA 78:4625–4629, 1981.

151. Kneisley L W, Moskowitz M H, Lynch H J. Cervical spinal cord lesions disrupt the rhythm in human melatonin excretion. J Neurol Transm, Suppl 13:311–323, 1978.

152. Vaughan G M, McDonald S D, Bell R, Stevens E A. Melatonin, pituitary function and stress in humans. Psychoneuroendocrinology 4:351–362, 1979.

153. Tetsuo M, Polinsky R J, Markey S P, Kopin I J. Urinary 6-hydroxymelatonin excretion in patients with orthostatic hypotension. J Clin Endocrinol Metab 53:607–610, 1981.

154. Vaughan G M, Pelham R W, Pang S F, Loughlin L L, Wilson K M, Sandock K L, Vaughan M K, Koslow S H, Reiter F J. Nocturnal elevation of plasma melatonin and urinary 5-hydroxy-indoleacetic acid: attempts at modification by brief changes in environmental lighting and sleep and by autonomic drugs. J Clin Endocrinol Metab 42:752–754, 1976.

155. Hanssen T, Heyden T, Sundberg T, Wetterberg L. Effect of propanolol on serum-melatonin. Lancet 2:309–310, 1977.

156. Lewy A J, Siever L, Uhde T W, Murphy D L, Post R A, Markey S P, Goodwin F K. Clonidine reduces human melatonin secretion. In preparation.

157. Siever L J, Cohen R M, Murphy D L. Antidepressants and alpha-adrenergic auto-receptor desensitization. Am J Psychiatry 138:681–682, 1981.

158. Lewy A J, Wehr T A, Gold P W, Goodwin F K. Melatonin secretion in manic-depressive patients. In preparation.

159. Wetterberg L, Beck-Friis J, Aperia B, Pettersen U. Melatonin/cortisol ratio in depression. Lancet 2:1361, 1979.

160. Jimerson D C, Lynch H J, Post R M, Wurtman R J, Bunney W E. Urinary melatonin rhythms during sleep deprivation in depressed patients and normals. Life Sci 20:1501–1508, 1977.

161. Carr D R, Reppert S M, Bullen B, Skrinar G, Beitins I, Arnold M, Rosenblatt M, Martin J B, McArthur J W. Plasma melatonin increases during exercise in women. J Clin Endocrinol Metab 53:224–225, 1981.

162. Lewy A J, Markey S P. Analysis of melatonin in human plasma by gas chromatography negative chemical ionization mass spectrometry. Science 201:741–743, 1978.

163. Arendt J. Current status of assay methods of melatonin. In Melatonin—Current Status and Perspectives, Advances in the Biosciences, vol 29, ed N Birau, W Schloot. Pergamon Press, New York, 1981, pp 3–7.

164. Rollag M D. Methods for measuring pineal hormones. In The Pineal Gland, Anatomy and Biochemistry, vol 1, ed R J Reiter. CRC Press, Boca Raton, Fla., 1981, pp 273–302.

165. Fellenberg A J, Phillipou G, Seamark R F. Specific quantitation of urinary 6-hydroxymelatonin sulphate by gas chromatography mass spectrometry. Biomed Mass Spec 7:84–87, 1980.

166. Tetsuo M, Markey S P, Kopin I J. Measurement of 6-hydroxymelatonin in human urine with its diurnal variation. Life Sci 27:105–109, 1980.

167. Lewy A J, Tetsuo M, Markey S P, Goodwin F K, Kopin I J. Pinealectomy abolishes plasma melatonin in the rat. J Clin Endocrinol Metab 50:204–205, 1980.

168. Pelham R W, Ralph C L, Campbell I M. Mass spectral identification of melatonin in blood. Biochem Biophys Res Commun 46:1236–1241, 1972.

169. Pelham R W. A serum melatonin rhythm in chickens and its abolition by pinealectomy. Endocrinology 96:543–546, 1975.

170. Arendt J, Forbes J M, Brown W B, Marston A. Effect of pinealectomy on immunoassayable melatonin in sheep. J Endocrinol 85:1P–2P, 1980.

171. Richter C P. Biological Clocks in Medicine and Psychiatry, Charles C Thomas, Publisher, Springfield, Ill., 1965.

172. Richter C P. Sleep and activity: their relation to the 24-hour clock. Proc Assoc Res Ner Ment Dis 45:8–27, 1967.

173. Moore R Y, Eichler V B. Loss of circadian adrenal corticosterone rhythm following suprachiasmatic lesions in the rat. Brain Res 42:201–206, 1972.

174. Stephan F K, Zucker I. Circadian rhythms in drinking behavior and locomotor activity of rats are eliminated by hypothalamic lesions. Proc Natl Acad Sci USA 69:1583–1586, 1972.

175. Ibuka N, Kawamura H. Loss of circadian rhythm in sleep-wakefulness cycle in the rat by suprachiasmatic nucleus lesions. Brain Res 96:76–81, 1975.

176. Rusak B. The role of the suprachiasmatic nuclei in the generation of circadian rhythm in the golden hamster, Mesocricetus auratus. J Comp Physiol 118:145–164, 1977.

177. Moore R Y, Klein D C. Visual pathways and the central neural control of a circadian rhythm in pineal serotonin N-acetyltransferase activity. Brain Res 71:17–33, 1974.

178. Nishino E, Koizumi K, Brooks C M. The role of the suprachiasmatic nuclei of the hypothalamus in the production of circadian rhythms. Brain Res 112:45–59, 1976.

179. Groos G A, Mason R. The visual properties of rat and cat suprachiasmatic neurones. J Comp Physiol 135:349–356, 1980.

180. Schwartz W J, Davidsen L C, Smith C B. In vivo metabolic activity of a putative circadian oscillator, the rat suprachiasmatic nucleus. J Comp Neurol 189:157–167, 1980.

181. Schwartz W J, Gainer H. Suprachiasmatic nucleus: use of ^{14}C-labeled deoxyglucose uptake as a functional marker. Science 197:1089–1091, 1977.

182. Moore R Y, Lenn N J. A retinohypothalamic projection in the rat. J Comp Neurol 146:1–14, 1972.

183. Hendrickson S E, Wagoner N, Cowan W M. Autoradiographic and electron microscopic study of retino-hypothalamic connections. Z Zellerforsch 125:1–26, 1972.

184. Ribak C E, Peters A. An autoradiographic study of the projections from the lateral geniculate body of the rat. Brain Res 92:341–368, 1975.

185. Swanson L W, Cowan W M, Jones E G. An autoradiographic study of the efferent connections of the ventral lateral geniculate nucleus in the albino rat and the cat. J Comp Neurol 156:143–164, 1974.

186. Aghajanian G K, Bloom F E, Sheard M H. Electron microscopy of degeneration within the serotonin pathway of rat brain. Brain Res 13:266–273, 1969.

187. Dark J G, Asdourian D. Entrainment of the rat's activity rhythm by cyclic light following lateral geniculate nucleus lesions. Physiol Behav 15:295–301, 1975.

188. Block M, Zucker I. Circadian rhythms of rat locomotor activity after lesions of the midbrain raphe nuclei. J Comp Physiol 109:235–247, 1976.

189. Kam L M, Moberg G P. Effect of raphe lesions on the circadian pattern of wheel running in the rat. Physiol Behav 18:213–217, 1977.

190. Klein D C, Reiter R J, Weller J L. Pineal N-acetyltransferase activity in blinded and anosmic rats. Endocrinology 89:1020–1023, 1971.

191. Ralph C L, Hull D, Lynch H J, Hedlund L. A melatonin rhythm persists in rat pineals in darkness. Endocrinology 89:1361–1366, 1971.

192. Halberg F. Physiologic 24-hour periodicity; general and procedural considerations with reference to the adrenal cycle. Z Vitamin Hormon Fermentforschung 10:225–296, 1959.

193. Pohl C R, Gibbs F P. Circadian rhythms in blinded rats: correlation between pineal activity cycles. Am J Physiol 234:110–114, 1978.

194. Tamarkin L, Reppert S, Anderson A, Pratt B, Goldman B D, Klein D C. Regulation of pineal melatonin in the Syrian hamster. Pharmacologist 20:151, 1978.

195. Aschoff J. Exogenous and endogenous components in circadian rhythms. Cold Spring Harbor Symp Quant Biol 25:11–28, 1960.

196. Aschoff J. Desynchronization and resynchronization of human circadian rhythms. Aerosp Med 40:844–849, 1969.

197. Pittendrigh C S. Circadian systems: entrainment. In Handbook of Behavioral Neurobiology Biological Rhythms, vol 4, ed J Aschoff. Plenum Press, New York, 1981, pp 95–124.

198. Binkley S, Muller G, Hernandez T. Circadian rhythm in pineal N-acetyltransferase activity: phase-shifting by light pulses (I). J Neurochem 37:798–800, 1981.

199. Vaněček J, Illnerová H. Changes of a rhythm in rat pineal serotonin N-acetyltransferase following a one-minute light pulse at night. In The Pineal Gland of Vertebrates Including Man, Progress in Brain Research, 52 ed J Ariëns Kappers, P Pévet. Elsevier Biomedical, New York, 1979, pp 245–248.

200. Minneman K P, Lynch H, Wurtman R J. Relationship between environmental light intensity and retina-mediated suppression of rat pineal serotonin-N-acetyltransferase. Life Sci 15:1791–1796, 1974.

201. Rollag M D, Niswender G D. Radioimmunoassay of serum concentrations of melatonin in sheep exposed to different light regimens. Endocrinology 98:482–489, 1976.

202. Perlow M J, Reppert S M, Boyar R M, Klein D C. Daily rhythms in cortisol and melatonin in primate cerebrospinal fluid. Effects of constant light and dark. Neuroendocrinology 32:193–196, 1981.

203. Illnerová H, Vaněček J. Response of rat pineal serotonin N-acetyltransferase to one min light pulse at different night times. Brain Res 167:431–434, 1979.

204. Hoffmann K, Illnerová H, Vaněček J. Effect of photoperiod and of one minute light at night-time on the pineal rhythm on N-acetyltransferase activity in the Djungarian hamster Phodopus syngorus. Biol Reprod 24:551–556, 1981.
205. Cardinali D P, Larin F, Wurtman R J. Control of the rat pineal gland by light spectra. Proc Natl Acad Sci USA 69:2003–2005, 1972.
206. Illnerová H, Vaňáček J. Pineal rhythm in N-acetyltransferase activity in rats under different artificial photoperiods and in natural daylight in the course of a year. Neuroendocrinology 31:321–326, 1980.
207. Rudeen P K, Reiter R J. Effect of shortened photoperiods on pineal serotonin N-acetyltransferase activity and rhythmicity. J Interdisc Cycle Res 8:47–54, 1977.
208. Grota L J, Brown G M, Pang S F. Dissociation of N-acetylserotonin and melatonin levels in serum of rats. 11th Annual Meeting, Society for Neuroscience, October 1981, Los Angeles, p 717 (abstract).
209. Hoffman K, Illnerová H, Vaněček J. Pineal N-acetyltransferase activity in the Djungarian hamster. Naturwissenschaften 67:408–409, 1980.
210. Tamarkin L, Reppert S M, Klein D C, Pratt B, Goldman B D. Studies on the daily pattern of pineal melatonin in the Syrian hamster. Endocrinology 107:1525–1529, 1980.
211. Zatz M, Brownstein M J. Intraventricular carbachol mimics the effects of light on the circadian rhythm in the rat pineal gland. Science 203:358–361, 1979.
212. Zatz M, Brownstein M J. Injection of alpha-bungarotoxin near the suprachiasmatic nucleus blocks the effects of light on nocturnal pineal enzyme activity. Brain Res 213:438–442, 1981.
213. Goldman B, Hall V, Hollister C, Reppert S, Roychoudhury P, Yellon S, Tamarkin L. Diurnal changes in pineal melatonin content in four rodent species: relationship to photoperiodism. Biol Reprod 24:778–783, 1981.
214. Petterborg L J, Richardson B A, Reiter R J. Effect of long or short photoperiod on pineal melatonin content in the white-footed mouse, Peromyscus leucopus. Life Sci 29:1623–1627, 1981.
215. Rollag M D, O'Callaghan P L, Niswender G D. Serum melatonin concentrations during different stages of the annual reproductive cycle in ewes. Biol Reprod 18:279–285, 1978.
216. Arendt J. Radioimmunoassayable melatonin: circulating patterns in man and sheep. *In* The Pineal Gland of Vertebrates Including Man, Progress in Brain Research, vol 52, ed J Ariëns Kappers, P Pévet. Elsevier/North-Holland, New York, 1979, pp 249–258.
217. Griffiths D, Seamark R F, Bryden M M. Summer and winter cycles in plasma melatonin levels in the elephant seal (Mirounga leonina). Aust J Biol Sci 32:581–586, 1979.
218. Bünning E. Biological clocks. Cold Spring Harbor Symp Quant Biol 25:1–10, 1960.
219. Pittendrigh C S, Minis D H. The entrainment of circadian oscillations by light and their role as photoperiodic clocks. Am Naturalist 98:261–294, 1964.
220. Pittendrigh C S. Circadian rhythms and the circadian organization of living systems. Cold Spring Harbor Symp Quant Biol 25:159–184, 1960.
221. US Naval Observatory. Tables of Sunrise, Sunset and Twilight, 2nd printing, Nautical Almanac Office. US Naval Observatory, Washington, DC, 0-639087, 1962.
222. Henderson S T. Daylight and Its Spectrum. Elsevier, New York, 1970, p 171.
223. Thorington L. Actinic effects of light and biological implications. Photochem Photobiol 32:117–129, 1980.
224. Jimerson D C, Lynch H J, Post R M, Wurtman R J, Bunny W E. Urinary melatonin rhythms during sleep deprivation in depressed patients and normals. Life Sci 20:1501–1508, 1977.

225. Lynch H J, Jimerson D C, Ozaki Y, Post R M, Bunney W E, Wurtman R J. Entrainment of rhythmic melatonin secretion in man to a 12-hour phase shift in the light dark cycle. Life Sci 23:1557–1564, 1977.

226. Arendt J. Melatonin assays in body fluids. J Neural Transm, Suppl 13:265–278, 1978.

227. Weitzman E D, Weinberg U, D'Eletto R, Lynch H J, Wurtman R J, Czeisler C A, Erlich S. Studies of the 24 hour rhythm of melatonin in man. J Neural Transm, Suppl 13:325–337, 1978.

228. Wetterberg L. Melatonin in humans: physiological and clinical studies. J Neural Transm, Suppl 13:289–310, 1978.

229. Akerstedt T, Froberg J E, Friberg Y, Wetterberg L. Melatonin secretion, body temperature and subjective arousal during 64 hours of sleep deprivation. Psychoneuroendocrinology 4:219–225, 1979.

230. Vaughan G M, Bell R, De La Pena A. Nocturnal plasma melatonin in humans: episodic pattern and influence of light. Neuroscience Letters 14:81–84, 1979.

231. Perlow M J, Reppert S M, Tamarkin L, Wyatt R J, Klein D C. Photic regulation of the melatonin rhythm: monkey and man are not the same. Brain Res 182:211–216, 1980.

232. Lewy A J, Wehr T A, Goodwin F K, Newsome D A, Markey S P. Light suppresses melatonin secretion in humans. Science 210:1267–1269, 1980.

233. Moore R Y. The anatomy of central neural mechanisms regulating endocrine rhythms. In Comprehensive Endocrinology, ed D T Krieger. Raven Press, New York, 1979, pp 63–87.

234. Lydic R, Schoene W C, Czeisler C A, Moore-Ede M C. Suprachiasmatic region of the human hypothalamus: homolog to the primate circadian pacemaker? Sleep 2:355–361, 1980.

235. Hollwich F. The Influence of Ocular Light Perception on Metabolism in Man and in Animal. Springer-Verlag, New York, 1979.

236. Sharp G W G. The effect of light on the morning increase in urine flow. J Endocrinol 21:219–223, 1960.

237. Hollwich F, Dieckhues B. Eosinopeniereaktion und Sehvermögen. Klin mbl Augenheilk 152:11–16, 1968.

238. Rivest R W, Lynch H J, Ronsheim P M, Wurtmann R J. Effect of light intensity on regulation of melatonin secretion and drinking behavior in the albino rat. In Melatonin—Current Status and Perspectives, Advances in the Biosciences, vol 29, eds N Birau, W Schloot. Pergamon Press, Oxford, 1981, pp 119–121.

239. Lynch H J, Rivest R W, Ronsheim P M, Wurtman R J. Light intensity and the control of melatonin secretion in rats. Neuroendocrinology 33:181–185, 1981.

240. Lewy A J, Newsome D A, Unusual melatonin secretion in some blind subjects. Submitted for publication.

241. Klein K E, Wegmann H-M. The resynchronization of psychomotor performance circadian rhythm after transmeridian flights as a result of flight direction and mode of activity. In Chronobiology, ed LE Scheving, F Halberg, JE Pauly. George Thieme Purl, Stuttgart, 1974, pp 564–570.

242. Wever R A. Phase shifts of human circadian rhythms due to shifts of artificial Zeitgebers. Chronobiologia 7:303, 1980.

243. Aschoff J, Wever R. The circadian system of man. In Handbook of Behavioral Neurobiology, vol 4, ed J Aschoff. Plenum Press, New York, 1981, pp 311–331.

244. Lewis P R, Lobban M C. Dissociation of diurnal rhythms in human subjects living on abnormal time routines. Q J Exp Physiol 42:371–376, 1957.

245. Orth D P, Island D P. Light synchronization of the circadian rhythm in plasma cortisol (17-OHCS) concentration in man. J Clin Endocrinol Metab 29:479–486, 1969.

246. Zulley J. Der Einfluss von Zeitgebern auf den Schlaf des Menschen. Rita G. Fischer, Verlag, Frankfurt, 1979.

247. Czeisler C A, Weitzman E D, Moore-Ede M C, Zimmerman J C, Knauer R S. Human sleep: its duration and organization depend on its circadian phase. Science 210:1264–1266, 1980.

248. Aschoff J. Annual rhythms in man. *In* Handbook of Behavioral Neurobiology, Biological Rhythms, vol 4., ed J Aschoff. Plenum Press, New York, 1981, pp 475–487.

249. Lewy A J, Kern H, Rosenthal N E, Wehr T A. Case report: Artificial light treatment of a manic-depressive patient with a seasonal mood cycle. Am. J. Psych., Nov. 1982.

250. Aschoff J. Circadian rhythms: general features and endocrinological aspects. *In* Comprehensive Endocrinology, ed D T Krieger. Raven Press, New York, 1979, pp 1–61.

251. Weitzman E D, Czeisler C A, Moore-Ede M C. Sleep-wake, neuroendocrine and body temperature circadian rhythms under entrained and non-entrained (free-running) conditions in man. *In* Biological Rhythms and Their Central Mechanisms, ed M Suda, O Hayaishi, H Nakagawa. Elsevier North Holland, New York, 1979, pp 199–227.

252. Czeisler C A, Moore-Ede M C, Regestein Q R, Kisch E S, Fang V S, Erhlich E N. Episodic 24-hour cortisol secretory rhythm during cardiac surgery. J Clin Endocrinol Metab 42:273–283, 1979.

253. Herbert D C, Reiter R J. Influence of protein-calorie malnutrition on the circadian rhythm of pineal melatonin in the rat. Soc Exp Biol Med 166:360–363, 1981.

254. Lynch H J, Eng J P, Wurtman R J. Control of pineal indole biosynthesis by changes in sympathetic tone caused by factors other than environmental lighting. Proc Natl Acad Sci USA 70:1704–1708, 1973.

255. Illnerová H. The effects of immobilization of the activity of serotonin N-acetyltransferase in the rat epiphysis. *In* Catecholamines and Stress, ed E Usdin, R Kvetnansky, I J Kopin. Pergamon Press, New York 1976, pp 129–136.

256. Vaughan G M, McDonald S D, Jordan R M, Allen J P, Bohm Falk A L, Abou-Samro M, Story J L. Melatonin concentration in human blood and cerebrospinal fluid. J Clin Endocrinol Metab 47:220–223, 1978.

257. Weinberg J, D'Eletto R D, Weitzman E D, Erlich S, Hollander C S. Circulatory melatonin in man: episodic secretion throughout the dark-light cycle. J Clin Endocrinol Metab 48:114–118, 1979.

258. Vaughan G M, Allen J P, Tullis U, Silar-Khodr T J, De La Pena A, Sackman J W. Overnight plasma profiles of melatonin and certain adenohypophysial hormones in men. J Clin Endocrinol Metab 47:566–571, 1978.

259. Wehr T A, Goodwin F K. Biological rhythms and psychiatry. *In* American Handbook of Psychiatry, vol 7, 2nd ed, ed S Arieti, H K H Brodie. Basic Books, New York, 1981, pp 46–74.

260. Lewy A J, Wehr T A, Goodwin F K, Newsome D A, Rosenthal N E. Manic-depressive patients may be supersensitive to light. Lancet 1:383–384, 1981.

261. Gaston S, Menaker M. Pineal function: the biological clock in the sparrow? Science 160:1125–1127, 1968.

262. Turek F W, McMillan J P, Menaker M. Melatonin: effects on the circadian locomotor rhythm of sparrows. Science 194:1441–1443, 1976.

263. Gwinner E, Benzinger I. Synchronization of a circadian rhythm in pinealectomized European starlings by daily injections of melatonin. J Comp Physiol 127:209–213, 1978.

264. Underwood H. Melatonin affects circadian rhythmicity in lizards. J Comp Physiol 130:317–323, 1979.

265. Ebihara S, Kawamura H. The role of the pineal organ and the suprachiasmatic nucleus in the control of circadian locomotor rhythms in the Java sparrow, Padda oryzivora. J Comp Physiol 141:207–214, 1981.

266. Underwood H. Circadian organization in the lizard Scelopurus occidentalis: the effects of pinealectomy, blinding, and melatonin. J Comp Physiol 141:537–547, 1981.

267. Tamarkin L, Westrom W K, Hamill A I, Goldman B D. Effect of melatonin on the reproductive systems of male and female Syrian hamsters: a diurnal rhythm in sensitivity to melatonin. Endocrinology 99:1534–1541, 1976.

268. Reiter R J, Blask D E, Johnson L Y, Rudeen P K, Vaughan M K, Waring P J. Melatonin inhibition of reproduction in the male hamster: its dependency on time of day of administration and on an intact and sympathetically innervated pineal gland. Neuroendocrinology 22:107–116, 1976.

269. Turek F W, Pappas P. Daily melatonin injections inhibit short day-induced testicular regression in hamsters (Mesocricetus auratus). Experientia 36:1426–1427, 1980.

270. Cheze G, Ali M A, Rôle de l'épiphyse dans la migration du pigment épithélial rétinien chez quelques Téleostéens. Can J Zool 54:475–481, 1976.

271. Gern W A, Gorell T A, Owens D W. Melatonin and pigment cell rhythmicity. In Melatonin—Current Status and Perspectives, Advances in the Biosciences, vol 29, ed N Birau, W Schloot. Pergamon Press, Oxford, 1981, pp 223–233.

272. Pang S F, Yew D T. Pigment aggregation by melatonin in the retinal pigment epithelium and choroid of guinea pigs, Cavia porcellus. Experientia 35:231–233, 1979.

273. Rudeen P K, O'Steen W K. The effects of the pineal gland on light-induced retinal photoreceptor damage. Exp Eye Res 28:37–44, 1979.

274. Bubenik G A, Purtill R A The role of melatonin and dopamine in retinal physiology. Can J Physiol Pharmacol 58:1457–1462, 1980.

275. Gern W A. Evolution of melatonin function: a hypothesis. In Melatonin—Current Status and Perspectives, Advances in the Biosciences, vol 29, ed N Birau, W Schloot. Pergamon Press, Oxford, 1981, pp 85–87.

NOTE ADDED IN PROOF

Regarding the question of the source of plasma melatonin (see pp. 94–96), the author and Dr. Edward Neuwalt recently studied a patient both before and following removal of a low-grade astrocytoma-pineoblastoma. Melatonin levels were normal preoperatively and undetectable postoperatively when measured by gas chromatographic-negative chemical ionization mass spectrometric assay.

HARRY J. LYNCH, Ph.D.

ASSAY METHODOLOGY

INTRODUCTION

The first practical application of a melatonin assay preceded the discovery of melatonin. In 1917, McCord and Allen (1), in seeking to establish the influence of pineal gland substances on growth and differentiation processes in tadpoles, discovered that 30 minutes after feeding pineal tissue, the tadpoles, which before feeding had been uniformly dark, became so translucent that their larger viscera were plainly visible through the dorsal body wall. Pineal tissue alone elicited such a response. The quantitative relations between tissue concentrations and the time interval needed for maximum blanching afforded a means for gauging the strength of various pineal tissue preparations. Tadpoles of the leopard frog, *Rana pipiens,* were identified as the animals of choice for such an assay because in the course of their development they briefly display a dense uniform dermal melanophore layer that is highly sensitive to the effects of pineal extracts. McCord and Allen showed that the growth-stimulating principle in the pineal is distinct from the principle con-

From the Laboratory of Neuroendocrine Regulation, Department of Nutrition and Food Science, Massachusetts Institute of Technology, Cambridge, Massachusetts 02139.

Author's studies were supported in part by a grant from the National Institutes of Health (HD 11722).

cerned with pigment changes. The pineal substance responsible for pigment changes is wholly extracted by acetone, whereas the residue after acetone extraction influences growth and differentiation. An obstacle to the continued study of the blanching phenomenon at that time was the fact that the appropriate test animals (larval *Rana pipiens*) were available only for a short time each spring.

Some four decades later, Lerner and his associates (2), hoping to identify a neurogenic agent that might be involved in the depigmentation characteristic of human vitiligo, undertook a search for the skin-lightening constituent of pineal extracts. To trace the melanophorotrophic constituent of pineal tissue through an exhaustive extraction procedure, they used the bioassay principle discovered by McCord and Allen, but they circumvented the problem of seasonal availability of tadpoles by using instead isolated pieces of frog skin in an in vitro system; and instead of a subjective visual assessment of color change, they measured changes in the skin's light absorption by means of a photoelectric photometer (3). Finally, in 1958, they identified melatonin (5-methoxy-N-acetyltryptamine) as the pineal compound responsible for skin lightening in amphibians (2). This compound was shown to be a derivative of serotonin, a widely distributed indole stored in very large quantities in mammalian pineals (4). Melatonin differed from all other indoles previously identified in mammals in that it contained a methoxy group.

Soon thereafter, Axelrod and Weissbach showed that the pineal contained all of the enzymes needed to synthesize melatonin from its amino acid precursor, tryptophan, and described for the first time the peculiar pineal enzyme that catalyzes the terminal step in melatonin biosynthesis, hydroxyindole-O-methyltransferase (HIOMT) (5). Because no method was then available that allowed direct measurement of melatonin in pineal glands or body fluids, investigators examined the effects of various experimental manipulations on pineal HIOMT activity, assayed in vitro, and hypothesized that treatments that changed the enzyme's activity also caused parallel changes in the rate at which melatonin was synthesized and secreted in vivo.

This technique for inferring changes in the rate of melatonin secretion was instrumental in a series of experiments that showed that environmental lighting suppresses mammalian pineal function (6), that melatonin synthesis varies rhythmically in parallel with the light-dark cycle (7), and that information about environmental lighting conditions reaches the nonphotoreceptive mammalian pineal via a pathway involving the eyes, central neural tracts independent of those that subserve vision, and the pineal's unusual sympathetic innervation (8,9).

Fiske and associates, in studying the mechanisms by which exposure of rats to continuous illumination accelerated the maturation of their gonads, discovered that the weights of pineals of female rats kept in a continuously lit environment decreased, whereas the weights of their ovaries increased and a "persistent vaginal estrus" syndrome was induced (10). These observations supported the notion that the function of the nonphotoreceptive mammalian pineal (which is homologous with the photoreceptive parietal structures in phylogenetically more primitive vertebrate classes) was somehow related to environmental illumination.

Wurtman and associates then showed that exposure of female rats to continuous light, or removal of their pineals, has similar but nonadditive effects on the weights of their ovaries; they further showed that administration of crude pineal extracts (11) or of melatonin (12) could exert antigonadal effects and reverse the effects of pinealectomy.

In 1963, Quay introduced the first assay method, based on differential extraction and spectrophotofluorometric measurement, that allowed estimation of the melatonin content of individual rat pineal glands (13). Using this assay method, he was able not only to affirm the daily rhythm in the rate of melatonin production but also to detect a rhythmic variation in pineal melatonin content corresponding to the estrous cycle (14).

In 1965, Wurtman and Axelrod published a "state of the art" paper on pineal research in *Scientific American* (15). In it, they summarized the observations just outlined and advanced the hypothesis that the pineal functions as a neuroendocrine transducer, responding to neural stimulation (norepinephrine release from its sympathetic innervation) by releasing more of a hormone (melatonin); they also posited a special role for the pineal in converting an external cycle (environmental light and darkness) into a humoral signal (variations in circulating melatonin levels) and proposed that a receptor for that signal is the brain—particularly brain regions that control gonadal rhythms.

This formulation has served well as a reference paradigm for much of the pineal research that has ensued. It has been significantly extended and embellished by various investigations: notably, Shein and Wurtman's development of an organ culture system that further demonstrated that norepinephrine accelerates melatonin's synthesis from tryptophan and that it works via a beta receptor and cyclic AMP (16); Klein's demonstration of the marked daily oscillations in rat pineal N-acetyltransferase activity and the qualitative similarity between this enzyme's responses and that of HIOMT to environmental light, pineal denervation, and other experimental manipulations (17); Reiter's demonstration that the pineal gland, through the agency of melatonin, is an important mediator of photoperiodically induced changes in the hamster's reproductive physiology (18); and Tamarkin et al.'s finding that the effectiveness of exogenous melatonin as an antigonadal agent depends on the timing of its administration (19).

In 1971, at the time of the Ciba Foundation Symposium on the Pineal Gland, attention was clearly focused on melatonin (20). In the view of many investigators, melatonin was the gonad-inhibiting product of the pineal. Over the next few years, the spectrophotofluorometric assay of melatonin was further refined (21) and several investigators advanced bioassay methods for the semiquantitative or quantitative estimation of pineal melatonin content (22–24). The next advance in pineal research, however, awaited the introduction in 1975 of the first radioimmunoassay for melatonin by Arendt (25). This assay made it possible to measure levels of circulating melatonin in humans and in experimental animals directly: a new age in pineal-melatonin research was born. Since then, several more radioimmunoassays for melatonin have been reported; gas chromatographic methods used to measure melatonin and to validate radioimmunoassays for melatonin have been developed and, to a considerable extent, the study of pineal function has become the measurement of melatonin.

Melatonin assay methodology is young and fallible. Our notions about where melatonin should be, when, how much, and why are based for the most part on indirect evidence amassed and variously interpreted over the years. It is not the purpose of this chapter to advocate any particular approach to melatonin measurement nor to advance any new discovery, but rather, to provide a brief review of melatonin assay methodology that might aid in the assimilation and interpretation of that which has been or will later be discovered.

MELATONIN ASSAYS

Approaches to the assay of melatonin include bioassay, spectrophotofluorometric assay, radioimmunoassay, and diverse modes of detection and quantitation used in conjunction with chromatographic isolation techniques. Each approach exploits a different biological, chemical, or physical property of melatonin, and each assay method has characteristic sensitivity and specificity. However, to the extent that the results they yield agree quantitatively and the changes they display after various experimental manipulations are similar, they tend to be mutually corroborative.

The various analytical methods that have been used to quantify melatonin will be addressed here in roughly the same order as they appeared chronologically. The principle upon which each assay method is based will be outlined, and each assay's contribution to our present knowledge of the natural history of melatonin will be summarized.

Bioassay

The phenomenon that provides the basis for all melatonin bioassay methods is the serendipitous discovery by McCord and Allen described earlier. In the presence of melatonin, the dark melanin pigment granules within the dermal melanophores of amphibian skin undergo a dose-dependent nucleocentric aggregation resulting in a net blanching or lightening of the skin.

Various methods have been used to quantify the response: (1) measurement of the time required to bring about maximum blanching as visually assessed in living tadpoles (1); (2) photometric measurement of changes in the reflectance or transmission of incident light by isolated pieces of frog skin (3,26); or (3) microscopic assessment of the extent of melanin aggregation within the melanophores of intact amphibian larvae as judged relative to an arbitrary scale of melanophore stages, the Hogbin index (27,28). The first method was used by McCord and Allen in their pioneering work on the fractionation of pineal tissue (1). The second method was refined by Lerner and associates and used to trace the isolation of melatonin from pineal tissue (3). The third method has proved most useful in the quantitative estimation of melatonin by bioassay (24).

To circumvent practical problems posed by the seasonal availability of the optimum test animal, larval *Rana pipiens*, Ralph and Lynch (24) instituted a tadpole culturing program in their laboratory. By maintaining adult frogs in states of protracted hibernation (refrigerated at 5°C), spawning could be induced at will, eggs inseminated, and tadpoles of the appropriate developmental stage made available continuously.

To use these animals in a quantitative melatonin bioassay, groups of light-adapted (melanin-dispersed) tadpoles are exposed to media containing either known concentrations of authentic melatonin or to aqueous extracts of pineal tissue or other biological material. A calibration curve is plotted relating the melanophore responses, in terms of the Hogbin index, to graded concentrations of melatonin (0.1–5.0 ng/ml). From this curve, melatonin concentrations in the various extracts are estimated.

This assay method is remarkably specific for melatonin in the presence of naturally occurring melatonin metabolites and analogues (29,30), and melatonin in pineal tissue homogenates can be measured by bioassay without prior purification. Similarly, melatonin in extracts of body fluids can be assayed readily if sufficient amounts of the hormone are concentrated to bring it within the sensitivity range of the assay. Although tadpole melanophores respond discernibly to as little as 100 pg/ml of melatonin, accuracy and precision in the bioassay of melatonin from natural sources require replicate sampling at various concentrations. Therefore, as the total melatonin content of a given sample approaches the melanophore's limit of sensitivity, the accuracy of quantitative estimates diminishes. Thus, while pineal melatonin content can be measured readily, the useful estimate of melatonin in small samples of blood or cerebrospinal fluid (CSF) is simply not feasible. Nevertheless, with this assay method, Pelham and associates (31), using 20-ml blood samples, successfully demonstrated diurnal variations with nocturnal increases in the concentration of a "melatonin-like substance" in human plasma. Using the same assay method, Vaughan et al. (32) reaffirmed the rhythmic nocturnal rise in human plasma melatonin, demonstrated that this daily rhythm persisted through $2^{1}/_{2}$ days of constant light, and postulated, on the basis of their observations, that melatonin might be secreted in pulses in humans.

To measure urinary melatonin, the limited sensitivity of the bioassay method necessitated development of a column chromatographic technique using Amberlite XAD-2 (33) to concentrate melatonin from 4- or 8-hour human urine collections. Such studies demonstrated the relationship between diurnal lighting and rhythmic melatonin excretion, with nocturnal increases, revealed that the rhythm persists through 28 hours of constant artificial light (34); and showed that 5–7 days were required to reentrain rhythmic melatonin excretion to a 12-hour phase shift in the lighting schedule (35). Studies of human urinary melatonin also showed that, in a "timeless environment," the rhythmic pattern of melatonin excretion can be dissociated from a "self-selected" wake-sleep schedule (36) and that blind human subjects exhibit a circadian rhythm in melatonin excretion, which is not phase-locked to their customary wake-sleep schedule (36).

Spectrophotofluorometric Assay

A distinctive characteristic of all 5-hydroxy- and 5-methoxyindoles is their fluorescence in strong mineral acid at 540–550 nm, when activated at 295 nm. This phenomenon, discovered by Udenfriend, Bogdanski, and Weissbach (37), facilitated development of a sensitive chemical method for measuring serotonin and studying its tissue distribution (4).

Quay (13) employed the fluorometric approach and described techniques for selective extraction (using different organic solvents and pH adjustments of the aqueous phase) and measurement of a variety of indoles, including melatonin. In 1964, he demonstrated, for the first time, daily and estrous rhythms in rat pineal melatonin content (14). Quay found that selective extraction of melatonin occurs with p-cymene and an alkaline solution. Because all 5-hydroxy and 5-methoxyindole derivatives have almost identical fluorescence characteristics, a truly selective extraction is necessary. Although p-cymene affords such selectivity, Quay also found that significant technical difficulties remain in the practical application of this method. For example, impurities in commercial reagent-grade solvents appear to affect the efficiency of recovery of the primary indole solutes much more than they do the specificity of the extraction (13).

Maickel and Miller (21) discovered that when indoles containing HO- or CH_3O-substituents on the fifth carbon are heated with O-phthalaldehyde (OPT) in 3 N hydrochloric acid, they yield highly fluorescent products and thus enhance the fluorometric assay's sensitivity. Again, the fluorescent spectra of the reaction products of OPT with serotonin, 5-methoxytryptamine, N-acetylserotonin, and melatonin are very similar. Therefore, a discriminating separation procedure is needed to measure the various compounds in each other's presence. The procedure developed by Maickel and Miller (21) uses multiple solvent extractions to separate the indoles; the final step in each preparation is reaction with OPT. The estimated sensitivity of this method permits accurate measurement of 10–20 ng of each compound.

Using the selective extraction technique, Quay pooled 4–6 rat pineal glands for each assay and estimated their pineal melatonin content to be about 1 ng/gland in the daytime and 3 ng/gland at night (14). Using multiple solvent extraction and OPT-enhanced fluorescence, Maickel and Miller worked with 4–5 mg of tissue for each assay and estimated the daytime melatonin concentration to be about 0.4 ng/mg in the rat pineal (21,38) and 0.17 ng/mg in the dog pineal (38). Ozaki and associates used the fluorometric melatonin assay with OPT enhancement to show that pretreatment of rats with chlorpromazine slows the disappearance of exogenous unlabeled melatonin from the plasma (39).

Although the data are few, fluorometric assays of melatonin are of more than historical significance. This assay method provided the first demonstration of circadian rhythms in rat pineal melatonin content and showed that the rhythms were correlated with light and dark periods and possibly were influenced to a lesser degree by the estrous cycle.

The early efforts to exploit the sensitivity of fluorometric detection in the assay of melatonin were frustrated by the inadequacy of available methods to separate the hormone from endogenous compounds with similar fluorescent spectra. The very recent development of high performance liquid chromatography (discussed later) may reinstate fluorescence as the detection mode of choice for the routine measurement of melatonin.

Radioimmunoassay

The principle of the radioimmunoassay (RIA) technique was described by Yalow and Berson in 1960 (40). All that is needed is a labeled ligand to be assayed, a protein containing the specific receptor for the ligand, and a way of separating bound from free ligand without disturbing the equilibrium. Constant amounts of free labeled antigen (Ag*) and a limited number of antibody sites (Ab) are in equilibrium with the labeled antigen-antibody (Ag*:Ab) complex. If unlabeled antigen (Ag), either in standard solutions or in the sample to be analyzed, is added, it competes for the limited number of Ab sites and, depending on its concentration, displaces different amounts of the labeled Ag* from the Ag*:Ab complex.

$$Ag \qquad Ag^*$$
$$Ag - Ab \; \underset{\rightarrow}{\leftharpoons} \; Ab \; \rightleftarrows \; Ag^*{:}Ab$$

After equilibration, free Ag* and Ag*:Ab are separated. Ag*:Ab (or free Ag*) is then measured by radioactive counting. The antigen concentration of the sample is then determined by comparing the diminished Ag* binding of the sample to that of a standard curve obtained by adding graded amounts of Ag to Ag* and Ab.

Organic molecules that are nonimmunogenic as such, but that produce an immune response when they are attached to a protein, are termed haptens. Melatonin is such a molecule. Since melatonin does not have intrinsic protein reactivity, an activating agent must be supplied to promote covalent bond formation. The resulting antigenic product is then used to immunize (i.e., to stimulate antibody production in) a rabbit. The useful specificity and potency of an antiserum grown to an antigen-hapten complex depends on several factors including the number and spatial distribution of immunogenically distinctive features of the hapten, the nature of its attachment to the carrier molecule, the immunization protocol, and, most significantly, the individual immune response of the animal that is "immunized."

Several methods for coupling melatonin or one of its analogues to different carrier molecules have been devised, and several relatively specific antisera have been produced for use in melatonin RIAs. In a recent review, Arendt (41) summarized the brief history of these RIAs, outlined some of the methods used to produce antimelatonin sera, and enumerated criteria that might be used in characterizing the specificity of a given antiserum.

Another prerequisite to the development of an RIA is the availability of a radioactive tracer with a sufficiently high specific activity to allow efficient estimation of bound or free antigen. Tritiated melatonin (26 Ci/mmole) supplied by The New England Nuclear Co. of Boston fills this requirement for most of the current melatonin RIAs.

A significant technical innovation in the melatonin RIA developed by Rollag and Niswender (42) is the use of a radioiodinated melatonin analogue as a tracer; the high specific activity obtainable with radioiodine (1620 Ci/mmol) allows roughly tenfold greater sensitivity than that obtained with tritiated melatonin. Several laboratories are now using adaptations of this procedure.

In 1974, Grota and Brown (43) reported that antibodies to indoles can be raised after conjugation of serotonin or N-acetyl-serotonin to antigenic protein by means of the formaldehyde condensation reaction. The resulting antisera were described and proposed as the basis for RIA and immunohistochemical localization of melatonin in brain structures.

The first report of a practical RIA for melatonin, validated by comparison with bioassay measurements and accompanied by data on human plasma melatonin levels, was that of Arendt and associates in 1975 (25). Within the next 2 years, at least five additional RIA methods were developed (42,44–47) and melatonin measurements in pineal tissue, blood, CSF, and urine from humans and various other animal species were reported internationally. Studies have affirmed and extended earlier ideas about the nature of rhythmic melatonin secretion and its control by environmental illumination, melatonin's role in reproductive physiology, and the clinical significance of changes in circulating melatonin levels.

In 1977, an international cross-validation study was conducted by Wetterberg (48) using a reference serum containing 0.86 nmol/l (200 pg/ml) melatonin. Results obtained in seven laboratories using six different antisera indicate that melatonin can be measured with reasonable accuracy by the various RIA methods. Estimates of the melatonin concentration in the reference samples ranged from 128 ± 15 to 239 ± 35 pg/ml; the mean value obtained was 176 pg/ml.

A year later, a second collaborative study was performed by Wetterberg and Eriksson (49) in which night and day sera from human donors were used. Samples of both night and day sera to which known amounts of authentic melatonin had been added were included in this study to permit estimates of recovery of exogenous melatonin. Six of the 12 participating laboratories reported results within 70–130% of the "true" value in the recovery test. In both collaborative studies, only laboratories using RIA methods participated. Results were not obtained from laboratories using the more sophisticated gas chromatography-mass spectrometric methods.

All of the RIA methods now in use involve initial extraction of melatonin from its biological source into a nonpolar solvent. It is then usually purified further by aqueous washes or by column (47) or thin-layer chromatography (42,50), according to the specificity of the anti-serum used and the challenge presented by the specific tissue or body fluid under study. The number of protocols for sample preparation and RIA of melatonin far exceed the number of different antisera used in studying melatonin levels. A given laboratory may employ entirely different methods for extracting melatonin from blood, urine, and tissue (50); also, different experimental questions impose different analytical constraints. Thus, studies designed to monitor entrainment of a melatonin secretion rhythm to an altered lighting schedule or to demonstrate suppression of rhythmic melatonin secretion under constant light, are far less demanding than studies aimed at detecting very subtle changes in the absolute amounts of melatonin secreted or slight phase shifts in its rhythmic pattern.

The contribution of melatonin RIA methodology to our present knowledge of the role of the pineal and melatonin in animal physiology vastly exceeds, at least in quantitative terms, the contribution of all previous melatonin assay methods. The evolution and elaboration of the RIA method together with the fruits of its application are summarized in the proceedings of recent symposia (51–53). A few of the salient observations that melatonin RIAs have made possible include:

1. Documentation of the near universality of the fixed relationship between rhythmic changes in the rate of melatonin secretion and environmental light and darkness, with peak values occurring in the dark (47).
2. Measurement of blood and CSF melatonin levels when the two compartments are sampled simultaneously (54–59).
3. Detection of changes in human blood melatonin levels that correspond to annual and menstrual periods as well as to daily and ultradian periods (41,60–62).
4. Documentation of characteristic temporal patterns of melatonin secretion in diverse animal species with respect to the daily photoperiod (for review see Lynch and Wurtman, 63).
5. Detection of melatonin in animals after pinealectomy (47,64).

Whether some of these observations have raised more questions than they have answered will be considered later.

Chromatographic Isolation and Quantification

Most current melatonin assay methods depend on some degree of isolation and concentration of melatonin from the biological matrix in which it occurs (blood, urine, CSF, tissue) in combination with a more-or-less specific, more-or-less sensitive detection modality. As the extent of isolation increases, the requirement for specificity in the detector decreases and its sensitivity becomes the limiting factor. The work outlined following represents the status of recent efforts to find a practical compromise between absolute isolation in sample preparation and absolute specificity in measurement.

HIGH PERFORMANCE LIQUID CHROMATOGRAPHY (HPLC)

Chromatography is probably the most effective technique available for analytical separation of chemical mixtures. All types of chromatography are based on the phenomenon that each component in a mixture ordinarily interacts with its environment differently from all other components under the same conditions. In liquid chromatography, separation of a chemical mixture is achieved by the differential distribution of its components between moving and stationary phases where the moving phase is a liquid. The HP of HPLC is sometimes read "high pressure" because the mobile phase is pumped through the column at high pressure; it is sometimes read "high performance" because the increased linear velocity of the developing solution through a column packing of small high-surface-area particles yields a smaller height equivalent theoretical plate, a narrower solute band, and better separation. In addition, HPLC methods allow continuous monitoring of column effluent by any of a variety of detectors (65,66).

Roth et al. (67) used the high resolving power of HPLC without an on-line detector. Instead, they used a sensitive melatonin RIA, analyzed 0.5-ml fractions of the column effluent, and thereby validated their demonstration of melatonin in the blood of alligators.

Goldman et al. (65) used a system that employed a citrate-acetate buffer and a cation exchange resin with electrochemical detection to obtain baseline resolution of melatonin from other indoles in pure solution. They concluded that the system possesses more than sufficient sensitivity to analyze melatonin in biological tissues and fluids.

In electrochemical (or amperometric) detection, the effluent of the HPLC column (containing chromatographically separated solutes) passes over a planar electrode held at a preset fixed potential. If the potential is greater than that required for the electrolysis of a solute, a measurable charge passes from the electrode to the solute. The resulting current is directly proportional to the concentration of the solute passing through the detector.

Mefford and Barchas (68) used reversed-phase HPLC (a nonpolar stationary phase used with a relatively more polar liquid mobile phase) and electrochemical detection to determine levels of tryptophan and several of its metabolites in rat brain and pineal tissue. They found detection limits for these compounds to be in the low picogram range, and they measured 1.35 ng of melatonin in the rat pineal.

Very recently, a report has appeared that describes the use of a reversed-phase HPLC column with a dual detector system (66). The column effluent is monitored first by a fluorometric and then by an amperometric detector. With this system, a centrifuged pineal tissue homogenate can be injected directly onto the column and the chromatographically resolved components identified on the basis of their retention time and their relative fluorometric and amperometric response. The detection limit for melatonin with the fluorometric and amperometric detectors in this system were estimated to be 25 pg and

50 pg, respectively. Thus, the combination of reversed-phase HPLC with fluorometric and amperometric detectors allows determination of indoles in the pineal to be made easily and with a great deal of specificity and sensitivity. For routine use, the elements of this system with fluorometric detection alone might afford the simplicity and sensitivity that would facilitate the assay of large numbers of samples. The method must still, of course, be validated for the measurement of melatonin in blood and other body fluids.

GAS CHROMATOGRAPHY

In gas-liquid chromatography, separation of a chemical mixture is achieved by the transient differential distribution of its components between a stationary liquid phase coated on an inert column packing material and a mobile gas phase forced through the column. Such a system is very rapid, yields exquisite resolution of the components of a mixture, and lends itself to continuous monitoring of the column effluent.

Gas chromatography (GC) has been used in combination with increasingly discriminating modes of detection to measure melatonin. Prerequisite to all such assays is an extraction step that affords partial isolation and concentration of melatonin from its biological source, as well as a chemical reaction that yields a derivative of melatonin with an appropriate vapor pressure for GC and that facilitates its detection.

Electron-capture Detection (GC-EC). Most ionization detectors operate by measuring an ion current; recombination of ions decreases the signal. The electron capture detector employs recombination of ions as its principle of operation. The detector is thus extremely sensitive to compounds of high electron affinity, e.g., a richly halogenated melatonin derivative.

An ion chamber containing an ionizable gas is held at a potential sufficient for the collection of all free electrons produced; this is the standing current of the detector. The introduction of an electron-capturing vapor results in a decrease in the standing current, which is recorded.

For electron-capture detection, melatonin is extracted from the biological matrix in which it occurs and a volatile, halogenated derivative is formed. In 1970, Degen and Barchas, using the extraction procedure of Miller and Maickel (38) followed by the derivitization procedure, found that melatonin could be measured in pineal tissue with 100 pg as the lower limit of detectable material (69). Grenier and Chan (70) used the method to measure melatonin contents of pineal glands collected at autopsy from 22 human subjects; melatonin values ranged from 0 to 71.1 ng/gland. A diurnal variation in pineal melatonin content, based on the times of death, was observed; the melatonin concentration increased in the evening and through the night and started to fall in the morning.

Mass Spectrometric Detection (GC-MS). A gas chromatograph inter-
faced with a mass spectrometer is used in mass spectrometric detection.
Of all the spectroscopic techniques available, only the mass spectrometer
is capable of giving information that can lead to an identification of a
solute band with the extremely small samples used in GC. Components
of a chemical mixture, resolved by GC, are concentrated and ionized;
the resulting charged fragments are accelerated through electric and
magnetic fields that separate them on the basis of their charge and mass.
They are then recorded as a spectrum of lines characteristic of the parent
compounds.

Chromatographically resolved components in the GC effluent are
quantified in the mass spectrometer by measuring the ion densities generated by specific fragments. Specificity in GC-MS assays is enhanced
because quantified substances are simultaneously identified by GC retention time and by the molecular weight of fragment ions. The method
has been used for the quantitation and absolute identification of melatonin in extracts of various tissues (47,71) and body fluids (47,72,73) and
to validate various RIAs for melatonin (42,47,73).

**Negative-chemical-ionization Mass Spectrometry (Negative CI GC-
MS).** Lewy et al. (74) used a recent innovation of GC-MS technology
that very significantly enhances the sensitivity of mass-spectrometric
measurement of melatonin.

Simple GC-MS methodology requires that extracted samples be de-
rivitized in order to increase their volatility and to facilitate passage of
the sample through the GC. The enhanced sensitivity afforded by operation of a mass spectrometer under negative chemical-ionization conditions is achieved by employing derivatives that allow the sample to
undergo efficient ionization, with reduced fragmentation, by resonance
capture of low, near-thermal energy electrons. Thus, negative ions are
formed by the interaction of electrons and sample molecules and the
sample ion current is greatly increased.

This analytical technique revealed daytime melatonin levels as low as
1.5 pg/ml and nighttime levels as high as 42.6 pg/ml in plasma from
human subjects (74). In rats, daytime plasma melatonin levels were 4
pg/ml; nighttime levels were 52 pg/ml; and, $2^1/_2$ hours after treatment
with 3 mg/kg isoproterenol in the daytime, 30 pg/ml (75).

An outstanding advantage of the GC-MS methods for melatonin measurement is the high-accuracy analyses that can be obtained through
isotope dilution-mass spectrometry. This technique was used in some
of the work described previously (47,74). The basic principle is that the
ratio between unlabeled melatonin and melatonin labeled with deuter-
ium, $[^2H_3]$ melatonin, can be determined with high accuracy and precision with use of mass spectrometry. The isotope labeled melatonin is
added in a fixed amount to a fixed volume of sample (e.g., serum, urine,
CSF). After extraction, derivitization, and eventual chromatographic purification, the ratio between the labeled and unlabeled molecules is determined with a mass spectrometer equipped with a multiple-ion de-

tector (MID). Because the labeled molecules have a mass that differs only very little from that of the unlabeled molecules, the ratio between the labeled and unlabeled molecules cannot be changed during sample preparation and chromatography. On the basis of the measured ratio, the concentration of the endogenous, unlabeled melatonin can be calculated with great accuracy.

FUNDAMENTAL UNRESOLVED ISSUES

A decade ago there were only about a dozen or so published reports that described the detection or quantitative estimation of melatonin in animals. These studies employed early bioassay and fluorometric methods and demonstrated the occurrence of melatonin in extracts of mammalian sciatic nerves and human urine (76); a daily rhythm in rat (22,77) and bird (23,77) pineal melatonin content; effects of continuous light or darkness (22,78), blinding and anosmia (79), and pineal denervation (22) on rat pineal melatonin content. These data, though fragmentary and of unsubstantiated accuracy, were eagerly embraced because they fairly established that the pineal organ is a gland; that in addition to synthesizing melatonin, it contains and secretes melatonin; and that rhythmic melatonin secretion is influenced by environmental light. In sum, the observations on melatonin tended to substantiate the basic tenets of the melatonin hypothesis (15).

Then the questions changed—or the old questions demanded more detail. Is the pineal gland the only source of melatonin? By what anatomical route is melatonin secreted? How exclusively, or to what extent and through what neural mechanism does environmental light control melatonin secretion? Over the past 5 years, increasingly sophisticated melatonin assay methodology has been brought to bear on these questions. The following sections outline the current status of some of these questions.

Occurrence of Melatonin in Pinealectomized Animals

The utility of pinealectomy for studying melatonin's physiologic effects requires that the operation either completely deprive animals of the methoxyindole or at least terminate diurnal and gonadal-dependent rhythms of melatonin secretion. It was believed initially that, among mammalian organs, only the pineal contained HIOMT activity and thus could synthesize melatonin (5,80); however, subsequent investigations demonstrated that there is HIOMT activity in the retina (81), Harderian gland (82), and erythrocytes (83). Melatonin is found in the rat digestive system (84), and it is synthesized from tryptophan in the mammalian retina (81). The extent to which these organs contribute to circulating melatonin remains controversial. There are numerous reports that melatonin continues to circulate after pinealectomy, but that its levels do not exhibit normal daily rhythms (47,64,71). At least one report (85) describes a significant reduction in the concentration of serum melatonin in rats after pinealectomy, but a persisting circadian rhythm. Melatonin has been detected in urines of pinealectomized rats by both bioassay and RIA (64); in blood of pinealectomized rats (64), sheep (47), and baboons (86) by RIA; and in hypothalamic tissue of pinealectomized rats by GC-MS (71). Other investigators failed to detect melatonin by bioassay (87) or GC-MS (75) in blood of pinealectomized rats. Melatonin production by extrapineal tissues is reviewed in detail by Ralph (88). The question remains open.

Locus of Melatonin Secretion

There are two potential routes for melatonin secretion in mammals. Since the pineal gland is an intracranial organ, it could secrete melatonin into the surrounding subarachnoid space; in mammals such as humans, where the pineal forms part of the roof of the third ventricle, it could also secrete melatonin directly into ventricular CSF. The alternative route of melatonin secretion, of course, would be into the circulation via the pineal's rich vascularization. Melatonin has been identified and measured in CSF obtained from calves (54), sheep (55), rhesus monkeys (56), and humans (57–59). Its reported CSF concentrations vary substantially among and within species (for a review, see Reppert et al., 56). In two studies, melatonin concentrations in CSF exceeded those in blood sampled simultaneously: the first involved calves (54); the other, children undergoing treatment for leukemia (58). Other studies have consistently shown blood melatonin levels to be greater than those of the CSF. Melatonin was measured in human daytime CSF samples presumably originating in the lumbar sac and basal cisterns. Since no gradient in melatonin concentration was detected, it was inferred that melatonin is not released directly from the pineal into the third ventricle (57). The most meticulous studies investigating the route of melatonin secretion have been done with sheep (55) and rhesus monkeys (56,89,90). The time courses of the appearance and disappearance of endogenous melatonin were monitored, as was the rate at which radioactively tagged melatonin was transferred from one compartment to the other. High frequency sampling revealed a lag time between increases and decreases in blood melatonin levels and corresponding changes in CSF melatonin levels. It was concluded from these studies that the primary route of secretion from the pineal gland was into the circulatory system. The tendency of circulating melatonin concentrations to be higher than those in the CSF could, of course, be due partly to melatonin's ability to bind to plasma albumin (91).

Control of Melatonin Secretion by Daily Photoperiods

Exhaustive studies by Moore and associates (92,93) have shown that the retinohypothalamic projection that terminates in the suprachiasmatic nuclei mediates visual influences in the entrainment of circadian rhythms. Details about how this neural apparatus, and possible interactions between visual input and other environmental influences, functions to entrain endogenous oscillating mechanisms await resolution. Clearly, the modulation of rhythmic melatonin secretion by environmental illumination is one manifestation of this process.

A recent review (63) summarized the efforts of investigators to document the precise temporal pattern, with respect to the daily photoperiod, of melatonin levels in various mammalian species. The studies included measurements of blood and CSF melatonin in cattle (54), sheep (55), humans (57–59), and rhesus monkeys (56,88,89); blood melatonin levels in sheep (42,94); and blood and urinary melatonin levels in humans (33–35,37,61). The time course of melatonin secretion in hamsters was estimated indirectly, by measuring pineal melatonin content at frequent intervals throughout the 24-hour day (95–99). Similar studies conducted with the laboratory rat measured blood and urinary melatonin levels (100,101) and the activity of melatonin-forming enzymes in the pineal (102,103).

Although the collated data (accumulated over the years by various investigators using different assay methods) revealed substantial inconsistency in the absolute amounts of melatonin estimated, the studies answered the experimental question that had been asked. The various mammalian species studied were found to exhibit characteristic but similar daily rhythms in melatonin concentration, with melatonin peaking during the daily dark period. The rhythms themselves persist when animals are kept in continuous darkness, but, with one interesting exception, are abruptly suppressed by the sudden onset of light in the midst of a normally dark period.

Studies involving human subjects have consistently shown *persistence* of cyclic oscillations in melatonin secretion when one or two darkness-sleep periods have been omitted and subjects have been kept awake in artificial light or when artificial light has been imposed during a normal darkness-sleep period. Both blood melatonin measurements by bioassay (31) or RIA (32,34,35,104) and urinary measurements by RIA (34,35,104) have documented this seeming independence of the human pineal of short-term changes in lighting. Very recently, Lewy and his associates (105) have shown that exposure to sunlight or to artificial light of sufficiently high intensity can suppress nocturnally elevated plasma melatonin levels in human subjects. In contrast to the results of previous experiments in which ordinary room light was used, these findings establish that the human response to light is similar to that of other animals when light is provided of an intensity similar to that which normally characterizes the human's ecological niche.

It should be noted that in this instance it was the experiment (testing the effect of increased light intensity) and not the merits of the assay method that resolved the conundrum. In a recent review (106), Reiter noted that a mistake early investigators made when testing for the endocrine capability of the pineal gland was the placement of the experimental rodents (e.g., hamsters) under long photoperiodic conditions. It has been found that such treatment (12–14 hours of light with no ability to burrow and escape the long days) results in what has been referred to as a physiological pinealectomy (18). Although this condition is relieved in some experimental contexts by the use of shorter daily photoperiods, even 8–10 hours of involuntary exposure to light constitutes an alien environment to a nocturnal, burrowing animal that normally shuns daylight.

It has been shown that hamster pineal melatonin content can be suppressed by as little as 0.186 μW/cm^2 of environmental illumination (107) and that the rat pineal can interpret an ambient light intensity of 0.1–0.3 μW/cm^2 presented for part of a day as either light or darkness depending on the light intensity provided for the rest of the day (108). These observations suggest that we have much more to learn about the "normal" relationship between melatonin secretion and environmental lighting among such animals. We should not hasten to judge the results of melatonin assays on the basis of what we imagine they should be.

At this time, to assign the cause of contradictory results either to assay inaccuracy or to our ignorance of the basic biological phenomena involved would be premature. We need both improved assay methodology and fundamental knowledge; achievement of the former will, no doubt, contribute to the latter.

QUALITY CONTROL IN MELATONIN ASSAY METHODOLOGY

The performance characteristics of melatonin assay methods fall into two categories: those that relate to reliability (specificity, precision, sensitivity, accuracy) and those that relate to practicability (speed, cost, technical skill requirements). In selecting a method for the pursuit of a particular research interest, neither category can be ignored and, inevitably, compromises must be made. Practicability is the concern of the individual laboratory. Reliability is the concern of those who publish research findings and those who seek understanding on the basis of published results.

One of the best means of maintaining and improving the reliability of melatonin measurements is the establishment of a system of quality control. The term quality with respect to melatonin assay methodology implies that:

☐ The method measures nothing but melatonin (specificity)

☐ The method permits the detection of physiologically significant changes in melatonin levels (sensitivity)

☐ The same result will be obtained if the same sample is analyzed repeatedly in a single assay run or in different runs (precision)

☐ The result corresponds to the "true" concentration of melatonin in the sample (accuracy)

Well-known procedures are available for the assessment of each of these quality control parameters. It should be remembered that sensitivity and precision have no numerical value and refer to a set of results obtained under stated conditions, not to single results, and that although with a given assay sensitivity and precision may be very good, measurements may be very wrong. It is also important to remember that specificity (assessed by testing individually potential interfering substances and demonstrating parallelism between the melatonin calibration curve and graded concentrations of sample) is a significant part of accuracy and that accuracy is a theoretical ideal.

Quality control programs have been developed specifically for RIA methods. Some of these have been tailored to aid in the optimization of variables in the assay procedure (109). Regardless of the assay method used, a quality control system makes it possible to evaluate the stability and reproducibility of the assay system and facilitates combining results from different assays (e.g., by pooling estimates of within-assay error). The quality control system also provides information indispensable to proper experimental design.

No doubt accuracy is the most important and elusive requirement of an assay method. A first approximation of accuracy is obtained with recovery data. In recovery experiments, assays are made on a pair of samples of a specimen, a known amount of melatonin having been added to one of the two samples. The difference between results within the pair is the amount recovered; the deviation of this value from the amount added is a measure of the accuracy or, more properly, the inaccuracy of the assay, but only in the range covered and for the sample used. The accuracy of melatonin assays can only be properly assessed with biological specimens for which the method is to be used; and, since the true value of these is not known, estimates must be made by a comparison method that ideally should give true values. Such a method is termed a definitive or absolute method (110), one that, after exhaustive investigation, is found to have no known source of inaccuracy or ambiguity. An obvious candidate for such an assay would be the isotope dilution-mass spectrometry method for determining melatonin. Once a definitive method is thoroughly tested and established, reference materials (e.g., serum and urine samples containing known concentrations of endogenous melatonin) can be made available for the maintenance of quality control in routine methods (e.g., RIA, HPLC).

The development of a definitive assay method usually involves complex, costly, and highly sophisticated instrumentation manned by highly skilled and trained scientific specialists. These considerations put the establishment of such a method for melatonin measurement beyond the means of most individual laboratories. The responsibility for such developments should properly be borne by agencies such as professional societies or instrument and diagnostic material manufacturers. With the increasingly apparent clinical significance of melatonin measurements (105,111,112), this may come to pass. In the meantime, volunteer quality control programs, including publication of pertinent quality control data together with experimental results, and interlaboratory collaborative studies, such as those conducted by Wetterberg and associates (48,49), are needed.

REFERENCES

1. McCord C P, Allen F P. Evidences associating pineal gland function with alterations in pigmentation. J Exp Zool 23:207–224, 1917.

2. Lerner A B, Case J D, Heinzelman R V. Structure of melatonin. J Am Chem Soc 81:6084–6087, 1959.

3. Lerner A B, Wright R M. In vitro frog skin assay for agents that darken and lighten melanocytes. Methods Biochem Anal 8:294–307, 1960.

4. Giarman N J, Day M. Presence of biogenic amines in the bovine pineal body. Biochem Pharmacol 1:235, 1959.

5. Axelrod J, Weissbach H. Purification and properties of hydroxyindole-O-methyl transferase. J Biol Chem 236:211–213, 1961.

6. Wurtman R J, Axelrod J, Phillips L S. Melatonin synthesis in the pineal gland: control by light. Science 142:1071–1073, 1963.

7. Axelrod J, Wurtman R J, Snyder S H. Control of hydroxyindole-O-methyl-transferase activity in the rat pineal by environmental light. J Biol Chem 240:949–954, 1965.

8. Wurtman R J, Axelrod J, Fisher J E. Melatonin synthesis in the pineal gland: effect of light mediated by the sympathetic nervous system. Science 143:1328–1330, 1964.

9. Moore R Y, Heller A, Bhatnagar R R. Central control of the pineal gland: visual pathways. Arch Neurol 18:208–218, 1968.

10. Fiske V M, Bryant G K, Putnam J. Effect of light on the weight of the pineal in the rat. Endocrinology 66:489–491, 1960.

11. Meyer C J, Wurtman R J, Altschule M D, Lazo-Wasem E A. The arrest of prolonged estrus in "middle-aged" rats by pineal gland extract. Endocrinology 68:795–800, 1961.

12. Wurtman R J, Axelrod J, Chu E W. Melatonin, a pineal substance: effect on rat ovary. Science 141:277–278, 1963.

13. Quay W B. Differential extraction for the spectrophotofluorometric measurement of diverse 5-hydroxy-and 5-methdoxyindoles. Anal Biochem 5:51–59, 1963.

14. Quay W B. Circadian and estrus rhythms in pineal melatonin and 5-hydroxyindole-3-acetic acid. Proc Soc Exp Biol Med 115:710–713, 1964.

15. Wurtman R J, Axelrod J. The pineal gland. Sci Am 213:50–60, 1965.

16. Shein H M, Wurtman R J. Cyclic adenosine monophosphate stimulation of melatonin and serotonin synthesis in cultured rat pineals. Science 166:519–520, 1969.

17. Klein D C, Berg G R. Pineal gland: stimulation of melatonin production by norepinephrine involves cyclic AMP-mediated stimulation of n-acetyl-transferase. Adv Biochem Psychopharmacol 3:241–263, 1970.

18. Reiter R J. Pineal regulation of hypothalamicopituitary axis: gonadotrophins. In Handbook of Physiology, vol 4 (part II), ed E Knobil, W H Sawyer. American Physiological Society, Washington, D.C., 1975, pp. 519–526.

19. Tamarkin L, Westrom W K, Hamill A I, Goldman B D. Effect of melatonin on the reproductive system of male and female Syrian hamsters: a diurnal rhythm in sensitivity to melatonin. Endocrinology 99:1534–1541, 1976.

20. Wolstenholme G E W, Knight J. The Pineal Gland, (a Ciba Foundation Symposium), Churchill, Livingstone, Edinburgh & London, 1971.

21. Maickel R P, Miller F P. The fluorometric determination of indolealkylamines in brain and pineal gland. Adv Pharmacol 6:71–77, 1968.

22. Tomatis M E, Orias R. Changes in melatonin concentration in pineal gland in rats exposed to continuous light or darkness. Acta Physiol Lat Am 17:227–233, 1967.

23. Ralph C L, Hedlund L, Murphy W A. Diurnal cycles of melatonin in bird pineal bodies. Comp Biochem Physiol 22:591–599, 1967.

24. Ralph C L, Lynch H J. A quantitative melatonin bioassay. Gen Comp Endocrinol 15:334–338, 1970.

25. Arendt J, Paunier L, Sizonenko P C. Melatonin radioimmunoassay. J Clin Endocrinol Metab 40:347–350, 1975.

26. Shizume K, Lerner A B, Fitzpatrick T B. *In vitro* bioassay for melanocyte stimulating hormones. Endocrinology 54:553–559, 1954.

27. Hogbin L, Slome D. The pigmentary effector system. VI. The dual character of endocrine coordination in amphibian colour change. Proc Roy Soc (London), Ser B B108:10–53, 1931.

28. Waring H. Color Change Mechanisms of Cold-Blooded Vertebrates. Academic Press, New York and London, 1963.

29. Quay W B, Bagnara J. Relative potencies of indolic and related compounds in the body-lightening reaction of larval Xenopus. Arch Int Pharmacodyn Ther 150:137–143, 1964.

30. Quay W B. Specificity and structure-activity relationships in the Xenopus larval melanophore assay for melatonin. Gen Comp Endocrinol 11:253–254, 1968.

31. Pelham R W, Vaughan G M, Sandock K L, Vaughan M K. Twenty-four-hour cycle of a melatonin-like substance in the plasma of human males. J Clin Endocrinol Metab 37:341–344, 1973.

32. Vaughan G M, Pelham R W, Pang S F, Loughlin L L, Wilson K M, Sandock K L, Vaughan M K, Koslow S H, Reiter R J. Noctural elevations of plasma melatonin and urinary 5-hydroxyindoleacetic acid in young men: attempts at modification by brief changes in environmental lighting and sleep and by autonomic drugs. J Clin Endocrinol Metab 42:752–764, 1976.

33. Lynch H J, Wurtman R J, Moskowitz M A, Archer M C, Ho M H. Daily rhythm in human urinary melatonin. Science 17:169–171, 1975.

34. Jimerson D C, Lynch H J, Post R M, Wurtman R H, Bunney W E. Urinary melatonin rhythms during sleep deprivation in depressed patients and normals. Life Sci 23:1501–1508, 1977.

35. Lynch H J, Jimerson D C, Ozaki Y, Post R M, Bunney W E, Wurtman R J. Entrainment of rhythmic melatonin secretion in man to a 12-hour phase shift in the light/dark cycle. Life Sci 23:1557–1564, 1978.

36. Lynch H J, Ozaki Y, Shakal D, Wurtman R J. Melatonin excretion of man and rats: effect of time of day, sleep, pinealectomy, and food consumption. Int J Biometeorol 19:267–279, 1975.

37. Udenfriend S, Bogdanski D F, Weissbach H. Fluorescence characteristics of 5-hydroxytryptamine (serotonin). Science 122:972–974, 1955.

38. Miller F P, Maickel R P. Fluorometric determination of indole derivatives. Life Sci 9:747–752, 1970.

39. Ozaki Y, Lynch H J, Wurtman R J. Melatonin in rat pineal, plasma, and urine: 24-hour rhythmicity and effect of chlorpromazine. Endocrinology 98:1418–1424, 1976.

40. Yalow R S, Berson S A. Immunoassay of endogenous plasma insulin in man. J Clin Invest 39:1157–1175, 1960.

41. Arendt J. Melatonin assays in body fluids. J Neural Transm Suppl 13:265–278, 1978.

42. Rollag M D, Niswender G D. Radioimmunoassay of serum concentrations of melatonin in sheep exposed to different lighting regimens. Endocrinology 98:482–489, 1976.

43. Grota L J, Brown G M. Antibodies to indolealkylamines: serotonin and melatonin. Can J Biochem 52:196–202, 1974.

44. Levine L, Riceberg L J. Radioimmunoassay for melatonin. Res Commun Pathol Pharmacol 10:693–702, 1975.

45. Pang S F, Brown G M, Grota L J, Rodman R L. Radioimmunoassay of melatonin in pineal glands, Harderian glands, retinas, and sera of rats or chickens. Fed Proc FASEB 35:691, 1976.

46. Wurtzberger R J, Kawashima K, Miller R L, Spector S. Determination of rat pineal gland melatonin content by radioimmunoassay. Life Sci 18:867–878, 1976.

47. Kennaway D J, Firth R G, Phillipou G, Matthews C D, Seamark R F. A specific radioimmunoassay for melatonin in biological tissue and fluids and its validation by gas chromatography-mass spectrometry. Endocrinology 101:119–127, 1977.

48. Wetterberg L. Melatonin in serum. Nature 269:646, 1977.

49. Wetterberg L, Eriksson O. Melatonin in human serum—a collaborative study of current radioimmunoassays. Advances in the Biosciences 29:15–20, 1981.

50. Lynch H J, Ozaki Y, Wurtman R J. The measurement of melatonin in mammalian tissues and body fluids. J Neural Transm Suppl 13:251–264, 1978.

51. Nir I, Reiter R J, Wurtman R J, ed. The Pineal Gland. (J Neural Transm, Suppl 13), Springer-Verlag, New York, 1978.

52. Birau N, Schloot W, ed. Melatonin: Current Status and Perspectives, (Advances in the Biosciences, 29), Pergamon Press, New York, 1981.

53. Pévet P, Tapp E, ed. Second Colloquium of the European Pineal Study Group. (EPSG Newsletter, Suppl 3), Giessen, West Germany, 1981.

54. Hedlund L, Lischko M M, Rollag M D, Niswender G D. Melatonin: daily cycle in plasma and cerebrospinal fluid of calves. Science 195:686–687, 1977.

55. Rollag M D, Morgan R J, Niswender G D. Route of melatonin secretion in sheep. Endocrinology 102:1–8, 1978.

56. Reppert S M, Perlow M J, Klein D C. Cerebrospinal fluid melatonin. In Neurobiology of Cerebrospinal Fluid, ed J H Wood. Plenum Press, New York, 1980, pp 579–589.

57. Brown G M, Young S N, Gauthier S, Tsui H, Grota L J. Melatonin in human cerebrospinal fluid in daytime: its origin and variation with age. Life Sci 25:929–936, 1979.

58. Smith J A, Mee T J X, Barns N D, Thronburn R J, Barnes J L C. Melatonin in serum and cerebrospinal fluid. Lancet 2:425, 1976.

59. Arendt J, Wetterberg L, Heyden T, Sizonenko P C, Paunier L. Radioimmunoassay of melatonin: human serum and cerebrospinal fluid. Horm Res 8:65–75, 1977.

60. Wetterberg L, Arendt J, Paunier L, Sizonenko P C, van Donselaar W, Heyden T. Human serum melatonin changes during the menstrual cycle. J Clin Endocrinol Metab 42:185–188, 1976.

61. Weitzman E D, Weinberg U, D'eletto R, Lynch H J, Wurtman R J, Czeisler C, Erlich S. Studies of the 24-hour rhythm of melatonin in man. J Neural Transm Suppl 13:325–337, 1978.

62. Weinberg U, D'eletto R D, Weitzman E D, Erlich S, Hollander C. Circulating melatonin in man: episodic secretion throughout the light-dark cycle. J Clin Endocrinol Metab 48:114–118, 1979.

63. Lynch H J, Wurtman R J. Melatonin levels as they relate to reproductive physiology. In The Pineal Gland: Reproductive Effects, vol 2, ed R J Reiter. CRC Press, Boca Raton, Fla, 1981, pp 103–123.

64. Ozaki Y, Lynch H J. Presence of melatonin in plasma and urine of pinealectomized rats. Endocrinology 99:641–644, 1976.

65. Goldman M E, Hamm H, Erickson C K. Determination of melatonin by high-performance liquid chromatography with electrochemical detection. J Chromatogr 190:217–220, 1980.

66. Anderson G M, Young J G, Batter D K, Young S N, Cohen D J, Shaywitz B A. Determination of indoles and catechols in rat brain and pineal using liquid chromatography with fluorometric and amperometric detection. J Chromatogr 223:315–320, 1981.

67. Roth J J, Gern W A, Roth E C, Ralph C L, Jacobson E. Nonpineal melatonin in the alligator (Alligator mississippiensis). Science 210:548–550, 1980.

68. Mefford I N, Barchas J D. Determination of tryptophane and metabolites in rat brain and pineal tissue by reversed-phase high performance liquid chromatography with electrochemical detection. J Chromatogr 181:187–193, 1980.

69. Degen P H, Barchas J D. Gas chromatographic assay for melatonin. Proc West Pharmacol Soc 13:34–35, 1970.

70. Greiner A C, Chan S C. Melatonin content of the human pineal gland. Science 199:83–84, 1978.

71. Koslow S H, Green A R. Analysis of pineal and brain indole alkylamines by gas chromatography mass-spectrometry. Adv Biochem Psychopharmacol 7:33–43, 1973.

72. Wilson B W, Snedden W, Silman R E, Smith I, Mullen P. A gas chromatography-mass spectrometry method for the quantitative analysis of melatonin in plasma and cerebrospinal fluid. Anal Biochem 81:283–291, 1977.

73. Wilson B W, Lynch H J, Ozaki Y. 5-methoxytryptophol in rat serum and pineal: detection, quantitation and evidence for daily rhythmicity. Life Sci 23:1019–1024, 1978.

74. Lewy A J, Markey S P. Analysis of melatonin in human plasma by gas chromatography: negative chemical ionization mass-spectrometry. Science 201:741–743, 1978.

75. Lewy A J, Tetsuo M, Markey S P, Goodwin J K, Kopin I J. Pinealectomy abolishes plasma melatonin in the rat. J Clin Endocrinol Metab 50:204–205, 1980.

76. Barchas J D, Lerner A B. Localization of melatonin in the nervous system. J Neurochem 11:489–491, 1964.

77. Lynch H J. Diurnal oscillations in pineal melatonin content. Life Sci 10:719–795, 1975.

78. Ralph C L, Mull D, Lynch H J, Hedlund L. A melatonin rhythm persists in rat pineals in darkness. Endocrinology 89:1361–1366, 1971.

79. Reiter R J, Sorrentino S Jr., Ralph C L, Lynch H J, Mull D, Jarrow E. Some endocrine effects of blinding and anosmia in adult male rats with observations on pineal melatonin. Endocrinology 88:895–900, 1971.

80. Weissbach H, Redfield B G, Axelrod J. Biosynthesis of melatonin: enzymatic conversion of serotonin to N-acetylserotonin. Biochem Biophys Acta 43:352–353, 1960.

81. Cardinali D P, Rosner J M. Serotonin metabolism by the rat retina in vitro. J Neurochem 18:1769–1770, 1971.

82. Vlahakes G, Wurtman R J. A Mg_2^+-dependent hydroxyindole-O-methyltransferase in rat Harderian gland. Biochim Biophys Acta 261:194–197, 1972.

83. Rosengarten H, Meller E, Friedhoff A J. In vitro enzymatic formation of melatonin by human erythrocytes. Res Commun Chem Pathol Pharmacol 4:457–465, 1972.

84. Bubenik G A, Brown G M, Grota L J. Immunohistochemical localization of melatonin in the rat digestive system. Experientia 33:262–263, 1977.

85. Yu H S, Pang S F, Tang P L, Brown G M. Persistence of circadian rhythms of melatonin and N-acetylserotonin in the serum of rats after pinealectomy. Neuroendocrinology 32:262–265, 1981.

86. Meyer A C, Wassermann W, Meyer B J, Joubert W S, Roux S, Biagio R. Melatonin rhythm in the chacma baboon (Pupio ursinus) and the effect of pinealectomy and superior cervical ganglionectomy on the rhythm. S Afr J Sci 77:39–41, 1981.

87. Pang S F, Ralph C L. Pineal and serum melatonin at midday and midnight following pinealectomy or castration in male rats. J Exp Zool 193:275–280, 1975.

88. Ralph C L. Melatonin production by extra-pineal tissues. Advances in the Biosciences 29:35–46, 1981.

89. Reppert S M, Perlow M J, Tamarkin L, Klein D C. A diurnal melatonin rhythm in primate cerebrospinal fluid. Endocrinology 104:295–301, 1979.

90. Perlow M J, Reppert S M, Tamarkin L, Wyatt R J, Klein D C. Photic regulation of the melatonin rhythm: monkey and man are not the same. Brain Res 182:211–216, 1980.

91. Cardinali D P, Lynch H J, Wurtman R J. Binding of melatonin to human and rat plasma proteins. Endocrinology 91:1213–1218, 1972.

92. Moore R Y, Eichler V B. Loss of circadian adrenal corticosterone rhythm following suprachiasmatic lesions in the rat. Brain Res 42:201–206, 1972.

93. Moore R Y, Klein D C. Visual pathways and the central neural control of a circadian rhythm in pineal serotonin N-acetyltransferase activity. Brain Res 71:17–33, 1974.

94. Rollag M D, O'Gallaghan P L, Niswender G D. Serum melatonin concentrations during different stages of the reproductive cycle in ewes. Biol Reprod 18:279–285, 1978.

95. Panke E S, Reiter R J, Rollag M D, Panke T W. Pineal serotonin-N-acetyltransferase activity and melatonin concentrations in prepubertal and adult Syrian hamsters exposed to short daily photo-periods. Endocrinol Res Commun 5:311–324, 1978.

96. Panke E S, Rollag M D, Reiter R J. Pineal melatonin concentrations in the Syrian hamster. Endocrinology 104:195–197, 1979.

97. Tamarkin L, Reppert S M, Klein D C. Regulation of pineal melatonin in the Syrian hamster. Endocrinology 104:385–389, 1979.

98. Rollag M D, Panke E S, Trakulrungsi W, Trakulrungsi S, Reiter R J. Quantification of daily melatonin synthesis in the hamster pineal gland. Endocrinology 106:231–236, 1980.

99. Tamarkin L, Brown S, Goldman B. Neuroendocrine regulation of seasonal reproductive cycles in the hamster. (Abstract) 5th Annual Meeting of the Society of Neuroscience, p 458, 1975.

100. Adler J, Lynch H J, Wurtman R J. Effect of cyclic changes in environmental lighting and ambient temperature on the daily rhythm in melatonin excretion by rats. Brain Res 163:110–120, 1979.

101. Lynch H J, Wurtman R J. Control of rhythms in the secretion of pineal hormones in humans and experimental animals. In Biological Rhythms and Their Central Mechanism (A Naito Foundation Symposium), ed M Suda, O Hayaishi, H Nakagawa. Elsevier North-Holland Biomedical Press, Amsterdam, 1979, pp 117–131.

102. Illnerova H, Vanacek J, Krecek J, Wetterberg L, Saaf J. Effect of one minute exposure to light at night on rat pineal serotonin-N-acetyltransferase and melatonin. J Neurochem 32:673–675, 1978.

103. Wilkinson M, Arendt J, Brodtke J, de Ziegler D. Determination of a dark-induced increase of pineal N-acetyltransferase activity and simultaneous radioimmunoassay of melatonin in pineal, serum, and pituitary tissue of the male rat. J Endocrinol 72:243–244, 1977.

104. Akerstedt T, Froberg J E, Friberg Y, Wetterberg L. Melatonin excretion, body temperature and subjective arousal during 64 hours of sleep deprivation. Psychoneuroendocrinology 4:219–225, 1979.

105. Lewy A J, Wehr T A, Goodwin F K, Newsome D A, Markey S P. Light suppresses melatonin secretion in humans. Science 210:1267–1269, 1980.

106. Reiter R J. The pineal and its hormones in the control of reproduction in mammals. Endocrine Rev 1:109–131, 1980.

107. Brainard G C, Richardson B A, Petterborg L J, Reiter R J. The effect of different light intensities on pineal melatonin content. Brain Res 233:75–81, 1982.

108. Lynch H J, Rivest R W, Ronsheim P M, Wurtman R J. Light intensity and the control of melatonin secretion in rats. Neuroendocrinology 33:181–185, 1981.

109. Rodbard D. Statistical quality control and routine data processing for radioimmunoassays and immunoradiometric assays. Clin Chem 20:1255–1270, 1974.

110. Bjorkhem I, Blomstrand R, Lantto O, Svensson L, Ohman G. Toward absolute methods in clinical chemistry: application of mass fragmentography to high-accuracy analyses. Clin Chem 22:1789–1801, 1978.

111. Wetterberg L. Melatonin in humans: physiological and clinical studies. J Neural Transm Suppl 13:289–310, 1978.

112. Birau N. Melatonin in human serum: progress in screening investigation and clinic. Advances in the Biosciences 29:297–326, 1981.

RUSSEL J. REITER, Ph.D.
BRUCE A. RICHARDSON, Ph.D.
THOMAS S. KING, Ph.D.

THE PINEAL GLAND AND ITS INDOLE PRODUCTS: THEIR IMPORTANCE IN THE CONTROL OF REPRODUCTION IN MAMMALS

The pineal gland is an azygous, midline structure that has captured the attention of philosophers and soothsayers for centuries. This, coupled with the early contradictory reports concerning its actions, severely stymied pineal research well into the twentieth century. Indeed, until recently there almost seemed to be a stigma associated with individuals who worked on this sometimes exasperating organ.

One of the most obvious features that characterize the pineal gland is its marked diversity, both morphological and physiological. The descriptions of the anatomy of the gland in vertebrates are numerous, with many reports describing substantial differences in the structure of the gland of even closely related species (1,2). Likewise, the actions of the pineal gland seem to differ even among mammals. Thus, although the interactions of the pineal gland with the neuroendocrine-reproductive axis are rather well defined in some species, in others the pineal may have little or no influence on reproduction (3). Because of this, however,

From the Department of Anatomy, The University of Texas, Health Science Center at San Antonio, 7703 Floyd Curl Drive, San Antonio, Texas 78284.

Work by the authors was supported by grants from the National Science Foundation. BAR is an NIH postdoctoral fellow 1F32 HD 05900. TSK is a postdoctoral fellow in the Center for Training in Reproductive Biology HD 07139.

it should not be concluded that the pineal is an inconsequential organ in these animals; rather, it is likely involved in other functions such as temperature regulation (4), behavioral adjustments (5), or general metabolic activity (6), to name only a few.

It appears that the function of the pineal gland is more varied than originally envisaged. To date, many of the studies on the gland have been concerned with its interactions with the neuroendocrine-reproductive axis. Although the results of these studies were highly informative, it rapidly became apparent that the manner in which the pineal gland influences the reproductive system varies among different animals. Thus what applies to one species may not be applicable to another, even though they may be closely related. This is an important point to remember when investigating pineal-reproductive relationships; the design of the experiment should be determined by the environmental circumstances to which the particular species is normally exposed and assumptions as to the possible interactions based on data from different species should be made with caution. Likewise, if results are obtained that appear contradictory to those reported by others, the answer may lie in the experimental design rather than represent bogus results.

It appears that the pineal monitors the photoperiod and sends a hormonal message, melatonin and possibly other indoles and polypeptides, to other organ systems. How the organism uses this information is possibly determined by the sensitivity of the particular target tissue to the hormone. Thus the actions of the pineal gland may depend more on organ responsiveness than on the fluctuation in the signal provided by the pineal. The pattern of melatonin secretion (high at night and low during the day) seems to be relatively uniform in all species in which it has been examined, yet there is a wide variety of responses that the organism may exhibit.

The following survey is concerned with the reproductive effects of the pineal gland and its indole products in mammals. For its influence on other organ systems, the reader should consult other sources as well as the chapters by Relkin in this book.

PHOTOPERIOD, PINEAL, AND REPRODUCTION

Historically, the function of the pineal gland has most frequently been linked to reproduction; however, the early evidence was not particularly compelling (7,8). Not until it was found that the daily light:dark cycle is critical in determining the inhibitory effects of the pineal gland on reproduction were pineal-reproductive interactions reliably demonstrated. Several rodent species have been particularly useful in illustrating the consequences of the darkness-activated pineal gland on the neuroendocrine-reproductive axis. A partial list of these include the Syrian hamster (*Mesocricetus auratus*) (9), the Djungarian hamster (*Phodopus sungorus*) (10), the white-footed mouse (*Peromycus leucopus*) (11,12), and the field vole (*Microtus agretis*) (13). Whereas the reproductive system of the rat is not particularly sensitive to inhibition by the pineal gland, there are certain perturbations that indirectly sensitize the system to the secretory products of the pineal gland (14).

Gonadal and Accessory Sex Organ Changes

In the mid-1960s it was found that increasing the percentage of darkness per 24-hour period to which Syrian hamsters are exposed caused gonadal atrophy in both males (15–18) and females (19,20). On the contrary, if the animals are either pinealectomized (15,16,19) or superior cervical ganglionectomized (20), their exposure to short days, or even total light deprivation, is not followed by gonadal involution (Figure 1). Regardless of the photoperiodic conditions, pinealectomized males are still capable of sperm production and insemination (21–23) and pineal-deprived females (24,25) continue to ovulate, exhibit normal vaginal cyclicity, become pregnant, and carry their young to term. The critical photoperiodic length in Syrian hamsters has been established at 12.5 hours of light daily; daylengths shorter than this promote an anatomical and functional collapse of the reproductive organs whereas daylengths in excess of 12.5 hours ensure a hightly functional neuroendocrine-reproductive axis (26). The critical daylength is probably different for every species.

An interesting and important sidelight at this juncture relates to the common usage of long daily photoperiods in small animal quarters. For years, most animal caretakers have routinely utilized light:dark schedules of 12–16 hours of light daily; these schedules were invariably se-

FIGURE 1. Testicular **(TES)** and accessory sex organ **(ASO)** weights (combined weights of the seminal vesicles and coagulating glands) in adult hamsters kept under either long or short daily photoperiods. **INT** = intact; **PINX** = pinealectomized; **SCGX** = superior cervical gangionectomized.

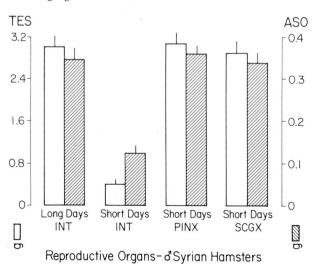

lected to suit the convenience of the caretakers rather than for the animals. The conventional use of long days severely retarded physiological research on the pineal gland. Under long-day conditions hamsters are, in essence, "pinealectomized" by the long daily periods of light; these animals are referred to as being either physiologically or functionally pinealectomized. Surgical removal of the pineal gland from such animals naturally has little or no effect on the sexual organs (9). However, this is not justification for concluding that the pineal gland is inconsequential in terms of reproductive physiology. Indeed, if the pineal gland is challenged by exposure of photoperiodic species to short days, the effects of surgical pinealectomy are readily apparent. It is frequently overlooked by both animal caretakers and researchers alike that animals in their natural habitat are exposed to marked seasonal variations in daylength; some of these are shorter than 12 hours (e.g., during the winter months) whereas others are longer (e.g., during the summer months).

As will be seen in a subsequent section of this report, seasonal fluctuations in daylengths are essential in determining the antigonadotrophic activity of the pineal gland (27). This brings up a second feature of most small animal quarters that has served to hamper physiological research on the pineal gland. There is a severe bias against having windows in rooms where small laboratory animals are maintained; thus, the animals are rarely if ever exposed to anything reminiscent of natural seasonal changes in daylength. When hamsters, for example, are kept in an environment where they experience the naturally occurring fluctuations in the photoperiod length, the status of the reproductive organs change accordingly (28).

Although in both male and female Syrian hamsters the gonads (the testes and ovaries, respectively) undergo a marked reduction in function in response to shortened days, the ovaries of light-deprived animals may actually increase in size (29). This is a consequence of the proliferation of the interstitial tissue in the ovaries; characteristically, they are devoid of corpora lutea, rare antral and preantral follicles are found, and the interstitial cells predominate (30). Thus, although grossly enlarged, on microscopic examination, the ovaries are clearly functionally depressed in terms of the processes related to ovulation. All the changes described are obviated if the animals are pinealectomized in advance of their exposure to short days (30).

In light-restricted hamsters, the accessory sex organs undergo changes similar to those experienced by the gonads. When the coagulating gland and seminal vesicle weights are recorded in males, the atrophy of these organs virtually parallels the drop in the weight of the testes (22). Indeed, the condition of the accessory sex glands in males can quite accurately be predicted from the status of the testes. Microscopically, the epithelium lining these organs is of the cuboidal variety; this is in contrast to the columnar cells lining the accessory sex organs in pinealectomized animals (31). When female hamsters are exposed to short-day conditions, the uteri undergo marked involutional changes and become infantile in appearance within a matter of weeks (29). At the light microscopic level, the uteri are seen to have thin muscular layers, atrophic endometrium, and few endometrial glands.

The specific length of short-day exposure required to force gonadal regression in hamsters is currently an issue of some interest to those investigators who use the hamster as the experimental animal in which to investigate the interactions of the photoperiod and the pineal gland with the reproductive system. In a report that appeared in 1964 it was shown that total testicular collapse was already evident in hamsters kept under short-day conditions for only 4 weeks (16). In subsequent studies the required duration of short-day exposure is becoming progressively longer. For example, in the late 1960s the treatment period had to be extended to 7–8 weeks in order to achieve the same degree of gonadal atrophy seen after 4 weeks just several years earlier (22). More recently, this time period has, on occasion, become even more prolonged. Reiter (3) has suggested several possible explanations for this apparent change in sensitivity of the pituitary-gonadal axis to the inhibitory influence of the pineal gland. The tentative explanations that were considered include the improved nutritional state of the animals and the perpetual inbreeding of hamsters by commercial breeders who undoubtedly select the most prolific animals as their breeding stock. It is unfortunate that the species that has provided such a wealth of information on pineal-gonadal interactions seems to be losing its propensity to respond to short daylengths.

As mentioned in a previous section of this report, the reproductive system of several other mammals also has been found to be highly sensitive to manipulation by the photoperiod. Without exception, in the species in which the daily light:dark cycle determines the reproductive state of the animal, the pineal gland is known to act as an intermediary between the prevailing photoperiod and the gonads. Hence, in the absence of the pineal gland these animals are incapable of exhibiting their normal reproductive responses to changing daylengths (11,32–36). Not all animals, however, are equally sensitive to photoperiodic manipulation of their reproductive system (37–39).

The laboratory rat is a rather poor animal of choice if pineal-reproductive relationships are to be investigated. For example, total (by bilateral orbital enucleation) or near total light deprivation has a relatively minor influence on the sexual capabilities of the species (37,40). Yet the rat has been frequently used to study the role of the pineal in controlling reproductive physiology. More often than not, these investigations yielded either equivocal or not particularly compelling data (7,41,42). Indeed, on the basis of such findings some workers prematurely concluded that the pineal is of no functional importance in terms of the mammalian reproductive system (43).

Experimental manipulations have been discovered that render the neuroendocrine-reproductive axis of the rat highly sensitive to inhibition by the pineal gland. These procedures, generally referred to as potentiating factors, include surgically induced anosmia, early neonatal steroid treatment, and reduced food intake (14,44). The mechanisms by which these perturbations increase the antigonadotrophic potential of the pineal gland remain enigmatic. When employed in conjunction with light deprivation, they cause pronounced atrophy of the reproductive organs of rats; these responses are prevented by pinealectomy. The potentiating factors have been useful in elucidating the mechanisms whereby the pineal gland and its secretory products alter sexual capability (45–47).

Hormonal Changes

When sensitive assays became available for measuring gonadotrophins, it was surmised that these hormones would be markedly depressed in hamsters with pineal-induced gonadal atrophy. Figure 2 summarizes the observed changes in plasma luteinizing hormone (LH) and follicle stimulating hormone (FSH) in male Syrian hamsters after the various types of treatment indicated. Hence, short-day exposure is often associated with a measurable drop in circulating levels of both LH (28,48–50) and FSH (48,49,51). Despite repeated reports documenting this change, there is the occasional publication that claims normal levels of gonadotrophins in the presence of severely depressed testicular weights (52). This unexpected finding led some authors to suspect that another hormone, in addition to LH and FSH, may be involved in the maintenance

FIGURE 2. Plasma luteinizing hormone **(LH)**, follicle stimulating hormone **(FSH)**, prolactin **(PRL)**, and testosterone **(TES)** levels in adult male hamsters kept under either long or short daily photoperiods. **INT** = intact; **PINX** = pinealectomized; **SCGX** = superior cervical ganglionectomized.

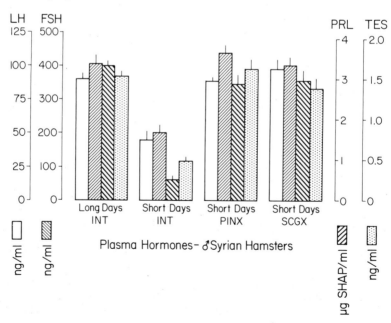

of normal gonadal size and function in the male hamster; it appears this hormone may be prolactin (PRL) (see below). Certainly, when male hamsters with atrophic gonads due to dark exposure are treated with twice daily injections of luteinizing hormone releasing hormone (LHRH), which in the hamster causes the discharge of both LH and FSH from the anterior pituitary, neither the growth of the testes nor of the accessory sex organs is stimulated (53). The changes in pituitary levels of LH seem somewhat more consistent than the alterations in circulating titers of the gonadotrophin; for example, pituitary levels of LH drop by 20–30% in male hamsters kept in less than 12.5 hours of light daily (52). The hormonal changes that occur as a result of light restriction are negated by removal of the pineal gland or by its sympathetic denervation (Figure 2).

The situation in female Syrian hamsters is somewhat different. Recall that, although the ovaries functionally regress in dark-exposed females, the organs actually become enlarged due to the proliferation of the interstitial cells. Since the integrity of the ovarian interstitial tissue depends on ample levels of circulating LH (54), it was predicted very early that light-restricted females would have at least normal levels of LH in their blood (55). This supposition was subsequently confirmed; rather than being depressed, female Syrian hamsters with pineal-induced gonadal atrophy experience a daily afternoon surge of LH and FSH (51,56). This is in contrast to the normally cycling female where hormonal surges occur only once every fourth afternoon. The daily rises are not associated with shedding of ova from the ovaries, and estrogen levels remain depressed judging from the infantile nature of the uterus. Pituitary reserves of LH are also increased (30). Again, pineal removal obviates the hormonal alterations induced by photoperiods of less than 12.5 hours of light daily.

Despite the very different patterns of gonadotrophin production and release in male and female Syrian hamsters maintained in restricted photoperiods, the end result of the exposure is regression of the sexual organs. In both cases, the changes are reversed either by surgical removal of the pineal or by destroying the sympathetic innervation to the gland (20). The mechanisms whereby the pineal intervenes in the control of the neuroendocrine-reproductive axis remain to be uncovered.

In a preceeding paragraph, PRL was alluded to as a potentially important hormone in the maintenance of testicular function in Syrian hamsters. The early studies revealed that pituitary and plasma levels of this constituent were often far below normal in hamsters kept under short-day conditions (3,52) (Figure 2). Following these observations, workers soon began testing PRL for its gonad-stimulating activity. Bartke and coworkers (57,58) found that the injection of PRL into male hamsters that exhibited pineal-induced atrophic reproductive organs promoted testicular growth as well as increased testosterone levels in the blood. Bex et al. (59) feel that the PRL-stimulating effects are possibly related to PRL's ability to maintain the LH receptors in the testes. Pituitary homografts at a site distant from the hypothalamus, i.e., under the kidney capsule, release copious amounts of PRL and also stimulate, although they do not fully maintain, the testes (60,61).

In the final analysis, it seems that all three hormones, i.e., LH, FSH, and PRL, are required to maintain normal testicular function in the Syrian hamster. This is certainly supported by a recent study of Chen and Reiter (62). Blinded male hamsters were given either twice daily injections of LHRH, received two pituitary homografts under their kidney capsule, or they were given both the peptide injections and received the implants. Neither LHRH (which releases both LH and FSH from the pituitary gland) nor the grafts (which secrete PRL) by themselves promoted testicular growth; however, when the treatments were combined, testicular function was completely restored. Hence, pineal-mediated testicular regression in this species is most likely a complex process that involves the suppression of not only LH and FSH but PRL as well.

PINEAL AND SEASONAL REPRODUCTION

The significance of the response of the reproductive system to daylength is realized in seasonal reproduction. Virtually all species that inhabit the temperate and polar regions of the earth reproduce during very specific times of the year. In photoperiodic species, of which there are many, the waxing and waning of reproductive competence depends on the changing photoperiod (63) acting by way of the pineal gland (15,28). The concept of the interaction of the light:dark cycle and the pineal gland with seasonal reproduction was first elaborated about 10 years ago (27,64); it has been tested on a variety of species in the intervening period.

Figure 3 summarizes what are believed to be the relationships among the photoperiod, the pineal gland, and seasonal reproduction in the Syrian hamster. For the purposes of discussion, the cycle has been divided into four more or less distinct phases: the inhibition phase, the sexually quiescent phase, the restoration phase, and the sexually active phase (65). This scheme has been devised for the purpose of describing the relationships in photoperiodic, long-day breeders.

Although 180° out of phase with each other, in both the southern and northern hemispheres the daylength becomes shorter after the summer solstice and eventually the days fall below the critical length required to maintain the gonads in the functional state. At the same time the pineal secretory products cause the collapse of the neuroendocrine-gonadal axis (inhibition phase) (Figure 3). During the late fall and early winter, the short days, acting by way of the pineal gland, maintain the gonads in the inactive state (sexually quiescent phase). Although in some species the restoration phase may be initiated and maintained by increasing daylengths, in the Syrian hamster this appears not to be the case. Rather, while the hibernating hamster is still confined to the darkness of its subterranean burrow, the neuroendocrine-gonadal axis becomes refractory to the inhibitory influence of the pineal gland and the

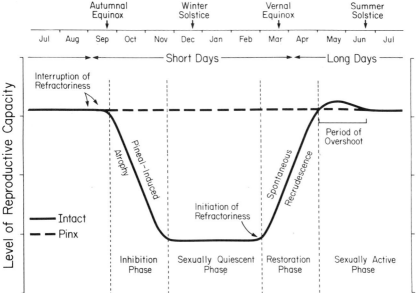

FIGURE 3. Circannual rhythm of reproductive competence in hamsters kept under natural photoperiodic and temperature conditions throughout the year. Pinealectomy **(PINX)** prevents the seasonal variation in sexual capability. The scheme may well apply to other photoperiodic, long-day breeders.

reproductive organs undergo what has been described and referred to as a spontaneous or endogenous regeneration (55,66–70).

The refractoriness is initiated roughly 8–10 weeks prior to the emergence of the hamsters from hibernation (Figure 3). This ensures that when they do terminate hibernation in the spring they are immediately capable of mating and bearing litters. The relationships are similar in both male and female hamsters. Early in the spring the gonads seem to exceed, somewhat, their normal size (period of overshoot, Figure 3); this probably coincides with the maximal reproductive capability of the animals. Throughout the long days of the summer the animals remain sexually competent (the sexually active phase) and the reproductive system retains its refractoriness to darkness and the pineal gland. The long days of the summer, however, eventually interrupt the refractory period so that the short days of the fall can again cause gonadal regression (67,71). This cycle is repeated on an annual basis. It requires both short days (to induce reproductive collapse, etc.) and long days (to interrupt the refractory period) and unquestionably involves the pineal gland. If the pineal is surgically removed, the gonads remain functional (28) and the animals reproduce (23) even during the winter months. The pineal gland continues to produce melatonin in a cyclic manner during all phases of the annual reproductive cycle (72); this is further evidence that the neuroendocrine system is refractory to the inhibitory influence of the pineal gland during certain seasons.

This explanation of the annual cycle of reproduction in photoperiodic, long-day breeders is based on data primarily collected from studies in which the Syrian hamster was the experimental subject. At least in part, however, the scheme probably applies to many other species (27,33,39,73). This area of research is currently very active, so new applications of these findings will no doubt be numerous in the years ahead.

MELATONIN

Indubitably, the isolation of the methoxyindole, N-acetyl-5-methoxytryptamine (melatonin) in 1958 by Lerner and colleagues (74) has been one of the significant events revolutionizing the study of pineal physiology. The prominence of this substance is perhaps best exemplified by the fact that in 1980 an entire symposium was devoted to the science of melatonin (75).

Although a multitude of actions in diverse physiological systems have been attributed to this pineal indole, the majority of research has dealt with the elucidation of its role in reproduction. The following sections review the effects of melatonin on mammalian reproductive physiology.

Evidence for the Presence of Melatonin in the Pineal

The earliest evidence for the presence of melatonin in the pineal gland was its isolation and identification in the bovine epiphysis by Lerner et al. (74,76). Following its discovery, further confirmation for melatonin's existence in the pineal was provided by a variety of physicochemical and immunochemical techniques. Included among the physicochemical procedures are gas chromatography (77,78), gas chromatorgraphy-mass spectrometry (78–83), and spectrofluoremetry (84–86).

With the recent availability of purified antisera to melatonin and melatonin analogs and the development of radioimmunoassay and immunohistochemical methods, there is no longer any question that melatonin is, indeed, present in the pineal (87,88). Through the utilization of specific radioimmunoassays it has been demonstrated that pineal melatonin undergoes a circadian rhythm with concentrations increasing during the dark phase and remaining low during the light phase of the light:dark cycle in several mammalian species (78,89–97).

Bubenik et al. in 1974 were the first to localize melatonin immunocytochemically within the pineal gland (98). They reported immunofluorescence and immunostaining in almost all the parenchymal cells of the rat pineal. This is in contrast to a later study by Freund et al. (99) who found specific fluorescence only in the parenchymal cells lying in a marginal zone of the rat pineal. However, a recent immunofluorescence study by Vivien-Roels et al. (88) on the pineal of rats, mice, and hamsters corroborates the initial report of Bubenik et al. (98). There are several possible explanations for the apparent discrepancies among these three studies. The most obvious is that in each of these reports a different antigen was used to generate the antisera. Bubenik et al. (98) used N-acetylserotonin, the precursor to melatonin (100), whereas Freund et al. (99) used 5-methoxy-N-acetyltryptophan and Vivien-Roels et al. (88) employed melatonin conjugated to a variety of haptens. Another possible source for the differing results was the time of day the animals were killed. Freund et al. (99) sacrificed their animals during the scotophase whereas Vivien-Roels et al. (88) killed theirs during the photophase. Bubenik et al. (98) did not report the time of sacrifice. It is also plausible that the discrepancy was a result of different strains of rats utilized. Finally, fixation artifact could possibly explain the apparent variation in localization of melatonin.

Although the pineal gland apparently represents the major source of melatonin, the indole continues to be detectable in the serum even after pinealectomy in the rat (101) and the ewe (102). Thus there appears to be a secondary source(s) of melatonin synthesis. Indeed, the retina (88,98,103), Harderian gland (88,103–105), and intestine (88,106) have been demonstrated to contain this indole and the melatonin-forming enzyme, hydroxyindole-O-methyltransferase (HIOMT) (107). The physiological significance of these extrapineal sources of melatonin has yet to be elucidated.

Prepubertal Effects of Melatonin

The effects of melatonin on the reproductive physiology of mammals prior to the onset of puberty have been the subject of a number of investigations (108). Wurtman et al. (109), in one of the first studies that provided evidence that this pineal autocoid could affect the reproductive axis, found that melatonin administration resulted in a decrease in ovarian growth in immature female rats. In another study, Sorrentino et al. (110) reported that melatonin, implanted in 7-day-old rats, inhibited the growth of the reproductive organs after 42 days of treatment. Banks and Reiter (111), however, demonstrated that chronic melatonin administration (i.e., via beeswax pellet implants) negated the repressive influence of combined androgen treatment and bilateral orbital enucleation on the maturation of the pituitary-gonadal axis of the rat. On the other hand, in juvenile male Djungarian hamsters (*Phodopus sungorus*), chronic melatonin treatment [via Silastic (polydimethyl-siloxane) capsule implants] for 39 days was found to inhibit testicular maturation (112). Thus in immature *Phodopus* melatonin implants mimic the consequences of exposure to short photoperiod (10). However, in the male Syrian hamster (*Mesocricetus auratus*), a species in which the onset of puberty appears to be a photic-independent phenomenon (39,113), similar treatment (i.e., Silastic implants of melatonin) had no apparent influence on gonadal development (114). Interestingly, if melatonin is administered as daily afternoon injections instead of Silastic implants, testicular maturation reportedly is delayed in the male Syrian hamster (115). Rissman has offered the different methods of melatonin treatment as one reason for the discrepancy between her and Turek's (114) results. This explanation seems plausible in view of the fact that in adult Syrian hamsters melatonin implants also can produce entirely different effects on reproductive physiology when compared to melatonin injections (see following). In addition, Silastic implants themselves seem to produce variable results in adult hamsters (116).

Martin and her colleagues (117–120) have conducted an eloquent series of experiments that have examined the influence of melatonin on the neonatal rat pituitary's response to LHRH. In organ cultures of neonatal rat anterior pituitaries, coincubation of LHRH with physiological concentrations of melatonin resulted in a marked depression in the LH response to LHRH (117,119). It was also shown that melatonin inhibited the in vivo pituitary response to LHRH in male and female neonatal rats (120). The ability of melatonin to curtail LHRH-stimulated LH release is apparently restricted to the neonatal period. As the rat approaches puberty, the pituitary may become relatively refractory to the inhibitory effects of this indole (117,120).

In addition to neonatal rats, the depressive effect of melatonin on the LH response of the anterior pituitary to LHRH was also found in prepubertal dogs in vivo (121). The dog, however, differs from the rat in that the response is not lost at the onset of puberty (122).

A very important interspecies difference has recently been reported by Bacon et al. (123) in the Syrian hamster. In this species, they were unable to detect any effect of this indole on the in vitro response of neonatal or adult anterior pituitary cells to exogenous LHRH. This was also the case for the in vivo response of adult hamsters.

As indicated in the studies just cited, the pituitary-gonadal axis of the neonate is responsive to exogenous melatonin, at least in the Djungarian hamster, rat, and dog. If one examines the ontogeny of endogenous melatonin production, it is seen that melatonin is probably not produced (e.g., in rats) during the first 10 days of life (124). This is approximately the time when the neonatal rat pituitary is beginning to lose its responsiveness to exogenous melatonin (117). Thus, it would seem that in order for melatonin to have physiological significance in the neonate it would have to be exogenously supplied. Not only is there evidence that maternal melatonin can be transported in the milk (although, in very low amounts) to suckling rats, but the apparent tissue distribution of this exogenously supplied melatonin is similar to that found in the mother (125). In addition, the fetus may also be exposed to maternal melatonin by placental transfer. When ^{3}H-acetyl-melatonin was injected into pregnant rats, it was found that each fetus examined contained 0.1% of the injected dose of the isotope (126). Further support for the placental transfer of melatonin has been provided by Vaughan et al. (127). They showed that rats treated with melatonin during the last 4 days of pregnancy gave birth to female offspring that had a significant reduction in pituitary weight. Thus transfer of maternal melatonin via the milk and/ or across the placenta may provide a possible mechanism by which environmental information could be conveyed from the maternal rat both to her fetuses and newborns.

Postpubertal Effects of Melatonin

The myriad of studies concerned with the effects of melatonin on the reproductive physiology of the adult renders it impossible to discuss them all in this brief review. Therefore, an attempt has been made to be selective in the references presented. This is in no way meant to imply that the papers excluded have not played an important role toward our understanding of this unique and often baffling substance.

The characterization of melatonin as being *the* pineal antigonadotrophic hormone (128) has been met with both staunch proponents and opponents in the scientific community. One of the principal reasons for this dichotomy is that the effects of melatonin under seemingly similar experimental conditions often vary in a diametrically opposed manner (108). This was observed to a certain degree in the previous section on the prepubertal effects of the indole.

ANTIGONADOTROPHIC ACTIONS

Perhaps one of the greatest contributing factors to the apparently inconsistent results of melatonin treatment, and thus the concomitant skepticism with regards to its being the pineal antigonadotrophic factor, has been the use of the albino rat as the experimental animal (108,129). Since these animals are highly inbred and have been particularly selected for their reproductive competence, it is not surprising that the laboratory rat is a relatively poor model for examining the ability of melatonin to alter reproductive function (130). In support of this view is the fact that the albino rat is also relatively unresponsive to pineal manipulations (108).

Many of the earlier studies on the reproductive effects of melatonin on rats examined its depressive influence on ovarian and uterine weights (109,131) and testicular and accessory organ development (132,133). Alterations in gonadotropin levels were often inconsistent. There were a few reports in which exogenously administered melatonin was found to inhibit ovulation and the LH surge associated with this event (134,135). However, not all investigators found this methoxyindole to have an inhibitory influence. In fact, some authors actually reported an enhancement of ovarian weights, numbers of corpora lutea, and seminal vesicle weights after daily melatonin treatment (136). Additionally, other investigators found no effect of daily injections of melatonin on the reproductive organs (137–139). The skepticism concerning the antigonadotrophic role of melatonin was further strengthened by the finding that in the Syrian hamster, which is overwhelmingly responsive to pineal manipulations, melatonin was initially found not to possess antigona-dotrophic properties (44).

It was not until 1976, when Tamarkin and colleagues (140) made the crucial observation that the Syrian hamster possesses a daily rhythm in its sensitivity to melatonin, that further support was gained for its acceptance as the pineal gonad-inhibiting factor. Prior to this, however, Fiske and Huppert (141) had reported that in the rat the circadian fluctuation in pineal serotonin could be abolished by melatonin injections 8 hours after the onset of the light phase of a 14:10 light:dark. This effect could be enhanced by injecting melatonin just prior to the onset of darkness. Therefore, the study of Fiske and Huppert (141) was perhaps the first report of a diurnal variation in an animal's sensitivity to melatonin.

In male and female hamsters maintained under long days (light:dark cycles of 14:10) Tamarkin et al. (140) found melatonin to be antigonadtrophic only when the injections were administered 6.5–13.75 hours after lights on (i.e., in the afternoon). Conversely, morning injections failed to inhibit sexual function. Interestingly, the degree of gonadal atrophy resulting from afternoon injections of melatonin was equivalent to that produced in hamsters exposed to short daily photoperiod (140,142). In males this included reductions in circulating levels of LH, FSH, and PRL that were of the same magnitude as those seen in animals with pineal-mediated gonadal regression (140,143). Tamarkin et al. (140) also found in females that daily afternoon, but not morning, injections of melatonin altered the pattern of gonadotrophin secretion such that the afternoon surge of LH and FSH occurred every day, resulting in the females becoming acyclic. Once again, the effects of melatonin given in the afternoon mimicked those in animals exposed to a short photoperiod (142,144).

Rollag et al. (95) have determined that the minimal effective dose of exogenously injected melatonin necessary to promote gonadal atrophy in the Syrian hamster is on the order of 1.6 µg/day. In addition, Sackman et al. (145) examined the specificity of the response and found that while daily afternoon injections of 5-methoxytryptophol (a product of serotonin metabolism) had an inhibitory effect on testicular and accessory sex organ weights, the magnitude of suppression was far below that for the same dose of melatonin. N-acetylserotonin (the immediate precursor of melatonin) and 5-hydroxytryptophol (a product of serotonin metabolism) did not possess any inhibitory activity under the same experimental paradigm.

Besides the requirement that exogenously administered melatonin be administered late in the afternoon in order for it to demonstrate antigonadotrophic activity, it was shown that the animals receiving the indole must also possess an intact and sympathetically innervated pineal gland (146). In other words, if either male or female Syrian hamsters had been pinealectomized or if their pineal was sympathetically denervated, then afternoon injections of melatonin were incapable of repressing the reproductive physiology of these animals.

The necessity of an intact pineal for exogenous melatonin to promote gonadal involution is open to a number of explanations. One is that under the experimental conditions just described melatonin itself may not be antigonadotrophic but instead acts on the pineal to cause the release of another substance(s) that induces the collapse of the reproductive system. Both biochemical (138,141) and morphological (147–150) data exist that demonstrate that exogenously administered melatonin has a direct effect on the pineal. Further support for this interpretation has been provided by the observations of Knigge and Sheridan (151) and Brown et al. (152), which show that gonadal atrophy can be caused

FIGURE 4. Similarities in the responses of the reproductive organs of Syrian hamsters to either short daily photoperiod exposure (top panel) or daily melatonin injections (bottom panel). In both cases, gonadal atrophy ensues (equivalent to the inhibition phase of the annual reproductive cycle); thereafter, the reproductive systems are maintained in an involuted state for a period of time reminiscent of the hibernatory interval of the hamster (sexually quiescent phase). If either treatment is continued indefinitely, the gonads eventually undergo a spontaneous recrudescence (restoration phase). During this period and for an interval thereafter, the reproductive systems are refractory (sexually active phase) to inhibition by either short photoperiodic exposure or melatonin injections. The refractory period is interrupted by exposure of the animals to long photoperiods throughout the "summer" months. The responses of both male and female Syrian hamsters are similar.

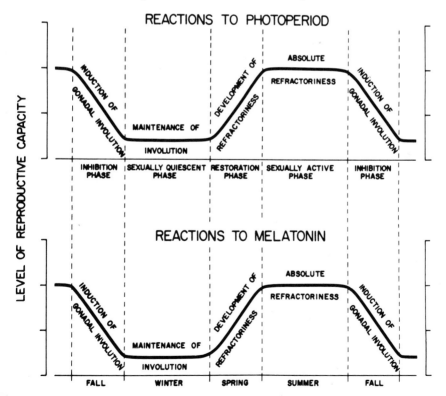

by darkness even in hamsters in which the endogenous melatonin has been neutralized by antibodies to the indoleamine. Also, in the cat, Pavel (153) found arginine vasotocin (AVT), a putative pineal substance, to be released into the CSF after melatonin treatment. An alternative interpretation of the data that would still allow for melatonin to be the antigonadotrophic factor is that the exogenously injected melatonin acts synergistically with endogenously produced pineal melatonin secreted during darkness to induce reproductive collapse. If this were the situation, then perhaps multiple daily injections of the indole into pinealectomized hamsters would also inhibit the neuroendocrine-reproductive axis. Hypothetically, the pattern of melatonin exposure experienced by intact hamsters receiving a pulse of melatonin in the afternoon (via injection) and another pulse at night (via the pineal) may be stimulated by a multiple daily injection paradigm. Data substantiating this hypothesis have been provided by Tamarkin et al. (154) and Goldman et al. (155). They found that when pinealectomized hamsters were subjected to three daily injections of melatonin (25 μg/injection; spaced at 3-hour intervals) testicular atrophy ensued and serum LH and FSH levels were depressed—in other words, changes that are observed when intact hamsters are exposed to short photoperiods. Finally, another plausible explanation is that the surgical manipulations employed by Reiter et al. (146) and by Tamarkin et al. (140) may have altered the sensitivity period to melatonin; that is, the sensitivity period was shifted to a time that did not coincide with the melatonin injections.

The reactions of the reproductive systems of Syrian hamsters to short photoperiods and melatonin treatment are graphically depicted in Figure 4. The fact that many, if not all, of the effects of short days on sexual function can be duplicated by appropriately administered melatonin provides strong support for this indole being the hormone responsible for mediating the effects of the pineal gland on reproduction. Albeit these findings do not prove that melatonin is the pineal constituent accountable for the entire antigonadotrophic capacity of the pineal, they do provide excellent substantiation. It is entirely possible, as indicated here, that melatonin works in conjunction with other compound(s) of pineal origin to regulate mammalian reproductive physiology.

COUNTERANTIGONADOTROPHIC ACTIONS

In view of the previous discussion on the suppressive actions of melatonin on reproduction, it seems inconsistent that the same indole can also thwart the antigonadal influence of a short photoperiod (156,157) and, even more interestingly, its own antigonadotrophic effects (142,143). This seemingly paradoxical action of melatonin has been referred to as its counterantigonadotrophic (158), or progonadal (159), influence.

In 1974, Hoffmann (156) and Reiter et al. (157), working independently and on different species of hamsters, observed that subcutaneous reservoirs of releasable melatonin could block the pineal-mediated effects of short photoperiod on gonadal regression. Hoffmann (156) employed the Djungarian hamster *(Phodopus sungorus)*, whereas the Syrian hamster was used as the experimental animal by Reiter et al. (157). In both these studies, melatonin (mixed with beeswax) was implanted subcutaneously into males exposed to what would normally be an inhibitory photoperiod. Presumably, the indole was continually released from these depots. With regard to the sexual parameters examined, melatonin administered in this manner actually prevented short photoperiods from exerting their inhibitory control over the sexual organs. Indeed, the chronically available melatonin released from these implants resulted in a "functional pinealectomy" (158). The counter antigonadotrophic actions of melatonin implants have also been demonstrated in short-day-exposed female hamsters (25,160) and male rats (161).

One of the possibilities that could account for the counterantigonadotrophic actions of melatonin was that they were a result of a pharmacological dosage of the indole. If all the melatonin from the beeswax implants (1 mg melatonin/24 mg beeswax) was absorbed by the animal, the daily dosage of the indole would have been roughly 143 µg/day. Hence experiments were conducted by Reiter et al. (162) in which hamsters received much lower quantities of melatonin. With all but the smallest amounts, melatonin was capable of preventing darkness-induced gonadal atrophy. Thus, as little as 3.6 µg (based on the same assumption above) of melatonin daily was able to prevent the suppressive effect of short daily photoperiods. It is important to recall that if this dosage is given as a single bolus injection late in the light period, reproductive involution takes place. Turek et al. (159) have also reported that continuously available melatonin in the Syrian hamster results in a counterantigonadotrophic influence. Their results were, however, somewhat more variable. This variability may have been a result of the mode by which the methoxyindole was administered. Silastic capsules were utilized by Turek et al. (159). However, Cutty et al. (163) recently reported that Silastic implants of melatonin into male Syrian hamsters prevented the decrease of plasma prolactin and LH associated with short photoperiod. There is no question that in the Syrian hamster melatonin can possess both anti- and counterantigonadotrophic activity contingent on its method of administration.

Not all species, however, respond to continually available melatonin in the same manner. For example, in the grasshopper mouse *(Onychomys torridus)* (130), the white-footed mouse *(Peromyscus leucopus)* (11), and the short-tailed weasel *(Mustela erimea)* (164), melatonin implants act the same as late afternoon injections in the Syrian hamster, i.e., in an antigonadotrophic manner. As discussed earlier, in Djungarian hamsters maintained in short photoperiods, melatonin implants acted in a counterantigonadotrophic manner (156). The reader should also recall that melatonin implants delayed the onset of puberty (antigonadotrophic) in juvenile *Phodopus* maintained in long photoperiods (112). To complicate the situation further, a similar retardation was found in adult winter animals exposed to long photoperiods after being implanted with melatonin (165,166), whereas this treatment had no effect if summer adults were utilized (167). It has also been reported by Turek et al. (130) that implants of melatonin in Syrian hamsters kept under long days induces gonadal involution. However, this latter effect has been difficult to repeat in the same laboratory (159) as well as by others (Petterborg and Reiter, unpublished observations) and may have been a spurious finding.

The next logical question to be answered with regard to these diametrically opposed observations was What would be the results of a combination of melatonin implants and daily afternoon melatonin injections? Reiter et al. (143) in male Syrian hamsters and Trakulrungsi et al. (144) in female Syrian hamsters found that the continuous-release reservoirs negated the effects normally observed with afternoon injections.

A number of plausible explanations for these seemingly paradoxical effects of melatonin in the Syrian hamster have been recently set forth (142–144). Although still hypothetical, the most interesting explanation involves the melatonin receptor and associated events. Reiter et al. (168) have postulated that as melatonin becomes available, either exogenously or endogenously, it interacts with its receptor. As a result of this interaction, the receptors are "down-regulated" or "desensitized" to additional melatonin. This phenomenon may be effected either by a diminution in the receptor-ligand affinity or by an actual decrease in the receptor population (169). Thus, since the synthesis and presumably the secretion of endogenously secreted melatonin occurs near the end of the dark period of the light:dark cycle in the Syrian hamster (8,96,170), the target organs become insensitive to additional melatonin given early in the light period. Not only would this hypothesis explain the apparent paradoxical effects of melatonin but it would also account for the findings of Tamarkin et al. (140) that only injections given late in the light phase result in gonadal regression. The continuously available melatonin afforded by implants would in essence extend the period of receptor refractoriness such that exogenously administered melatonin given in the afternoon or the endogenously produced melatonin secreted late in the dark phase would not have any effect. On the other hand, the afternoon injections by themselves would provide melatonin at a time when the receptors were available; therefore, reproductive collapse would occur.

Although direct proof is presently not available in corroboration of the down-regulation hypothesis, evidence for a diurnal variation in the number of melatonin receptors has been provided by Vacas and Cardinali (171). They reported that the number of melatonin binding sites in hamster and rat brains was 34–56% higher 1 hour before lights off (200 h) than at the time of lights on (0700 h). Furthermore, a hormone regulating the physiological state or the number of its own receptors is not without precedent. A number of hormones, including LH (172), LHRH (173), insulin (174), and thyrotropin releasing hormone (175), have been demonstrated to regulate the density of their own receptors in their target tissue.

Several experiments have recently been reported to test the "down-regulation" hypothesis. If melatonin does indeed regulate its own receptors, then an injection of a large dose of the indole (i.e., 1 mg) in Syrian hamsters late in the morning may prolong the period of refractoriness of the receptors and thereby prevent the normally suppressive effects of afternoon injections of melatonin. On the other hand, large doses of melatonin in the afternoon may block the pineal-mediated gonadal atrophy caused by short days. As predicted by the hypothesis, the large dose of melatonin injected late in the morning (1100 h) blocks the inhibitory actions of afternoon injections of the indole in both male (176) and female (176,177) Syrian hamsters (Figures 5 and 6). Interestingly, the large dose of melatonin administered in the afternoon (1600 h) to hamsters kept under long days was without influence on the reproductive capacity of the male (178) and female Syrian hamster (Richardson and Reiter, unpublished data). Richardson and colleagues (unpublished data) were also able to prevent short photoperiodic-induced

FIGURE 5. Effect of morning (1100 h) and/or afternoon (1700 h) injections of either saline **(Sal)** or melatonin **(Mel)** on absolute **(clear bars)** and relative **(hatched bars)** testicular and accessory organ weights of adult Syrian hamsters. Vertical lines signify standard errors. *$p < 0.001$; **$p < 0.01$ vs untreated controls. *From Richardson et al. (176).*

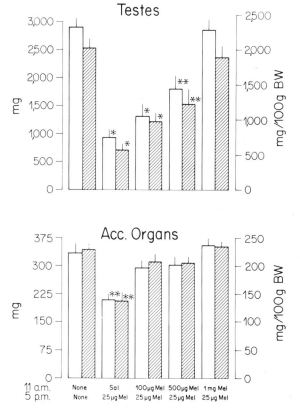

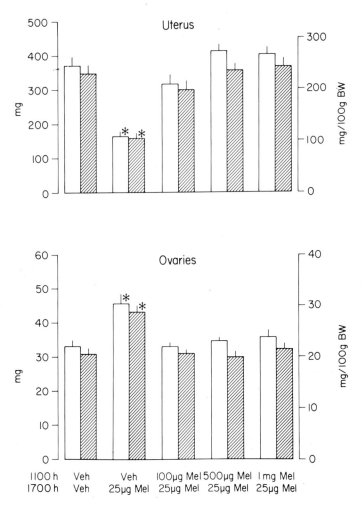

FIGURE 6. Effect of morning (1100 h) and/or afternoon (1700 h) injections of either vehicle **(Veh)** or melatonin **(Mel)** on absolute **(clear bars)** and relative **(hatched bars)** uterine and ovarian weights of adult Syrian hamsters. Vertical lines signify standard errors. *$p < 0.001$ vs Veh (1100 and 1700 h) treated controls. *From Richardson et al. (176).*

reproductive collapse with a large bolus of melatonin given daily in the afternoon (Figure 7). All these findings can be explained if we assume melatonin has the ability to down-regulate its receptors. Definitive proof for the hypothesis awaits further experimental evidence. The findings leading up to the formulation of the hypothesis have been described in greater depth elsewhere (3,179).

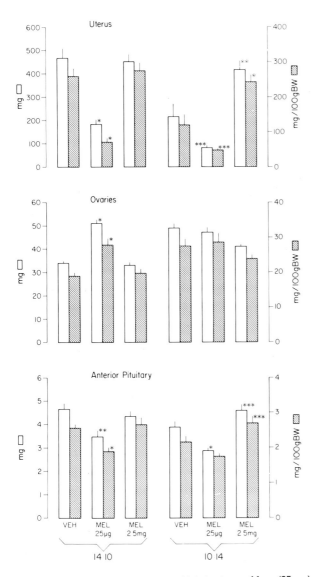

FIGURE 7. Effect of daily (at 1600 h) injections of low (25 μg) and high (2.5 mg) doses of melatonin **(MEL)** on absolute **(clear bars)** and relative **(hatched bars)** uterine, ovarian, and anterior pituitary weights of adult Syrian hamsters maintained in either a 14:10 or 10:14 LD cycle. Verticle lines signify standard errors. *$p < 0.001$, **$p < 0.01$, ***$p < 0.05$ vs respective 10:14 vehicle **(VEH)** treated controls.

Potential Sites of Action of Melatonin

Although there is no longer any question that melatonin has definitive effects on mammalian reproduction, the target site for this pineal indole still remains a mystery. The available literature on the primary target for melatonin has implicated each of the components of the neuroendocrine-reproductive axis as potential sites of action. Thus melatonin may possess multiple interactions within the brain, anterior pituitary, and reproductive organs.

Seeing that the central control and integrative locus for the neuroendocrine regulation of reproduction is the hypothalamus, it would seem to be the most logical choice to be considered as the potential site of action for melatonin; as such, it has received a great deal of attention.

The hypothalamus has been indirectly and directly implicated as the primary site of action of melatonin in a number of studies (108). It was noted earlier that melatonin, when appropriately administered during the neonatal period in a number of species, delays the growth and function of the reproductive tract (110,112,115). When consideration is given to the fact that the sexual differentiation of the hypothalamic center controlling gonadotrophin release is almost achieved by postnatal day 10, it is feasible that melatonin might interfere with the normal development and functioning of hypothalamic-steroidal feedback mechanisms (180). In this way, it is possible that the mechanisms that control hypothalamic sensitivity to steroids at the time of puberty as well as the pubertal surge of steroids are altered (181).

Fraschini et al. (182) has provided more direct evidence that melatonin effects the gonadotrophin control center of the hypothalamus. They reported that melatonin implanted stereotaxically into the median eminence resulted in a depression of both the pituitary stores and plasma titers of LH. Fraschini et al. (182) also observed that if pineal fragments were implanted into the median eminence, pituitary LH was likewise decreased. Therefore, these investigators concluded that melatonin inhibits LH synthesis and secretion by acting on specific receptors in the median eminence. Several studies have also demonstrated that intraventricular injections of melatonin result in a significant depression in LH and FSH levels whereas prolactin secretion was enhanced (182–185).

Radiolabeled uptake studies have provided additional support for a hypothalamic site of action for melatonin. Both Anton-Tay and Wurtman (186) and Cardinali et al. (187) found that the hypothalamus concentrates exogenously administered ^{3}H-melatonin more selectively than any other brain region. Furthermore, gas chromatographic-mass spectrophotometric techniques have demonstrated significant levels of melatonin in the rat hypothalamus (188).

Recently, Fishback et al. (189) reported that melatonin treatment resulted in enhanced levels of hypothalamic LHRH. However, this observation appears to be an inconsistent finding because melatonin has also been shown to depress hypothalamic LHRH or have no effect at all on the levels of this peptide in the hypothalamus (Richardson and Reiter, unpublished observations). Moreover, Kao and Weisz (190) found that 10–15-minute pulses of melatonin consistently caused release of LHRH from perifused medial basal hypothalami.

As suggested by Fraschini et al. (182), if melatonin does in fact act on the hypothalamus, then specific receptors for this indole should be present. Apparently, as alluded to earlier in the discussion of the down-regulation hypothesis, this is indeed the case. Recently, Cardinali et al. (191) and Niles et al. (192) provided direct evidence for high-affinity binding sites for melatonin in membrane or cytosol preparations of bovine, rat, and hamster brain, suggesting the presence of melatonin receptors in the mammalian CNS. In these studies, melatonin binding was maximal in the medial basal hypothalamus. Interestingly, Vacas and Cardinali (171) also found a diurnal variation in the number of melatonin receptors in the rat and hamster brain with maximal concentration occurring at a time during the lighting cycle when exogenous melatonin injections are most effective in causing gonadal atrophy.

Numerous investigations have also provided support for extrahypothalamic sites of action for melatonin within the CNS. These sites include the mesencephalic reticular formation (182,186,193,194) and, as previously discussed, the pineal gland itself (141,146,147).

Direct interference with the secretion of gonadotrophic hormones from the anterior pituitary by melatonin may be affected by at least two possible mechanisms. These are alterations in either the basal and/or releasing hormone-stimulated release of pituitary gonadotrophins (195). There exists little evidence for the former. Intrapituitary implants or the infusion of melatonin have no effect on pituitary LH, FSH, or PRL release (184,185,194). In addition, direct effects of melatonin on basal LH or prolactin in vitro have not been observed (119,196,197). However, melatonin may alter the responsiveness of the anterior pituitary to LHRH (123,120).

As a result of the marked gonadal and accessory organ regression associated with increased pineal activity, it has been suggested that the gonads may represent a principal site of action of melatonin (195). Melatonin injections into hypophysectomized rats or mice was found to inhibit gonadal and accessory organ stimulation by human chorionic gonadotrophin (132,198). The findings of Trentini et al. (199) suggest that this may be due to an inhibition of the gonadal uptake of gonadotrophins. They demonstrated that the ovarian uptake of ^{3}H-LH is reduced in rats pretreated with melatonin, implying that the binding of LH to its receptors may be inhibited. Further substantiation for a peripheral site of action for melatonin comes from several papers that report the ability of this indole to impede the synthesis of testicular androgens (200,201).

If melatonin does indeed act at the level of the gonads, then the uptake by the tissue of the indole and an interaction with its specific receptor is suggested. However, studies related to the uptake of ^{3}H-melatonin by the ovary are conflicting. Uptake in certain species has been shown to be significant whereas in others it is all but nonexistent (202–204). Cohen et al. (205) have described the presence of alleged cytoplasmic melatonin receptors in the ovary and uterus of several species.

Generally, it appears that melatonin may act at all levels of the neuroendocrine-reproductive hierarchy (Figure 8). Even though the evidence suggests primarily a CNS site of action, melatonin may also influence the endocrine activity and responsiveness of secondary sites outside the CNS.

Of some note is that the rat has been used as the experimental subject in many of the studies designed to locate the site of action of melatonin. Yet this species is not particularly responsive to the inhibitory influence of either the pineal or melatonin. In the hamster, there is a consensus that the primary site of action of melatonin is within the CNS, possibly at the level of the suprachiasmatic nuclei (SCN) (206–208).

In summary, the similarities between the pineal-mediated regulation of the reproductive capacity of many mammals, particularly the Syrian hamster, and that of melatonin strongly intimates that this substance is the pineal antigonadotrophic factor. Even the apparent paradoxical ef-

FIGURE 8. Diagrammatic representation of the potential sites of action of pineal melatonin. **Thick solid arrow** is directed toward the primary effector site whereas **thin solid arrows** are directed toward secondary and tertiary sites of action. **Open arrows** represent activity within the hypothalamo–pituitary–reproductive axis.

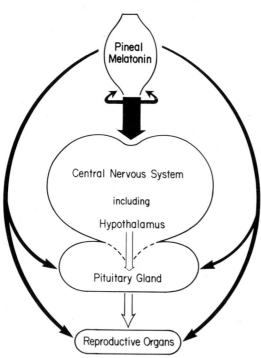

fects of this substance provides support for its role as the pineal constituent governing the reproductive process in that the neuroendocrine-reproductive axis of seasonal breeders (e.g., Syrian hamster) enters a state of refractoriness to the pineal and exogenously administered melatonin (Figure 4). It appears that the regulation of reproduction by melatonin may take place at the level of its receptors (3,179).

OTHER INDOLES

Serotonin

The mammalian pineal gland contains inordinately high concentrations of serotonin (86). This amine serves as a pivotal precursor for nearly all other pineal indoleamines, many of which may be secreted as pineal hormones (Figure 9). Although no evidence presented to date suggests systemic release of pineal serotonin, various laboratories have examined from time to time this rather ubiquitously distributed indoleamine for

FIGURE 9. Metabolic pathway for the biosynthesis of the various pineal indole alkylamines. All pineal indoles isolated to date originate from tryptophan, which is hydroxylated to form 5-hydroxytryptophan. The decarboxylated derivative of the latter is 5-hydroxytryptamine (serotonin), which serves as a precursor to most pineal indole products including melatonin. The various enzymes involved in pineal indole biosynthesis include (1) tryptophan hydroxylase, (2) L-amino acid decarboxylase, (3,4,7,10,11) hydroxyindole-O-methyltransferase, (5) monoamine oxidase, (8,9) aldehyde dehydrogenase, and (6) N-acetyltransferase.

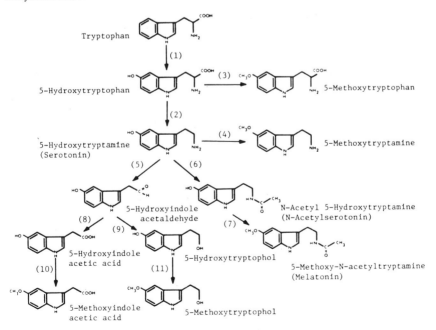

antigonadotrophic potential. Implants of serotonin, placed in the rat median eminence, significantly depressed pituitary FSH, but not LH, levels (182). This effect was similar to that following median eminence implantation of 5-methoxytryptophol.

Intraventricular injection of serotonin (or melatonin) in male rats resulted in a reduction in both LH and FSH levels (182–185) and increased plasma PRL levels (183,185). However, no changes in PRL or FSH titers were noted following hypophyseal-portal infusion of the indoles, suggesting that these substances may effect pituitary gonadotrophin and PRL stores by suppressing the action of gonadotrophic releasing hormone and prolactin inhibiting factor.

In apparent conflict with earlier reports from the same laboratory (184), Porter et al. (209) reported that intraventricular infusion of serotonin increased pituitary LH release in male rats although melatonin and N-acetylserotonin did not seem to affect levels of this gonadotrophin. No explanation for this discrepancy was offered. The authors also reported that serotonin, N-acetylserotonin, and melatonin increased pituitary PRL release.

Incubation of neonatal (but not postpubertal) rat pituitary glands with LHRH and physiological concentrations of serotonin or 5-methoxytryptamine significantly reduced LHRH-induced LH release (119). When the animal reaches puberty, the pituitary gland becomes refractory to the influence of these pineal indoles; this presumably correlates developmentally with the decrease in hypothalamic responsiveness to steroidal inhibition. The net effect is the pubescent gonadotropin increase.

Intraventricular injection of serotonin had no apparent influence on bioassayable hypothalamic LHRH activity in immature rats (210). If these animals also received an injection of the monoamine oxidase inhibitor, nialamide, then hypothalamic LHRH activity was significantly depressed. The authors suggested that administration of serotonin may have acted synergistically with nialamide-augmented hypothalamic serotonin content to decrease hypothalamic gonadotrophin releasing activity.

Thus intraventricular administration of serotonin as well as other pineal indoleamines can influence gonadotrophin release at the level of both hypothalamus and neonatal pituitary gland. However, in spite of various reports that exogenously administered serotonin may act as an antigonadotrophin, this indoleamine is not generally considered a pineal hormone. Considering the large amounts of serotonin present in the peripheral circulation, it is difficult to conceive of the idea that serotonin of pineal origin is important in normally regulating the neuroendocrine axis.

N-Acetylserotonin

N-Acetylserotonin is an intermediate product in the conversion of serotonin to melatonin (N-acetyl-5-methoxytryptamine). Pineal concentrations of this indole are generally low (100), presumably due to the instability and rapid turnover of the compound. The few reports concerning the potential of this compound to exert an influence on the neuroendocrine-reproductive axis are contradictory. Administration of N-acetylserotonin inhibited compensatory ovarian hypertrophy (COH) in unilaterally ovariectomized mice (Figure 10) (211) but stimulated the number of ova released in immature rats treated with pregnant mare's serum (PMS) (212). Intraventricular injection of N-acetylserotonin into male rats had little or no effect on plasma LH levels but increased pituitary PRL release (209). N-acetylserotonin had no influence on the release of LH from neonatal rat pituitary glands incubated with LHRH (119).

5-Hydroxytryptophol

5-Hydroxytryptophol has been identified in bovine (213) and rat (214) pineal glands. The formation of 5-hydroxyindole acetaldehyde from serotonin is catalyzed by monoamine oxidase. This unstable product is rapidly oxidized to form 5-hydroxyindole 3-acetic acid or reduced to form 5-hydroxytryptophol. 5-Hydroxytryptophol serves as a precursor in the formation of 5-methoxytryptophol (215).

Although little information is available concerning the antigonadotrophic potential of this indoleamine, current evidence suggests that this compound is not particularly important as a pineal hormone. Injection of microgram quantities of 5-hydroxytryptophol daily resulted in no changes in ovarian maturation or in the subsequent estrous cycles but did inhibit COH in unilaterally ovariectomized mice (Figure 10) (211). Subcutaneous injection of the indole was also shown to reduce the percentage of immature rats in which first ovulation was induced by the administration of PMS (212). Median eminence implants of 5-hydroxytryptophol depressed pituitary levels of LH but not FSH (182).

5-Methoxytryptophol

5-Methoxytryptophol has been identified in bovine (215), sheep (216), rat (81,82,217,218), and human (219) pineal gland as well as rat plasma (81,82) and human CSF (220,221). Although more than one pathway for its synthesis in the pineal gland is possible, formation of this methoxyindole requires the catalytic activities of both hydroxyindole-O-methyltransferase and monoamine oxidase. 5-Methoxytryptophol may be produced either by the methylation of 5-hydroxytryptophol or by the methylation of serotonin to form 5-methoxytryptamine, which is then deaminated. Smith et al. (222) have suggested that pineal 5-hydroxytryptophol is primarily metabolized to form O-acetyl-5-methoxytryptophol. They propose that the isolation of 5-methoxytryptophol from pineal tissue may be artifactual, presumably due to rapid, plasma-associated hydrolysis of O-acetyl-5-methoxytryptophol in the course of routine extraction procedures. Further evidence in support of this hypothesis would be provided by the isolation of acetyl-hydroxytryptophol, an interme-

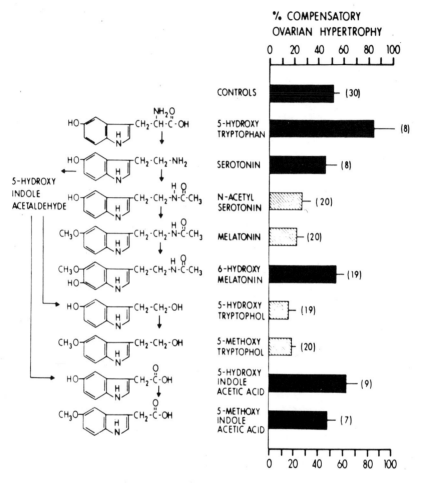

FIGURE 10. Effect of various pineal indole alkylamines on the percentage of compensatory ovarian hypertrophy following unilateral ovariectomy in mice. N-acetylserotonin, melatonin, 5-hydroxytryptophol, and 5-methoxytryptophol **(hatched bars)** produced significant inhibition of compensatory ovarian hypertrophy ($p < 0.005$). Numbers in parentheses indicate the number of mice per group. *From Vaughan et al. (211).*

diate product in the pathway from 5-hydroxytryptophol to O-acetyl-5-methoxytryptophol, in the pineal gland.

Measured by gas chromatography-mass spectrometry, pineal levels of 5-methoxytryptophol are substantially lower (max 340 pg/gland) than those of serotonin or melatonin (72 and 2 ng/gland, respectively) (217,218). The level of 5-methoxytryptophol was significantly elevated during darkness in comparison to that during the light period in the rat pineal gland, suggesting the existence of a well-defined circadian rhythm in the formation of this methoxyindole (217). On the other hand, plasma levels of 5-methoxytryptophol were substantially greater (max 684 pg/ml) than pineal levels and exhibited a daytime peak and low or undetectable nighttime levels. Similar circadian fluctuations in human plasma 5-methoxytryptophol levels have been reported (221,223). The authors could not readily explain the difference between circadian fluctuations in plasma and pineal levels of 5-methoxytryptophol but suggested that the difference could be due to the release of this indole from extrapineal sources having significant hydroxyindole-O-methyltransferase activity, e.g., the retina or Harderian gland (224). This difference could also be explained as a result of increased peripheral conversion of 5-methoxytryptophol nocturnally.

Although most radioactively labeled 5-methoxytryptophol is excreted in urine as 5-methoxyindole 3-acetic acid, high levels of radioactivity were also localized in thyroid, adrenal, ovarian, and uterine tissues (225). The specificity of this apparent binding activity was not determined.

Plasma 5-methoxytryptophol levels were highest during the first two-thirds of the human menstrual cycle (226). Those women receiving oral contraceptives demonstrated consistently lower plasma levels of 5-methoxytryptophol throughout the cycle. No correlations between 5-methoxytryptophol and FSH/LH levels were evident. In contrast, melatonin decreased with the approach of ovulation (227), illustrating a lack of correlation between plasma melatonin and 5-methoxytryptophol in humans. A similar difference between plasma levels of these two methoxyindoles relative to the estrous cycle could be expected in other mammalian species.

Systemic administration of microgram quantities of 5-methoxytryptophol inhibited normal ovarian maturation, delayed pubertal onset (182), and reduced the incidence of estrus in adult rats (213). 5-Methoxytryptophol appeared to be more effective than melatonin in inhibiting human chorionic gonadotrophin-induced uterine growth in mice and rats (198). COH was inhibited when measured 9 days after unilateral ovariectomy and 5-methoxytryptophol injection in mice (Figure 10) (211). Adult male rats injected daily with this indole exhibited decreased sexual activity and reduced spermatogenesis (228). Like melatonin, a single, daily injection of 5-methoxytryptophol near the end of the light period reduced gonadal and accessory sex organ weights in adult male hamsters (145). Subcutaneous implants of 5-methoxytryptophol prevented testicular and accessory sexual organ regression in light-deprived male hamsters (53). In this respect, the effects of 5-methoxytryptophol were identical to those of melatonin.

5-Methoxytryptophol, but not melatonin, has been shown to inhibit the postcastration rise in plasma and pituitary FSH in adult male rats (229). These authors further demonstrated that administration of 5-methoxytryptophol enhanced the increase in pituitary PRL levels accompanying postcastration hypertrophy of the rat pituitary gland. The inhibitory influence of median eminence implants of 5-methoxytryptophol on FSH secretion in rats had been reported previously (182).

O-Acetyl-5-methoxytryptophol

Smith et al. (222,230) have identified this methoxyindole in the rat pineal gland by gas chromatography-mass spectrometry. They have proposed that O-acetyl-5-methoxytryptophol represents the primary conversion product of 5-hydroxytryptophol (5-hydroxytryptophol→O-acetyl-5-hydroxytryptophol→O-acetyl-5-methoxytryptophol), the presence of 5-methoxytryptophol in the pineal gland being an artifact of tissue extraction techniques. Although O-acetyl-5-methoxytryptophol is normally produced in both male and female rat pineal glands, the functional significance of this newly discovered indole has yet to be determined.

5-Methoxytryptamine

5-Methoxytryptamine is formed by the HIOMT-catalyzed methylation of serotonin, a pathway present in the pineal gland (231). 5-Methoxytryptamine has been identified in rat (79,232) and human (233) pineal glands. Although small amounts of the indole are normally found in human CSF samples, elevated levels are usually seen only in manic and acutely schizophrenic patients (234,235), emphasizing pathologically the demonstrable psychomimetic properties of this compound (236). Although information concerning the influence of this compound on the reproductive system are scant, 5-methoxytryptamine injections have been shown to duplicate the effects of afternoon injections of melatonin in inducing gonadal regression in hamsters (237). Intraventricular injection of 5-methoxytryptamine has also been shown to increase plasma prolactin levels in urethane-anesthetized male rats (183).

INFLUENCE OF HORMONES ON THE PINEAL

The influence of the pineal gland on reproductive function in numerous species is obviously well established. An increasing body of evidence supports the contention that the pineal gland does not represent an open-ended loop within the neuroendocrine-reproductive axis. Rather, pineal secretion(s) is (are) controlled by "endocrine-endocrine" and "endocrine-neuronal" feedback mechanisms. The former mechanism refers to the direct interactions between reproductive hormones and pineal hormone-generating pathways; the latter, to the indirect interactions between these systems via the influence of reproductive hormones on various components of the pineal sympathetic innervation. Reproductive hormones that influence pineal activity include gonadal steroids, pituitary gonadotrophins, and hypothalamic gonadotrophic releasing factors (128).

Changes in the estrous cycle reportedly influence various constituents and pathways in the pineal gland. For example, norepinephrine-induced activation of adenyl cyclase (238), adenosine 3',5'-monophosphate (cAMP) concentrations (239), HIOMT activity (240–243), 5-hydroxytryptamine (serotonin), 5-hydroxindole-3-acetic acid and N-acetyl-5-methoxytryptamine (melatonin) content (244,245), plasma 5-methoxytryptophol concentrations (226), and urinary melatonin concentrations (246) all seem to vary with the estrous cycle.

HIOMT activity and melatonin levels decrease in the rat pineal gland with the approach of the estrous (periovulatory) stage and increase during the luteal stages of the cycle (244). A similar decrease in plasma melatonin levels in women occurs during the proliferative and up to the ovulatory stage (Figure 11) (226). Interestingly, plasma levels of another putative pineal hormone, 5-methoxytryptophol, are generally increased during the proliferative stages (226,247).

Ozaki et al. (246) reported a decrease in urinary melatonin concentrations during proestrus in the rat. Insofar as the estrus-related changes in melatonin were paralleled by changes in urinary norepinephrine concentrations, the reduction in excreted melatonin during proestrus was presumed due, in part, to a similar reduction in norepinephrine-stimulated pineal melatonin production. Estrus-related changes in melatonin were also attributed to the inhibitory influence of ovarian steroids on pineal activity. Because administration of melatonin throughout the estrous cycle did not affect changes in urinary melatonin levels relative to the estrous cycle, they concluded that changes in urinary melatonin concentrations were due to changes in the rate of pineal secretion of

FIGURE 11. Plasma melatonin **(MEL)** and serotonin **(HT)** levels during the human menstrual cycle compared to plasma prolactin **(PRL)**, luteinizing hormone **(LH)**, follicle stimulating hormone **(FSH)**, estradiol **(E)**, and progesterone **(P)** levels.

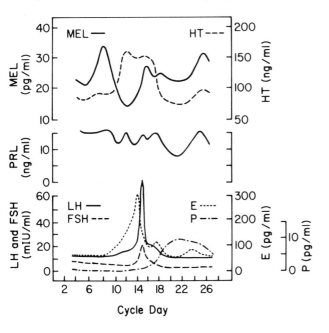

melatonin and not to changes in peripheral metabolism and renal clearance of this indole. However, it should be cautioned that peripheral concentrations of melatonin may also be affected by extrapineal release of melatonin such as the retina, Harderian gland, and intestinal mucosa (104,248). HIOMT activity in these extrapineal tissues varies during the estrous cycle, after castration, or after treatment with gonadal steroids (248).

Endocrine-Endocrine Interaction: Influence of Gonadal Steroids

Castration of male or female rats depresses pineal melatonin synthesis. This effect can be reversed by the administration of low doses (e.g., 0.05–2 µg/day), but not high doses (e.g., greater than 5 µg/day), of testosterone or estrogen (240,249–252).

In correlation with peak plasma levels of estradiol, the concentration of nuclear receptor estrogen complexes in the rat pineal gland is highest during proestrus (253). Administration of 2 µg of estradiol to ovariectomized rats produced a translocation of pineal estrogen receptor complexes from cytoplasm to nucleus in amounts identical to those of intact, untreated rats during proestrus (253). Incubation of rat pineal glands in the presence of presumed physiological levels (i.e., 1–15 nM) of estradiol, which represents the concentration range for the K_d of cytoplasmic and nuclear binding of the steroid, led to an increase in HIOMT activity and melatonin production in a dose-dependent fashion (254). The addition of excess clomiphene, a nonsteroidal competitor for estradiol binding sites, blocked estradiol stimulation of pineal HIOMT activity. Addition of α-amanitin, actinomycin D, cycloheximide, or puromycin blocked estradiol-induced increases in O-methylation of 5-hydroxyindoles, indicating involvement of RNA and protein synthesis in the pineal response to low levels of estradiol. Thus the effects of low doses of estradiol to increase O-methylation of pineal 5-hydroxyindoles are the result of cytoplasmic estrogen receptor binding, nuclear translocation of the receptor complex, and transcription/translation to synthesis proteins leading to increased enzymatic (e.g., HIOMT) activity.

The inhibitory effects of high doses of estradiol on the formation of pineal methoxyindoles may be explained by O-methylation of this steroid itself within the pineal gland (255). These authors described the formation of a 3-methylether derivative of estradiol, catalyzed by a partially purified preparation of HIOMT from bovine pineal glands. The similarity between the K_m values for estradiol and N-acetylserotonin (3.13 × 10^{-5} M and 1.41 × 10^{-5} M, respectively) in concert with the lower K_m value for S-adenosylmethionine in the presence of estradiol versus N-acetylserotonin suggest that the inhibitory influence of high doses of estradiol on pineal methoxyindole synthesis is a result of competitive O-methylation of this steroid catalyzed by HIOMT. How high doses of estradiol can also inhibit HIOMT activity has yet to be determined.

Certainly the biphasic, dose-dependent response of HIOMT activity to estradiol provides an explanation for the seemingly contradictory reports that low doses of estradiol increased (251), and high doses decreased (256), pineal HIOMT activity. A similar explanation could be postulated for the effects of testosterone treatment of castrated rats, low doses of which stimulate pineal HIOMT activity (257) and high doses of which inhibit the activity of this enzyme (249,257,258). It is possible that these results could reflect pineal aromatization of testosterone to form estrogens. Such a possibility could be tested by the use of the nonaromatizable androgen dihydrotestosterone.

Endocrine-Neuronal Interactions: Influence of Gonadal Steroids

Administration of 2 μg of estradiol for 3 days to ovariectomized rats significantly reduced the amount of ^{3}H-norepinephrine taken up by the pineal gland 60 and 20 minutes after pulse injection of the isotope (259). Estrogen treatment did not alter pineal norepinephrine concentrations but enhanced the turnover (i.e., synthesis, release, and inactivation) rate of the neurotransmitter (260). This effect of estradiol could occur by interaction of this steroid with components of the superior cervical ganglia or their axonal terminals within the pineal gland. A site of action excluding central descending pathways leading to these ganglia was assumed on the basis of a persistence of the steroid-mediated effects following interruption of preganglionic fibers (i.e., decentralization) to the superior cervical ganglia. That this steroid could directly affect the ganglia in contrast to an indirect effect mediated by gonadotrophins was determined by the identification of high affinity binding sites for estradiol within the rat superior cervical ganglia and significant nuclear translocation of steroid receptor complexes from the cytoplasm after injection of 2 μg of estradiol (260). Additionally, microelectrophoretic injection of testosterone or estrone into guinea pig pineal glands increases electrical activity, presumably related to an increase in norepinephrine turnover (261).

The effect of isoproterenol in increasing pineal synthetic activity in intact or ganglionectomized rats can be blocked by subsequent estradiol or testosterone injection (262). Because nuclear translocation of estrogen receptor complexes from the cytoplasm are inhibited by isoproterenol (263), another site of action for the inhibitory effects of estradiol must be the pineal beta-adrenergic receptor. In addition, gonadal steroids have been shown to influence the receptor-associated cAMP mechanism as demonstrated by reduced adenyl cyclase activity and cAMP concentrations in the rat pineal gland during proestrus (238,239) and by the observation that ovariectomy increased norepinephrine-induced activation of adenyl cyclase activity (238). Administration of estradiol for 3 days to ovariectomized rats decreased norepinephrine stimulation of adenyl cyclase activity. The effectiveness of steroids to modulate pineal norepinephrine-related synthetic activity varies as a function of time of day in a fashion paralleling circadian changes in norepinephrine levels in the rat pineal gland (262).

Pineal norepinephrine levels regulate the synthesis of pineal androgen and estrogen receptor proteins. Uptake and high affinity binding of gonadal steroids is substantially diminished in chronically ganglionectomized rats (262,263). Administration of norepinephrine or isoproterenol to ganglionectomized rats resulted in a return of receptor sites for androgens and estrogens to normal levels. This restorative effect was blocked by pretreatment with propranolol or actinomycin D, but not by phentolamine. A similar, stimulatory effect of isoproterenol on cytoplasmic steroid receptors was observed in vitro. These results support the idea that steroid receptors are found in pinealocytes and not pineal nerve terminals.

Various studies have reported the presence of progesterone receptor binding sites in the pineal gland having properties similar to those of this steroid's receptor complexes in the uterus, hypothalamus, and pituitary gland (252,264–266). Incubation of rat pineal glands with progesterone (10 µg/ml) decreased the stimulatory effect of isoproterenol to increase melatonin synthesis and secretion (267). In contrast, progesterone had no effect on norepinephrine-induced increases in pineal adenyl cyclase activity or on estradiol inhibition of noradrenergic activity within the castrate rat pineal gland (268). Thus the pineal gland represents an exception to the premise that progesterone acts jointly with estrogens to affect neuroendocrine target organs in castrated females.

Because of the strong interactions between gonadal steroids and pineal noradrenergic innervation, these hormones might also be expected to exert a strong influence on pineal serotonin N-acetyltransferase activity considering the close relationship between pineal beta-adrenergic receptors and this enzyme. However, daily changes in the activity of this enzyme are apparently independent of changes in the rat estrous cycle (241,168). NAT activity was not influenced by injection of estradiol (10 µg/day) for 3 days into ovariectomized rats (269). This study reported further that estradiol treatment was unable to alter isoproterenol-stimulation of pineal NAT activity. Thus, whereas pineal HIOMT activity responds readily to changes in the hormonal milieu, pineal NAT activity does not (270).

Influence of Pituitary Gonadotrophins

The changes in pineal synthetic activity following castration could obviously involve reduced gonadal steroid levels or increased pituitary gonadotrophin levels. Hypophysectomy of male rats has been shown to decrease pineal HIOMT activity (271,272). However, subsequent treatment with human chorionic gonadotrophin failed to restore the reduced activity of this enzyme. Gonadotrophin (FSH/LH) treatment can influence pineal cAMP content (273), MAO activity (274), serotonin and nor-

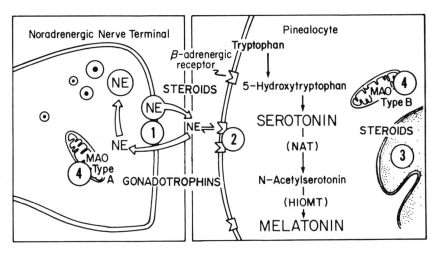

FIGURE 12. Proposed sites of action by which reproductive steroids and gonadotrophins influence pineal melatonin biosynthesis. Gonadal steroids may regulate norepinephrine turnover (1), norepinephrine stimulation of beta-adrenergic receptors (2), nuclear expression leading to protein synthesis (3), and monoamine oxidase activity (4). Gonadotrophins may affect cyclic AMP levels (2) and monoamine oxidase activity (4). Other sites of action for these hormones could also exist within the pineal gland. The net effect of steroids (low doses) or gonadotrophins is to increase HIOMT activity and, thereby, melatonin production. Paradoxically, NAT activity does not seem to be affected by these hormones.

epinephrine turnover (171), and HIOMT activity (262,275). Treatment with 400 μg/day of LH, FSH, or PRL for 4 days of acutely or chronically castrated rats substantially increased pineal HIOMT activity (262,275). This effect was nullified by prior superior cervical ganglionectomy (275) or by bretylium or guanethidine administration (274) suggesting that the pituitary hormones influence HIOMT activity by altering norepinephrine metabolism. Obviously, the effects of castration and steroid treatment may be mediated by related changes in pituitary gonadotrophin levels. The various sites whereby gonadal steroids and pituitary gonadotrophins may influence melatonin production are summarizied in Figure 12.

Melatonin and Other Antigonadotrophins

Because melatonin and related methoxyindoles may be secreted by extra-pineal tissues such as the retinas, Harderian glands, and intestinal mucosa (104,248), these compounds should be considered potential hormones capable of influencing pineal synthetic activity. Melatonin injections, depending on the time of day at which they are given, inhibit the daily rhythms in rat pineal serotonin levels (141). In contrast, twice daily (morning/afternoon) injections of melatonin into male rats for 2 weeks produced dose-dependent increases both in pineal NAT and HIOMT activity (147). The lack of an effect on norepinephrine turnover by melatonin injection suggested that exogenously injected melatonin acted directly on the pinealocyte (247,248).

Single injection of adult male rats either at 1100 h or 2300 h (12:12 LD; lights on 0600 h) with 100 μg melatonin, 100 μg N-acetylserotonin, or 5 μg arginine vasotocin reportedly failed to elicit changes in pineal melatonin levels measured during either the light (1200 h) or the dark period (2400 h) (276). Although passive immunization against circulating melatonin likewise failed to alter pineal melatonin levels, active immunization against this methoxyindole slightly augmented the normal rise in pineal melatonin levels at night.

CONCLUDING REMARKS

At this point it may be well to reiterate that, although the pineal gland has potent effects on the reproductive system of some species, its overall influence in the organism may be somewhat broader than merely a regulator of sexual physiology. The pineal gland, because it has the capability of responding to seasonal changes in daylength, keeps the organism properly synchronized with the external environment. Most animals exhibit various physiological adjustments throughout the course of a year, e.g., there may be changes in temperature regulation, metabolism, endocrine activity. Many of these functions may depend on the photoperiod acting by way of the pineal gland.

In specific reference to reproduction, the changing activity of the pineal allows the animals not only to respond to a given season but, in fact, to anticipate the environmental conditions in the future months and respond accordingly. Since in some species a chief function of the pineal gland seems to be mediation of seasonal reproduction, in these animals the gland may well ensure survival of the species by, in essence, guaranteeing that the young are born at the optimal times of the year (the spring and early summer). Without the pineal to signal them as to the prevailing photoperiod, animals would indiscriminately breed without regard to the environment; some young would be born at times (e.g., winter) not conducive to their survival.

Although the hormonal envoy of the pineal gland has been debated for years, melatonin has captured much of the investigative effort. This relates to the fact that this indole is an extremely potent regulator of reproduction. In fact, it is capable of duplicating many of the effects of short-day exposure on the neuroendocrine-reproductive axis. Some workers continue to investigate other indoles and polypeptides in reference to their reproductive consequences. This is a wise decision considering the multitude of actions of the pineal gland; it would seem likely that the pineal produces and secretes more than one hormonal constituent.

REFERENCES

1. Bardasano Rubio J L. *In* La Glandula Pineal, H Blieme, Madrid, 1979, pp 111–164.
2. Vollrath L. *In* The Pineal Organ. Springer, Berlin, 1981, pp 12–44.
3. Reiter R J. The pineal and its hormones in the control of reproduction in mammals. Endocrinol Rev 1:109–131, 1980.
4. Ralph C F, Firth B, Gern W A, Owens D W. The pineal complex and thermoregulation. Biol Rev 54:47–72, 1979.
5. Armstrong S, Ng K T, Coleman G J. Influence of the pineal gland on brain-behavior relationships.*In* The Pineal Gland, Vol. 3. Extra-Reproductive Effects, ed R J Reiter. CRC Press, Boca Raton, Florida, 1982.
6. Milcu I, Nanu L. Glanda Pineala ca Organ Metabolic, Editura Academiei Republicu Socialiste Românìa, Bucharest, 1979.
7. Kitay J I, Altschule M D. The Pineal Gland, Harvard University Press. Cambridge, Massachusetts, 1954.
8. Thieblot L, Le Bars H. La Glande Pinéale ou Épiphyse, Librarie Malein, Paris, 1955.
9. Reiter R J. Interaction of photoperiod, pineal and seasonal reproduction as exemplified by findings in the hamster.*In* The Pineal and Reproduction, ed R J Reiter. Karger, Basel, 1978, pp 169–190.
10. Hoffmann K. Effects of short photoperiods on puberty, growth and moult in the Djungarian hamster *(Phodopus sungorus)*. J Reprod Fertil 54:29–35, 1978.
11. Lynch G R, Epstein A L. Melatonin induced changes in gonads, pelage and thermogenic characters in the white-footed mouse, *Peromycus leucopus*. Comp Biochem Physiol 53C:67–68, 1977.
12. Petterborg L J, Reiter R J. Effect of photoperiod and melatonin on testicular development in the white footed mouse, *Peromycus leucopus*. J Reprod Fertil 60:209–212, 1980.
13. Grocock C A. Effects of age on photo-induced testicular regression, recrudescence, and refractoriness in the short-tailed field vole Microtus agrestis. Biol Reprod 23:15–20, 1980.
14. Reiter R J, Sorrentino S Jr. Factors influential in determining the gonad-inhibiting activity of the pineal gland.*In* The Pineal Gland, eds GEW Wolstenholme, J Knight. Churchill Livingstone, London, 1971, pp. 329–340.
15. Czyba J C, Girod C, Durand N. Sur l'antagonisme épiphysohypophysaire et les variations saisonnieres de la spermatogénèse chez le hamster doré *(Mesocricetus auratus)*. C R Seanc Soc Biol 158:742–745, 1964.
16. Hoffman R A, Reiter R J. Pineal gland: influence on gonads of male hamsters. Science 142:1609–1611, 1965.
17. Hoffman R A, Reiter R J. Influence of compensatory mechanisms and the pineal gland on dark-induced gonadal atrophy in male hamsters. Nature 203:658–659, 1964.
18. Hoffman R A, Hester R J, Towns C. Effect of light and temperature on the endocrine system of the golden hamster *(Mesocricetus auratus*, Waterhouse). Comp Biochem Physiol 15:525–533, 1965.
19. Hoffman R A, Reiter R J. Responses of some endocrine organs of female hamsters to pinealectomy and light. Life Sci 5:1147–1151, 1966.
20. Reiter R J, Hester R J. Interrelationships of the pineal gland, the superior cervical ganglia and the photoperiod in the regulation of the endocrine systems of hamsters. Endocrinology 79:1168–1170, 1966.
21. Gaston S, Menaker M. Photoperiodic control of hamster testes. Science 158:925–928, 1967.
22. Reiter R J. Morphological studies on the reproductive organ of blinded male hamsters and the effects of pinealectomy or superior cervical ganglionectomy. Anat Rec 160:13–24, 1968.

23. Reiter R J. Influence of pinealectomy on the breeding capability of hamsters maintained under natural photoperiodic and temperature conditions. Neuroendocrinology 13:366–370, 1973–74.

24. Sorrentino S Jr, Reiter R J. Pineal-induced alteration of estrous cycles in blinded hamsters. Gen Comp Endocrinol 15:39–42, 1970.

25. Reiter R J, Rudeen P K, Vaughan M K. Restoration of fertility in light-deprived female hamsters by chronic melatonin treatment. J Comp Physiol 111:7–13, 1976.

26. Elliott J. Circadian rhythms and photoperiodic time measurement in mammals. Fed Proc 35:2339–2346, 1976.

27. Reiter R J. Circannual reproductive rhythms in mammals related to photoperiod and pineal function: a review. Chronobiologia 1:365–395, 1974.

28. Reiter R J. Pineal control of a seasonal reproductive rhythm in male golden hamsters exposed to natural daylight and temperature. Endocrinology 92:423–430, 1973.

29. Reiter R J. Changes in the reproductive organs of cold-exposed and light-deprived female hamsters. J Reprod Fertil 16:217–222, 1968.

30. Reiter R J, Johnson L Y. Pineal regulation of immunoreactive luteinizing hormone and prolactin in light-deprived female hamsters. Fertil Steril 25:958–964, 1974.

31. Reiter R J. The effect of pinealectomy, pineal grafts and denervation of the pineal gland on the reproductive organs of male hamsters. Neuroendocrinology 2:138–146, 1967.

32. Herbert J. The role of the pineal gland in the control by light of the reproductive cycle of the ferret.In The Pineal Gland, eds GEW Wolstenholme, J Knight. Churchill Livingstone, London, 1971, pp 303–320.

33. Lincoln G A, Short R V. Seasonal breeding: nature's contraceptive. Recent Prog Horm Res 36:1–52, 1980.

34. Hoffmann K. Pineal involvement in the phosoperiodic control of reproduction and other functions in the Djungarian hamster Phodopus sungorus. In The Pineal Gland, Vol. 2. Reproductive Effects, ed R J Reiter. CRC Press, Boca Raton, Florida, 1981, pp 83–102.

35. Petterborg L J, Reiter R J, Brainard G C. Ovarian response of pinealectomized and intact white-footed mice kept under naturally short photoperiods. Experientia 37:247, 1981.

36. Plotka E D, Seal U S, Verme Y J. Morphologic and metabolic consequences of pinealectomy in deer.In The Pineal Gland, Vol. 3. Extra-Reproductive Effects, ed R J Reiter. CRC Press, Boca Raton, Florida, 1982.

37. Relkin R. Pineal function relation to absolute darkness and sexual maturation. Am J Physiol 213:999–1002, 1967.

38. Turek F W, Campbell C S. Photoperiodic regulation of neuroendocrine-gonadal activity. Biol Reprod 20:32–50, 1979.

39. Zucker I, Johnston P G, Frost D. Comparative, physiological and biochronometric analyses of rodent seasonal reproductive cycles.In Seasonal Reproduction in Higher Vertebrates, eds R J Reiter, B K Follet. Karger, Basel, 1980, pp 102–133.

40. Reiter R J. The pineal gland and gonadal development in male rats and hamsters. Fertil Steril 19:1009–1017, 1968.

41. Relkin R. The pineal gland. N Engl J Med 274:944–950, 1966.

42. Relkin R. The Pineal. Eden, Montreal, 1976.

43. Wragg L E. Effects of pinealectomy in the newborn female rat. Am J Anat 120:391–402, 1967.

44. Reiter R J. Pineal regulation of the hypothalamicopituitary axis: gonadotrophins.In Handbook of Physiology, Endocrinology IV, Part 2, ed E Knobil, W H Sawyer. American Physiological Society, Washington, D.C., 1974, pp 519–550.

45. Blask D E, Nodelman J C. Antigonadotrophic and prolactin-inhibitory effects of melatonin in anosmic male rats. Neuroendocrinology 29:406–409, 1979.

46. Reiter R J, Petterborg L J, Trakulrungsi C, Trakulrungsi W K. Surgical removal of the olfactory bulbs increases sensitivity of the reproductive system of female rats to the inhibitory effects of late afternoon melatonin injections. J Exp Zool 212:47–52, 1980.

47. Nelson R J, Zucker I. Photoperiodic control of reproduction in olfactory-bulbectomized rats. Neuroendocrinology 32:266–271, 1981.

48. Berndtson W E, Desjardins C. Circulating LH and FSH levels and testicular function in hamsters during light deprivation and subsequent photoperiodic stimulation. Endocrinology 95:195–205, 1974.

49. Tamarkin L, Hutchinson J S, Goldman B D. Regulation of serum gonadotrophins by photoperiod and testicular hormone in the Syrian hamster. Endocrinology 99:1528–1533, 1976.

50. Turek F W, Alvis J D, Elliott J A, Menaker M. Temporal distribution of serum levels of LH and FSH in adult male golden hamsters exposed to long or short days. Biol Reprod 14:630–631, 1976.

51. Goldman B, Brown S. Sex differences in serum LH and FSH patterns in hamsters exposed to short photoperiod. J Steroid Biochem 11:531–535, 1979.

52. Reiter R J, Johnson L Y. Depressant action of the pineal gland on pituitary luteinizing hormone and prolactin in male hamsters. Horm Res 5:311–320, 1974.

53. Reiter R J, Vaughan M K, Blask D E, Johnson L Y. Pineal methoxyindoles: new evidence concerning their function in the control of pineal-mediated changes in the reproductive physiology of male golden hamsters. Endocrinology 96:206–213, 1975.

54. Greenwald G S. Histological transformation of the ovary of the lactating hamster. Endocrinology 77:641–647, 1965.

55. Reiter R J. Pineal function in long term blinded male and female golden hamsters. Gen Comp Endocrinol 12:460–468, 1969.

56. Seegal R F, Goldman B D. Effects of photoperiod on cyclicity and serum gonadotrophins in the Syrian hamster. Biol Reprod 12:233–239, 1975.

57. Bartke A, Craft B T, Dalterio S. Prolactin restores plasma testosterone levels and stimulates testicular growth in hamsters exposed to short day-length. Endocrinology 97:1601–1604, 1975.

58. Bartke A, Smith M S, Dalterio S. Reversal of short photoperiod-induced sterility in male hamsters by ectopic pituitary homografts. Int J Androl 2:257–265, 1979.

59. Bex F J, Bartke A, Goldman B D, Dalterio S. Prolactin, growth hormone, luteinizing hormone receptors, and seasonal changes in testicular activity in the golden hamster. Endocrinology 103:2069–2074, 1978.

60. Matthews M J, Benson B, Richardson D A. Partial maintenance of testes and accessory organs in blinded hamsters by homoplastic anterior pituitary grafts or exogenous prolactin. Life Sci 23:1311–1317, 1978.

61. Reiter R J, Ferguson B N. Delayed-reproductive regression in male hamsters bearing intrarenal pituitary homografts and kept under natural winter photoperiods. J Exp Zool 209:175–180, 1979.

62. Chen H J, Reiter R J. The combination of twice daily luteinizing hormone-releasing factor administration and renal pituitary homografts restores normal reproductive organ size in male hamsters with pineal-mediated gonadal atrophy. Endocrinology 106:1382–1385, 1980.

63. Sadlier R M F S. The Ecology of Reproduction in Wild and Domestic Mammals. Methuen, London, 1969.

64. Reiter R J. Comparative physiology: pineal gland. Annu Rev Physiol 35:305–328, 1973.

65. Reiter R J. The pineal gland and seasonal reproductive adjustments. Int J Biometeorol 19:282–288, 1975.

66. Reiter R J. Evidence for refractoriness of the pituitary-gonadal axis to the pineal gland in golden hamsters and its possible implications in annual reproductive rhythms. Anat Rec 173:365–372, 1972.

67. Reiter R J. Exogenous and endogenous control of the annual reproductive cycle in the male golden hamster: participation of the pineal gland. J Exp Zool 191:111–120, 1975.

68. Turek F W, Elliott J A, Alvis J D, Menaker M. Effect of prolonged exposure to non-stimulatory photoperiods on the activity of the neuroendocrine testicular axis of golden hamsters. Biol Reprod 13:475–481, 1975.

69. Zucker I, Morin L P. Photoperiodic influence on testicular regression, recrudescence and the induction of scotorefractoriness in male golden hamsters. Biol Reprod 17:493–498, 1977.

70. Bittman E L. Hamster refractoriness: Role of insensitivity of pineal target tissues. Science 202:648–649, 1978.

71. Stetson M H, Matt K S, Watson-Whitmyre M. Photoperiodism and reproduction in golden hamsters: circadian organization and the termination of photorefractoriness. Biol Reprod 14:531–542, 1976.

72. Rollag M D, Panke E S, Reiter R J. Pineal melatonin content in male hamsters throughout the seasonal reproductive cycle. Proc Soc Exp Biol Med 165:330–334, 1980.

73. Goodwin R L, Karsch F J. Control of seasonal breeding in the ewe: importance of changes in response to sex-steroid feedback.In Seasonal Reproduction in Higher Vertebrates, ed R J Reiter. Karger, Basel, 1980, pp 134–154.

74. Lerner A B, Case J D, Takahashi Y, Lee T H, Mori W. Isolation of melatonin, the pineal gland factor that lightens melanocytes. J Am Chem Soc 80:2587, 1958.

75. Birau N, Schloot W. Melatonin—Current Status and Perspectives. Pergamon, New York, 1981.

76. Lerner A B, Case J D, Heinzelman R V. Structure of melatonin. J Am Chem Soc 81:6084, 1959.

77. Lewy A J, Markey S P. Analysis of melatonin in human plasma by gas chromatography negative chemical ionization mass spectrometry. Science 201:741–743, 1978.

78. Greiner A C, Chan S C. Melatonin content of the human pineal gland. Science 199:83–84, 1978.

79. Cattabeni F, Koslow S H, Costa E. Gas chromatographic-mass spectrometric assay of four indole alkylamines of rat pineal. Science 178:166–168, 1972.

80. Smith I, Mullen P F, Silman R E, Snedden W, Wilson B. The absolute identification of melatonin in human plasma and CSF. Nature 260:718–719, 1976.

81. Wilson B W. The application of mass spectrometry to the study of the pineal gland. J Neural Transm Suppl 13:279–288, 1978.

82. Wilson B W, Snedden W, Silman R E, Smith I, Mullen P. A gas chromatographic mass spectrometry method for the quantitative analysis of melatonin in plasma and cerebrospinal fluid. Anal Biochem 81:283–291, 1977.

83. Silman R E, Leone R M, Hooper R J L, Preece M A. Melatonin, the pineal gland and human puberty. Nature 282:301–303, 1979.

84. Cole E R, Crank G. Tryptamines III: the estimation of melatonin in blood serum. Biochem Med 8:37–43, 1973.

85. Miller F P. Maickel R P. Fluorometric determination of indole derivatives. Life Sci 9:747–752, 1970.

86. Quay W B. Differential extractions for the spectrophotofluorometric measurement of diverse 5-hydroxy- and 5-methoxyindoles. Anal Biochem 5:51–59, 1963.

87. Rollag M D. Methods for measuring pineal hormones.In The Pineal Gland, vol. 1. Anatomy and Biochemistry, ed R J Reiter. CRC Press, Boca Raton, Florida, 1981, pp 273–299.

88. Vivien-Roels B, Pévet P, Dubois M P, Arendt J, Brown G M. Immunohistochemical evidence for the presence of melatonin in the pineal gland, the retina and the Harderian gland. Cell Tiss Res 217:105–115, 1981.

89. Panke E S, Rollag M D, Reiter R J. Pineal melatonin concentrations in the hamster. Endocrinology 104:194–197, 1979.

90. Petterborg L J, Richardson B A, Reiter R J. Effect of long or short photoperiod on pineal melatonin content in the white-footed mouse, Peromyscus leucopus. Life Sci 29:1623–1627, 1981.

91. Reiter R J, Rudeen P K, Banks A F, Rollag M D. Acute effects of unilateral or bilateral superior cervical ganglionectomy on rat pineal N-acetyltransferase activity and melatonin content. Experientia 35:691–692, 1979.

92. Reiter R J, Johnson L Y, Steger R W, Richardson B A, Petterborg L J. Pineal biosynthetic activity and neuroendocrine physiology in the aging hamster and gerbil. Peptides 1:69–77, 1980.

93. Reiter R J, Richardson B A, Hurlbut E C. Pineal, retinal and Harderian gland melatonin in a diurnal species, the Richardson's ground squirrel (Spermophilus richardsonii). Neurosci Lett 22:285–288, 1981.

94. Rollag M D, Chen H J, Ferguson B N, Reiter R J. Pineal melatonin content throughout the hamster estrous cycle. Proc Soc Exp Biol Med 162:211–213, 1979.

95. Rollag M D, Panke E S, Trakulrungsi W K, Trakulrungsi C, Reiter R J. Quantitation of daily melatonin synthesis in the hamster pineal gland. Endocrinology 106:231–236, 1980.

96. Tamarkin L, Reppert S M, Klein D C. Regulation of pineal melatonin in the Syrian hamster. Endocrinology 104:385–389, 1979.

97. Tamarkin L, Reppert S M, Klein D C, Pratt B, Goldman, B D. Studies on the daily pattern of pineal melatonin in the Syrian hamster. Endocrinology 107:1525–1529, 1980.

98. Bubenik G A, Brown G M, Uhlir I, Grota L J. Immunohistological localization of N-acetylindolalkylamines in pineal gland, retina and cerebellum. Brain Res 81:233–242, 1974.

99. Freund D, Arendt J, Vollrath L. Tentative immunohistochemical demonstration of melatonin in the rat pineal gland. Cell Tiss Res 181:239–244, 1977.

100. Quay W B. Pineal Chemistry. Charles C Thomas, Springfield, Illinois, 1974.

101. Ozaki Y, Lynch H J. Presence of melatonin in plasma and urine of pinealectomized rats. Endocrinology 99:641–644, 1976.

102. Kennaway D J, Frith R G, Phillipou G, Matthews C D, Seamark R F. A specific radioimmunoassay for melatonin in biological tissue and fluids and its validation by gas chromatography-mass spectrometry. Endocrinology 101:119–127, 1977.

103. Pang S F, Brown G M, Grota L J, Chambers J W, Rodman R L. Determination of N-acetylserotonin and melatonin activities in the pineal gland, retina, Harderian gland, brain and serum of rats and chickens. Neuroendocrinology 23:1–13, 1977.

104. Bubenik G A, Brown G M, Grota L J. Differential localization of N-acetylated indolealkylamines in CNS and the Harderian gland using immunohistology. Brain Res 118:417–427, 1976.

105. Bubenik G A, Brown G M, Grota L J. Immunohistochemical localization of melatonin in the rat Harderian gland. J Histochem Cytochem 24:1173–1177, 1976.

106. Bubenik G A, Brown G M, Grota L J. Immunohistological localization of melatonin in the rat digestive system. Experientia 33:662–663, 1977.

107. Cardinali D P, Wurtman R J. Hydroxyindole-O-methyl transferases in rat pineal, retina and Harderian gland. Endocrinology 91:247–252, 1972.

108. Reiter R J, Vaughan M K, Vaughan G M, Sorrentino S Jr, Donofrio R J. The pineal gland as an organ of internal secretion.In Frontiers of Pineal Physiology, ed M D Altschule. MIT Press, Cambridge, Massachusetts, 1975, pp 54–174.

109. Wurtman R J, Axelrod J, Chu E W. Melatonin, a pineal substance: effect on the rat ovary. Science 141:277–278, 1963.

110. Sorrentino S, Reiter R J, Schalch D S. Hypotrophic reproductive organs and normal growth in male rats treated with melatonin. J Endocrinol 51:213–214, 1971.

111. Banks A F, Reiter R J. Melatonin inhibition of pineal antigonadotrophic activity in male rats. Horm Res 6:351–356, 1975.

112. Brackmann M. Melatonin delays puberty in the Djungarian hamster. Naturwissenschaften 64:642–643, 1975.

113. Reiter R J, Sorrentino S, Hoffman R A. Early photoperiodic conditions and pineal antigonadic function in male hamster. Int J Fertil 12:163–170, 1970.

114. Turek F. Effect of melatonin on photic-independent and photic-dependent testicular growth in juvenile and adult male golden hamsters. Biol Reprod 20:1119–1122, 1979.

115. Rissman E F. Prepubertal sensitivity to melatonin in male hamsters. Biol Reprod 22:277–280, 1980.

116. Turek F. Antigonadal effect of melatonin in pinealectomized and intact male hamsters. Proc Soc Exp Biol Med 155:31–34, 1977.

117. Martin J E, Sattler C. Developmental loss of the acute inhibitory effect of melatonin on the in vitro pituitary LH and FSH responses to LH-releasing hormone. Endocrinology 105:1007–1012, 1979.

118. Martin J E, Klein D C. Melatonin inhibition of the neonatal pituitary response to luteinizing hormone-releasing factor. Science 191:301–302, 1976.

119. Martin J E, Engel J N, Klein D C. Inhibition of the in vitro pituitary response to luteinizing hormone-releasing hormone by melatonin, serotonin, and 5-methoxytryptamine. Endocrinology 100:675–680, 1977.

120. Martin J E, McKellar S, Klein D C. Melatonin inhibition of the in vivo pituitary response to luteinizing hormone-releasing hormone in the neonatal rat. Neuroendocrinology 31:13–17, 1980.

121. Mieno M, Yamashita Er, Iimori M, Yamashita K. An inhibitory effect of melatonin on the luteinizing hormone releasing activity of luteinizing hormone releasing hormone in immature male dogs. J Endocrinol 78:283–284, 1978.

122. Yamashita K, Mieno M, Shimizu T, Yamashita Er. Inhibition by melatonin of the pituitary response to luteinizing hormone releasing hormone in vivo. J Endocrinol 76:487–491, 1978.

123. Bacon A, Sattler C, Martin J E. Melatonin effect on the hamster pituitary response to LHRH. Biol Reprod 24:993–999, 1981.

124. Klein D C, Lines S V. Pineal hydroxyindole-O-methyl transferase activity in the growing rat. Endocrinology 84:1523–1525, 1969.

125. Reppert S M, Klein D C. Transport of maternal [^{3}H]melatonin to suckling rats and the fate of [^{3}H]melatonin in the neonatal rat. Endocrinology 102:582–588, 1978.

126. Klein D C. Evidence for the placental transfer of ^{3}H-acetyl-melatonin. Nature 237:117–118, 1972.

127. Vaughan M K, Vaughan G M, O'Steen W K. Pituitary, adrenal, pineal and renal weights in offspring of rats treated with testosterone and/or melatonin during pregnancy. J Endocrinol 51:211–212, 1971.

128. Cardinali D P. Melatonin and the endocrine role of the pineal gland. In Current Topics in Experimental Endocrinology, Vol 2, eds VHT James, L Martini. Academic, New York, 1974, pp 107–128.

129. Wurtman R J, Axelrod J, Kelly D E. The Pineal. Academic, New York, 1968.

130. Turek F, Desjardins C, Menaker M. Differential effects of melatonin on the testes of photoperiodic and nonphotoperiodic rodents. Biol Reprod 15:94–97, 1976.

131. Motta M, Fraschini F, Martini L. Endocrine effects of pineal gland and of melatonin. Proc Soc Exp Biol Med 126:431–435, 1967.

132. Debeljuk L. Effect of melatonin on the gonadotrophic function of the male rat under constant illumination. Endocrinology 84:937–939, 1969.

133. Kinson G A, Robinson S. Gonadal function of immature male rats subjected to light restriction, melatonin administration and removal of the pineal gland. J Endocrinol 47:391–392, 1970.

134. Longenecker D E, Gallo D G. The inhibition of PMSG-induced ovulation in immature rats by melatonin. Proc Soc Exp Biol Med 137:623–625, 1971.

135. Reiter R J, Sorrentino S Jr. Inhibition of luteinizing hormone release and ovulation in PMS-treated rats by peripherally administered melatonin. Contraception 4:385–392, 1971.

136. Thiéblot L, Blaise S. Étude biochimique du principe pinéal antigonadotrope. Probl Actuels Endocrinol Nutr 10:257–275, 1966.

137. Tilstra B, Prop N. On the possible function of melatonin. Acta Morphol Neerl Scand 5:289–290, 1962.

138. Ebels I, Prop N. A study of the effect of melatonin on the gonads, the oestrous cycle and the pineal organ of the rat. Acta Endocrinol (Kbh) 49:567–577, 1965.

139. Kunkel A. The influence of melatonin on the male gonad in Sprague-Dawley rats. Pol Endocrinol 20:32–35, 1969.

140. Tamarkin L, Westrom W K, Hamill A I, Goldman B D. Effect of melatonin on the reproductive systems of male and female Syrian hamsters: a diurnal rhythm in sensitivity to melatonin. Endocrinology 99:1534–1541, 1976.

141. Fiske V M, Huppert L C. Melatonin action on pineal varies with photoperiod. Science 162:279, 1978.

142. Trakulrungsi C, Reiter R J, Trakulrungsi W K, Vaughan M K, Waring-Ellis P J. Interaction of daily injections and subcutaneous reservoirs of melatonin on the reproductive physiology of female Syrian hamsters. Acta Endocrinol 91:59–69, 1979.

143. Reiter R J, Rudeen P K, Sackman J W, Vaughan M K, Johnson L Y, Little J C. Subcutaneous melatonin implants inhibit reproductive atrophy in male hamsters induced by daily melatonin injections. Endocrinol Res Commun 4:35–44, 1977.

144. Trakulrungsi C, Reiter R J, Trakulrungsi W K, Vaughan M K, Johnson L Y. Effects of injections and/or subcutaneous implants of melatonin on pituitary and plasma levels of LH, FSH and PRL in ovariectomized Syrian hamsters. Ann Biol Biochem Biophys 19:1647–1654, 1979.

145. Sackman J W, Little J C, Rudeen P K, Waring P J, Reiter R J. The effects of pineal indoles given late in the light period on reproductive organs and pituitary prolactin levels in male golden hamsters. Horm Res 8:84–92, 1977.

146. Reiter R J, Blask D E, Johnson L Y, Rudeen P K, Vaughan M K, Waring P J. Melatonin inhibition of reproduction in the male hamster: its dependency on time of day of administration and on an intact and sympathetically innervated pineal gland. Neuroendocrinology 22:107–116, 1976.

147. Freire F, Cardinali D P. Effects of melatonin treatment and environmental lighting on the ultrastructural appearance, melatonin synthesis, norepinephrine turnover and microtubule protein content of the rat pineal gland. J Neural Transm 37:237–257, 1975.

148. El-Domeiri A A, Das Gupta T K. The influence of pineal ablation and administration of melatonin on growth and spread of hamster melanoma. J Surg Oncol 8:197–205, 1976.

149. Barrat G F, Nadakavukaren M J, Frehn J L. Effect of melatonin implants on gonadal weight and pineal gland fine structure of the golden hamster. Tiss Cell 9:335–345, 1977.

150. Benson B, Krasovich M. Circadian rhythms in the number of granulated vesicles in mouse pinealocytes. Anat Rec 187:536, 1977.

151. Knigge K M, Sheridan M N. Pineal function in hamsters bearing melatonin antibodies. Life Sci 19:1235–1238, 1976.

152. Brown G M, Basinska J, Bubenik G, Sibony D, Grota L J, Stancer H C. Gonadal effects of pinealectomy and immunization against N-acetylindole-alkylamines in the hamster. Neuroendocrinology 22:289–297, 1976.

153. Pavel S. Arginine vaosotocin as a pineal hormone. In The Pineal Gland, eds I Nir, R J Reiter, R J Wurtman. Springer, Vienna, 1978, pp 135–156.

154. Tamarkin L, Hollister C W, Lefebvre N G, Goldman B D. Melatonin induction of gonadal quiescence in pinealectomized Syrian hamsters. Science 198:953–955, 1977.

155. Goldman B, Hall V, Hollister C, Roychoundbury P, Tamarkin L, Westrom W. Effects of melatonin on the reproductive system in intact and pinealectomized male hamsters maintained under various photoperiods. Endocrinology 104:82–88, 1979.

156. Hoffmann K. Testicular involution in short photoperiods inhibited by melatonin. Naturwissenschaften 61:364–365, 1974.

157. Reiter R J, Vaughan M K, Blask D E, Johnson L Y. Melatonin: its inhibition of pineal antigonadotrophic activity in male hamsters. Science 185:1169–1171, 1974.

158. Reiter R J. Anti- and counter antigonadotrophic effects of melatonin: an apparent paradox. *In* Brain-Endocrine Interaction III, Neural Hormones and Reproduction, eds D E Scott, G P Kozlowski, A Weindl. Karger, Basel, 1978, pp 344–355.

159. Turek F W, Desjardins C, Menaker M. Melatonin: antigonadal and progonadal effects in male golden hamsters. Science 190:280–282, 1975.

160. Reiter R J, Vaughan M K, Rudeen P K, Vaughan G M, Waring P J. Melatonin-pineal relationships in female golden hamsters. Proc Soc Exp Biol Med 149:290–293, 1975.

161. Chen H J, Reiter R J. Influence of subcutaneous deposits of melatonin on the antigonadotrophic effects of blinding and anosmia in male rats. A dose-response study. Neuroendocrinology 30:169–173, 1980.

162. Reiter R J, Vaughan M K, Waring P J. Studies on the minimal dosage of melatonin required to inhibit pineal antigonadotrophic activity in male golden hamsters. Horm Res 6:258–267, 1975.

163. Cutty G B, Goldman B D, Doherty P, Bartke A. Melatonin prevents decrease in plasma Prl and LH levels in male hamsters exposed to a short photoperiod. Int J Andrology 4:281–290, 1981.

164. Rust C C, Meyer P K. Hair color, molt, and testis size in male short-tailed weasels treated with melatonin. Science 165:921–922, 1969.

165. Hoffmann K. Melatonin inhibits photoperiodically induced testis development in a dwarf hamster. Naturwissenschaften 59:218–219, 1972.

166. Hoffmann K. The influence of photoperiod and melatonin on testis size, body weight, and pelage colour in the Djungarian hamster *(Phodopus sungorus).* J Comp Physiol 95:267–282, 1973.

167. Hoffmann K. The action of melatonin on testis size and pelage color varies with the season. Int J Chronobiol 1:333, 1973.

168. Reiter R J, Rollag M D, Panke E S, Banks A F. Melatonin: reproductive effects. J Neural Transm Suppl 13:209–223, 1978.

169. Catt K J, Dufau M L. Peptide hormone receptors. Ann Rev Physiol 39:529–557, 1977.

170. Panke E S, Reiter R J, Rollag M D, Panke T W. Pineal serotonin N-acetyltransferase activity and melatonin concentrations in prepubertal and adult Syrian hamsters exposed to short daily photoperiods. Endocrinol Res Commun 5:311–324, 1978.

171. Vacas M I, Cardinali D P. Diurnal changes in melatonin binding sites of hamster and rat brains. Correlation with neuroendocrine responsiveness to melatonin. Neurosci Lett 15:259–263, 1979.

172. Hsueh A J W, Dufau M L, Catt K J. Gonadotropin-induced regulation of luteinizing hormone receptors and desensitization of testicular 3':5'-cyclic AMP and testosterone responses. Proc Natl Acad Sci USA 74:592–595, 1977.

173. Belchetz P E, Plant T M, Nakai Y, Keogh E J, Knobil E. Hypophysial responses to continuous and intermittent delivery of hypothalamic gonadotropin-releasing hormone. Science 202:631–633, 1978.

174. Gavin J R III, Roth J, Neville D M Jr, De Meyts P, Buell D N. Insulin-dependent regulation of insulin receptor concentrations: a direct demonstration in cell culture. Proc Natl Acad Sci USA 71:84–88, 1974.

175. Hinkle P M, Tashjian A H Jr. Thyrotropin-releasing hormone regulates the number of its own receptors in the GH$_3$ strain of pituitary cells in culture. Biochemistry 14:3845–3851, 1975.

176. Richardson B A, Vaughan M K, Brainard G C, Huerter J J, de los Santos R, Reiter R J. Influence of morning melatonin injections on the antigonadotrophic effects of afternoon melatonin administration in male and female hamsters. Neuroendocrinology 33:112–117, 1981.

177. Chen H J, Brainard G C III, Reiter R J. Melatonin given in the morning prevents the suppressive action on the reproductive system of melatonin given in late afternoon. Neuroendocrinology 31:129–132, 1980.

178. Chen H J. Melatonin: failure of pharmacological doses to induce testicular atrophy in the male golden hamster. Life Sci 28:767–771, 1981.

179. Reiter R J. The pineal gland: a regulator of regulators. Psychol 9:323–356, 1980.

180. Vaughan M K. Sexual differentiation of the rat hypothalamus: interaction of pineal amines and steroids. Ph.D. thesis, The University of Texas Medical Branch, Galveston, 1970.

181. Ramaley J A. Development of gonadotropin regulation in the prepubertal mammal. Biol Reprod 20:1–24, 1979.

182. Fraschini F, Collu R, Martini L. Mechanisms of inhibitory action of pineal principles on gonadotropin secretion.*In* The Pineal Gland, eds GEW Wolstenholme, J Knight. Churchill Livingstone, London, 1971, pp 259–273.

183. Iwasaki Y, Kato Y, Ohgo S, Abe H, Imura H, Hiruta F, Senoh S, Tokuyama T, Hayashi D. Effects of indoleamines and their newly identified metabolites on prolactin release in rats. Endocrinology 103:254–258, 1978.

184. Kamberi I A, Mical R S, Porter J C. Effect of anterior pituitary perfusion and intraventricular injection of catecholamines and indoleamines on LH release. Endocrinology 87:1–12, 1970.

185. Kamberi I A, Mical R S, Porter J C. Effects of melatonin and serotonin on the release of FSH and prolactin. Endocrinology 88:1288–1293, 1971.

186. Anton-Tay F, Wurtman R J. Regional uptake of ^{3}H-melatonin from blood or cerebrospinal fluid by rat brain. Nature 221:474–475, 1969.

187. Cardinali D P, Hyyppa M T, Wurtman R J. Fate of intracisternally injected melatonin in the rat brain. Neuroendocrinology 12:30–40, 1973.

188. Green A R, Koslow S H, Costa E. Identification and quantification of a new indolealkylamine in rat hypothalamus. Brain Res 51:371–374, 1973.

189. Fishback J B, Gerall A A, Arimura A, King J C. Effect of photoperiod and melatonin on hypothalamic luteinizing hormone releasing hormone (LH-RH) and on serum gonadotrophin concentrations in intact and castrated male hamsters. Biol Reprod Suppl 1:28A, 1978.

190. Kao L W L, Weisz J. Release of gonadotrophin-releasing hormone (Gn-RH) from isolated, perifused medial-basal hypothalamus by melatonin. Endocrinology 100:1723–1726, 1977.

191. Cardinali D P, Vacas M I, Boyer E E. Specific binding of melatonin in bovine brain. Endocrinology 105:437–441, 1979.

192. Niles L P, Wong Y-W, Mishra R K, Brown G M. Melatonin receptors in brain. Eur J Pharmacol 55:219–220, 1979.

193. Cotzias B C, Tang L C, Miller S I, Ginos J Z. Melatonin and abnormal movements induced by L-dopa in mice. Science 173:450–452, 1971.

194. Fraschini F, Mess B, Piva F, Martini L. Brain receptors sensitive to indole compounds: function in control of luteinizing hormone secretion. Science 159:1104–1105, 1968.

195. Blask D E. Potential sites of actions of pineal hormones within the neuroendocrine-reproductive axis.*In* The Pineal Gland, Vol 2, Reproductive Effects, ed R J Reiter. CRC Press, Boca Raton, Florida, 1981, pp. 189–216.

196. Blask D E, Vaughan M K, Reiter R J, Johnson L Y, Vaughan G M. Prolactin-releasing and release-inhibiting factor activities in the bovine, rat, and human pineal gland: *in vitro* and *in vivo* studies. Endocrinology 99:152–161, 1976.

197. Padmanabhan V, Convey E M, Tucker E A. Pineal compounds alter prolactin release from bovine pituitary cells. Proc Soc Exp Biol Med 160:340–343, 1979.

198. Hipkin L J. Effect of 5-methoxytryptophol and melatonin on uterine weight responses to human chorionic gonadotrophin. J Endocrinol 48:287–288, 1970.

199. Trentini G P, Botticelli A R, Sannicola B C, Barbanti Silva C. Decreased ovarian LH incorporation after melatonin treatment. Horm Metab Res 8:234–236, 1976.

200. Ellis L C. Inhibition of rat testicular androgen synthesis *in vitro* by melatonin and serotonin. Endocrinology 90:17–28, 1972.

201. Peat F, Kinson G A. Testicular steroidogenesis *in vitro* in the rat in response to blinding, pinealectomy and to the addition of melatonin. Steroids 17:251–263, 1971.

202. Kopin I J, Pare C M B, Axelrod J, Weissbach H. The fate of melatonin in animals. J Biol Chem 236:3072–3075, 1964.

203. Wurtman R J, Axelrod J, Potter L T. The uptake of ^{3}H-melatonin in endocrine and nervous tissue and the effects of constant light exposure. J Pharmacol Exp Ther 143:314–318, 1964.

204. Younglai E V. *In vitro* effects of melatonin on HCG stimulation of steroid accumulation by rabbit ovarian follicles. J Steroid Biochem 10:714–715, 1979.

205. Cohen H, Rosselle D, Chabner B, Schmidt T J, Lippman M. Evidence for a cytoplasmic melatonin receptor. Nature 274:894–895, 1978.

206. Rusak B. Suprachiasmatic lesions prevent an antigonadal effect of melatonin. Biol Reprod 22:148–154, 1980.

207. Turek F W, Jacobsen C D, Gorski R A. Lesions of the suprachiasmatic nuclei affect photoperiod-induced changes in the sensitivity of the hypothalamic-pituitary axis to testosterone feedback. Endocrinology 107:942–947, 1980.

208. Reiter R J, Dinh D T, de los Santos R, Guerra J C. Hypothalamic cuts suggest a brain site for the antigonadotrophic actions of melatonin in the Syrian hamster. Neurosci Lett 23:315–318, 1981.

209. Porter J C, Mical R S, Cramer O M. Effect of serotonin and other indoles on the release of LH, FSH, and prolactin. Gynecol Invest 2:13–22, 1971-72.

210. Moskowska A, Scemama A, Lombard M N, Héry M. Experimental modulation of hypothalamic content of the gonadotropic releasing factors by pineal factors in the rat. J Neural Transm 34:11–18, 1973.

211. Vaughan M K, Reiter R J, Vaughan G M, Bigelow L, Altschule M D. Inhibition of compensatory ovarian hypertrophy in the mouse and vole: a comparison of Altschule's pineal extract, pineal indoles, vasopressin and oxytocin. Gen Comp Endocrinol 18:372–377, 1972.

212. Pomerantz G, Reiter R J. Influence of intraocularly-injected pineal indoles on PMS-induced ovulation in immature rats. Int J Fertil 19:117–120, 1974.

213. McIsaac W M, Taborsky R G, Farrell G. 5-methoxytryptophol: effect on estrus and ovarian weight. Science 145:63–64, 1964.

214. Klein D C, Notides A. Thin-layer chromatographic separation of pineal gland derivatives of serotonin-^{14}C. Anal Biochem 31:480–483, 1969.

215. McIsaac W M, Farrell G, Taborsky R G, Taylor A N. Indole compounds: isolation from pineal tissue. Science 148:102–103, 1965.

216. Ebels I, Horwitz-Bresser A E M. Separation of pineal extracts by gel filtration-IV. Isolation, localization and identification from sheep pineals of three indoles. J Neural Transm 38:31–41, 1976.

217. Carter S J, Laud C A, Smith I, Leone R M, Hooper R J, Silman R E, Finnie M D, Mullen P E, Larson-Carter D L. Concentration of 5-methoxytryptophol in pineal gland and plasma of the rat. J Endocrinol 83:35–40, 1979.

218. Carter S J, Laud C A, Smith I, Leone R M, Silman R E, Hooper R J, Larson-Carter D L, Finnie M D, Mullen P F. 5-methoxytryptophol in rat pineal glands and other tissues. Progr Brain Res 52:267–269, 1979.

219. Mullen P E, Leone R M, Hooper J, Smith I, Silman R E, Finnie M, Carter S, Linsell C. Pineal 5-methoxytryptophol in man. Psychoneuroendocrinology 2:117–126, 1979.

220. Curtius H C, Wolfensberger M, Redweik V, Leimbocher W, Mailbach R A, Isler W. Gas fragmentography of 5-hydroxytryptophol and 5-methoxytryptophol in human CSF. J Chromatogr 112:523–531, 1975.

221. Linsell C, Mullen P, Silman R, Leone R, Finney M, Carter S, Hooper R, Smith I, Francis P. The measurement of the daily fluctuations of 5-methoxytryptophol in human plasma. Progr Brain Res 52:501–505, 1978.

222. Smith I, Francis P, Leone R, Mullen P E. Identification of O-acetyl-5-methoxytryptophol in the pineal gland by gas chromatography-mass spectrometry. Biochem J 185:537–540, 1980.

223. Silman R, Hooper R, Leone R, Edwards R, Grudzinskas J, Gordon Y, Chard T, Savage M, Smith I, Mullen P. 5-methoxytryptophol and pituitary function in man. Progr Brain Res 52:507–511, 1978.

224. Cardinali D P, Rosner J J. Retinal localization of HIOMT in the rat. Endocrinology 89:301–310, 1971.

225. Delvigs P, McIsaac W M, Taborsky R G. The metabolism of 5-methoxytryptophol. J Biol Chem 240:348–350, 1965.

226. Hooper R, Silman R, Leone R, Finnie M, Carter S, Grudzinskas J, Gordon Y, Holland D, Chard T, Mullen P, Smith I. Changes in the concentration of circulating 5-methoxytryptophol at different stages of the menstrual cycle. J Endocrinol 82:269–274, 1979.

227. Wetterberg L, Arendt J, Paunier L, Sizonenko P, Van Donselaar W, Heyden T. Human serum melatonin changes during the menstrual cycle. J Clin Endocrinol Metab 42:185–188, 1976.

228. Mas M, Oaknin S. Effects of pineal methoxyindoles on male sex behaviour and spermatogenesis. J Neural Transm Suppl 13:376, 1977.

229. Talbot J A, Reiter R J. Influence of melatonin, 5-methoxytryptophol and pinealectomy on pituitary and plasma gonadotropin and prolactin levels in castrated adult male rats. Neuroendocrinology 13:164–172, 1973-74.

230. Smith I, Larson-Carter D, Laud C, Leone R, Silman S, Carter S, Francis P, Mullen P, Hooper R, Finnie M. O-acetyl-5-methoxytryptophol-tenative identification in pineal glands. Progr Brain Res 52:259–261, 1978.

231. Guchart R. Biogenesis of 5-methoxy-N, N-dimethyltryptamine in human pineal gland. J Neurochem 26:187–190, 1976.

232. Miller F, Maickel R. Fluorometric determination of indole derivatives. Life Sci 9:747–752, 1970.

233. Bosin T, Beck O. 5-methoxytryptamine in the human pineal gland: identification and quantification by mass fragmentography. J Neurochem 32:1853–1855, 1979.

234. Koslow S, Post R, Goodwin F, Gillin C. Mass fragmentographic identification and quantification of 5-methoxytryptamine (5-MT) in human cerebrospinal fluid (CSF). Neurosci Abstr 1:361, 1975.

235. Koslow S. The biochemical and biobehavioral profile of 5-methoxytryptamine. In Trace Amines and the Brain, eds E Usdin, M Sandler. Marcel Dekker, New York, 1976, pp 103–130.

236. DeMontigny C, Aghajanian G. Preferential action of 5-methoxytryptamine and 5-methoxydimethyltryptamine on presynaptic serotonin receptors: a comparative iontophoretic study with LSD and serotonin. Neuropharmacology 16:811–818, 1977.

237. Rollag M D, Irino D S, Litwak A B. Induction of gonadal regression by selected 5-methoxyindole and 5-methoxytryptoline cognates of melatonin. Anat Rec 199:215A, 1981.

238. Weiss B, Crayton J. Gonadal hormones as regulators of pineal adenyl cyclase activity. Endocrinology 87:527–533, 1970.

239. Davis G A. The response of adenosine 3',5'-monophosphate to norepinephrine in the hypothalamus and pineal organ of female rats in proestrus or diestrus. Endocrinology 103:1048–1053, 1978.

240. Wurtman R J, Axelrod J, Snyder S H. Changes in enzymatic synthesis of melatonin in the pineal during the estrous cycle. Endocrinology 76:798–800, 1965.

241. Cardinali D P, Nagle C A, Rosner T M. Changes in the pineal indole metabolism and plasma progesterone levels during the estrous cycle in ewes. Steroids Lipids Res 5:308–315, 1974.

242. Wallen E P, Yochim J M. Pineal HIOMT activity in the rat: effect of ovariectomy and hormone replacement. Biol Reprod 10:474–479, 1974.

243. Shivers B D, Fix J A, Yochim J M. Effect of 6-hydroxydopamine on pineal norepinephrine content and enzyme activity in the cyclic female rat. Biol Reprod 21:393–399, 1979.

244. Quay W B. Circadian rhythm in rat pineal serotonin and its modification by estrous cycle and photoperiod. Gen Comp Endocrinol 3:473–479, 1963.

245. Quay W B. Circadian and estrous rhythms in pineal melatonin and 5-hydroxyindole-3-acetic acid. Proc Soc Exp Biol Med 115:710–712, 1964.

246. Ozaki Y, Wurtman R J, Alonso R, Lynch H J. Melatonin secretion decreases during the proestrous stage of the rat estrous cycle. Proc Natl Acad Sci USA 75:531–534, 1978.

247. Silman R E, Edwards R. 5-methoxytryptophol and human menstrual cycle. Proc. 1st Colloq. Europ. Pineal Study Group, Amsterdam, pp 32–33, 1976.

248. Cardinali D P, Wurtman R J. Hydroxyindole-O-methoxy-transferases in rat pineal, retina and Harderian gland. Endocrinology 91:247–252, 1972.

249. Houssay A B, Barcela A C. Effects of testosterone upon the biosynthesis of melatonin by the pineal gland. Acta Physiol Lat Am 22:274–275, 1972.

250. Houssay A B, Barcela A C. Effects of estrogens and progesterone upon the biosynthesis of melatonin by the pineal gland. Experientia 28:478–479, 1972.

251. Cardinali D P, Nagle C A, Rosner J M. Effect of estradiol on melatonin and protein synthesis in the rat pineal organ. Horm Res 5:304–310, 1974.

252. Cardinali D P, Nagle C A, Rosner J M. Gonadal steroids as modulators of the function of the pineal gland. Gen Comp Endocrinol 26:50–58, 1975a.

253. Cardinali D P. Nuclear receptor estrogen complex in the pineal gland. Modulation by sympathetic nerves. Neuroendocrinology 24:333–346, 1977.

254. Mizobe F, Kurokawa M. Enhancement of hydroxyindole-O-methyltransferase and DNA dependent RNA polymerase activities induced by oestradiol in rat pineals in culture. Eur J Biochem 66:193–199, 1976.

255. Weisz J, O'Brien L V, Lloyd T. Methylation of estradiol-17β by a partially purified preparation of bovine pineal hydroxyindole-O-methyltransferase. Endocrinology 102:330–333, 1978.

256. Nagle C A, Neuspiller N R, Cardinali D P, Rosner J M. Uptake and effect of 17-estradiol on pineal hydroxy-indole-O-methyl transferase (HIOMT) activity. Life Sci 12:1109–1116, 1972.

257. Nagle C A, Cardinali D P, Rosner J M. Effects of castration and testosterone administration on pineal and retinal hydroxyindole-O-methyltransferase of male rats. Neuroendocrinology 14:14–23, 1974.

258. Nagle C A, Cardinali D P, Rosner J M. Testosterone effects on protein synthesis in the rat pineal gland. Modulation by the sympathetic nervous system. Life Sci 16:81–91, 1975.

259. Cardinali D P, Nagle C A, Gomez E, Rosner J M. Norepinephrine turnover in the rat pineal gland. Acceleration by estradiol and testosterone. Life Sci 16:1717–1724, 1975.

260. Cardinali D P, Vacas M I, Valenti C E, Gonzalez-Solveyra C. Pineal gland and sympathetic cervical ganglia as sites for steroid regulation of photosensitive neuroendocrine pathways. J Steroid Biochem 11:951–955, 1979.

261. Semm P, Demaine C, Vollrath L. The effects of microelectrophoretically applied melatonin, putative transmitters, thyroxine and sex hormones on the electrical activity of pineal cells in the guinea pig.In Melatonin—Current Status and Perspectives, Vol. 29, eds N Birau, W Schloot. Pergamon, Oxford, 1980, pp 129–134.

262. Cardinali D P, Nagle C A, Rosner J M. Pineal-gonads relationships. Nature of the feedback mechanism at the level of the pineal gland.In Neuroendocrine Regulation of Fertility, ed T C Anad-Kumar. Karger, Basel, 1975, pp 206–214.

263. Cardinali D P, Nagle C A, Rosner J M. Control of estrogen and androgen receptors in the rat pineal gland by catecholamine transmitter. Life Sci 16:81–91, 1975.

264. Luttge W G, Wallis C G. In vitro accumulation and saturation of H^3-progestins on selected brain regions and in the adenohypophysis, uterus and pineal of the female rat. Steroids 22:493–502, 1973.

265. Hanukoglu I, Karavolas H J, Goy R W. Progesterone metabolism in the pineal gland, brain stem, thalamus and corpus callosum of the female rat. Brain Res 125:313–324, 1977.

266. Karavolas H J, Hodges D R, O'Brien D J, Harnkoglu I. Progesterone and 5α-dihydroprogesterone uptake and metabolism in the pineal of female rats. J Neural Transm Suppl 13:370–371, 1978.

267. Wilkinson M, Arendt J. Effect of oestrogen and progesterone on rat pineal N-acetyltransferase activity and melatonin production. Experientia 34:667–669, 1978.

268. Cardinali D P, Vacas M I. Progesterone-induced decrease of pineal protein synthesis in rats. Possible participation in estrous-related changes of pineal function. J Neural Transm 42:193–205, 1978.

269. Illnerova H. Effect of estradiol on the activity of serotonin N-acetyl-transferase in the rat epiphysis. Endocrinol Exp 9:141–148, 1975.

270. Axelrod J. The pineal gland: a neurochemical transducer. Science 184:1341–1348, 1974.

271. Urry R L, Barfuss D W, Ellis L C. Hydroxyindole-O-methyl transferase activity of male rat pineal glands following hypophysectomy and HCG treatment. Biol Reprod 6:238–243, 1972.

272. Urry R L, Dougherty K A, Frehn J L, Ellis L C. Factors other than light affecting the pineal gland. Hypophysectomy, testosterone, dihydrotestosterone, estradiol, cryptorchidism and stress. Am Zool 16:79–91, 1976.

273. Karasek M, Karasek E. Effect of gonadotropic hormones on the concentration of adenosine 3',5'-monophosphate in the rat pineal organ. Endokrinologie 71:204–205, 1978.

274. Trentini G P, Gaetam C F, Barbieri-Palmeiri F. The role of sympathetic innervation in pineal-pituitary feedback. Ann Endocrinol 34:261–270, 1973.

275. Cardinali D P, Nagle C A, Rosner J M. Gonadotrophin- and prolactin-induced increase in rat pineal hydroxyindole-O-methyltransferase. Involvement of the sympathetic nervous system. J Endocrinol 68:341–342, 1976.

276. Niles L P, Brown G M, Pang S F, Grota L D. Pineal melatonin synthesis following neutralization of circulating N-acetyl-indolealkylamines. Int J Immunopharm 1:213–217, 1979.

DAVID E. BLASK, M.D., Ph.D.

MARY K. VAUGHAN, Ph.D.

RUSSEL J. REITER, Ph.D.

PINEAL PEPTIDES
AND REPRODUCTION

A second school of workers advocates the idea that, other than the indoles, the pineal gland produces and secretes primarily peptidic hormones. Although the two schools are not mutually exclusive, some investigators have been rather insistent that only one chemical family of hormones is produced within the pineal. The view of the present authors is somewhat less restrictive. Considering the plethora of effects of the pineal gland in the mammalian organism (1–3), it would seemingly be naive to assume that there is only one active pineal constituent. Although it may be unduly optimistic to predict that there are as many hormones from the pineal gland as from the anterior pituitary (4), it is equally unwise to attribute all known influences of the pineal gland to a single secretory envoy. If there are more that are pineal hormones, they could have different chemical compositions.

This chapter considers the pineal peptides that have been extracted and partially or totally characterized and reviews their reproductive consequences. The relative scarcity (compared to the commercially available

From the Department of Anatomy, University of Arizona School of Medicine, Tucson, Arizona 85724 (D.E.B.), and the Department of Anatomy, The University of Texas Health Science Center at San Antonio, San Antonio, Texas 78284 (M.K.V. and R.J.R.)

Work by the authors was supported by grants from the National Science Foundation.

inexpensive indoles) of most of the pineal peptides has often made long-term studies either impractical or prohibitively expensive. Thus, as readers peruse this survey, they will readily become aware of the different experimental approaches that have been used to investigate the diverse actions of the peptides. Whereas many of the studies with the indoles required their long-term administration, in the case of the peptides, the majority of the experiments are of the short-term variety.

ARGININE VASOTOCIN (AVT)

Evidence for Its Presence in the Pineal

From an evolutionary standpoint, AVT is perhaps the oldest neuropeptide and represents the archetypical molecule of the principle posterior pituitary hormones of mammalian species, vasopressin (AVP) and oxytocin (OT) (5,6). Whereas the existence of AVT in the pineal gland of nonmammalian vertebrates is uncontested, its presence or absence in the mammalian pineal gland is one of the most controversial and vigorously debated issues in modern pinealology.

It was clear from early studies that bovine and porcine pineal extracts contained a substance with chromatographic as well as bioassay characteristics similar to synthetic AVT (7,8). However, it was not until the early 1970s that the first biochemical and mass spectroscopic evidence emerged indicating that a factor in the bovine pineal gland not only possessed antigonadotrophic activity but was structurally identical with AVT (9). Notwithstanding the lack of the isolation and structural characterization of AVT in the pineals of other species, these findings represented the best argument for the presence of vasotocin in the mammalian pineal gland. Thus, for almost a decade, AVT has enjoyed serious consideration as a putative pineal antigonadotrophic hormone.

With the advent of immunological techniques for detecting vasotocin, it appeared that the confirmation of AVT's existence in the mammalian pineal gland was assured. For example, Bowie and Herbert (10) were the first to immunocytochemically detect the peptide in rat pineal parenchymal cells with an antiserum generated specifically against AVT. Other laboratories have since attempted to measure radioimmunoassayable levels of AVT in rat pineal glands with antisera generated against AVP or OT but showing significant cross-reactivity with AVT. Unfortunately, this indirect immunoassay approach has yielded both positive (11,12) and negative results (13).

In a further attempt to clarify this issue through more refined immunoassay methods, Pévet and colleagues (14) have performed studies with several antisera that are highly specific for AVT and show minimal cross-reactivity with AVP or OT. They have consistently failed to demonstrate the presence of immunoassayable vasotocin in either bovine, rat, hamster, rabbit, or ovine pineal glands. Surprisingly, however, in the pineals of several of these species they were able to detect small quantities of both AVP and OT with antisera specific for these peptides (15). They contend that extrahypothalamic AVP- and OT-containing nerve fibers entering the pineal stalk via the subcommissural organ and/or habenular commissure terminate in the anterior region of the pineal gland (16). Furthermore, immunocytochemical studies revealed that only one out of four AVT-specific antibodies produced a reaction product in rat pineal parenchymal cells (17). It was concluded that this particular antibody recognized an "AVT-like" peptide rather than authentic AVT. Interestingly, the same pineal cells evincing AVT-like immunocytochemical activity also showed a similar reaction product in the presence of antisera to either luteinizing hormone releasing hormone (LHRH), α-melanocyte stimulating hormone (α-MSH), somatostatin, or sheep pineal fraction UM-05R (17).

On the basis of their results, Pévet and colleagues (17) do not endorse AVT as a hormone of the mammalian pineal gland. Instead, they have postulated that a larger molecular weight compound, perhaps a precursor molecule or prohormone, is responsible for any bioassayable or immunodetectable AVT-like activity in the pineal gland. In this regard, it is of interest to recall a report some years ago by Neascu (18) that the bovine pineal gland contained a tetradecapeptide, termed E5, exhibiting AVT-like bioassayable activity and containing the nine amino acid residues of AVT; however, the compound, unfortunately, was not characterized. It has been suggested that this peptide or a similar one may be a prohormone that can be enzymatically cleaved to yield other biologically active peptides (17).

Corroborating the results of the European group, Fernstrom and cohorts (19) and Fisher and Fernstrom (20) recently published immunoassay data that are perhaps the most damaging to AVT's credibility as a mammalian pineal hormone. With a highly specific antiserum to AVT, they measured significant quantities of vasotocin in bovine and rat pineal glands. However, when the pineal extracts were further subjected to reverse-phase, ion-pair, high performance liquid chromatography (HPLC) fractionation, followed by postcolumn radioimmunoassay, they were able to detect only negligible amounts of AVT that were barely above background values. Like Pévet, they too found small, albeit significant, quantities of both AVP and OT in pineal extracts following HPLC fractionation. AVT's niche as a pineal substance appears to be at least partially vindicated, however, by a recent report (21) of its presence in both male and female adult human pineal glands. Although immunoassayable AVP and OT were also detected in much larger quantities than AVT, apparently the AVT immunoreactivity was quite specific and could not be accounted for by cross-reactivity with either AVP or OT.

On the basis of their AVT-bioassay (rat antidiuretic assay, frog bladder hydroosmotic assay) results, Pavel (22) has championed the idea that AVT is in fact the pineal antigonadotrophic hormone of mammals. Compared to adult bovine and rat pineal glands in which vasotocin is localized primarily to the basal region (14), fetal bovine and rat pineal glands contain relatively high levels of the peptide throughout the entire gland

(23,24). Since the majority of cells in the fetal pineal gland are ependymal in nature, they reasoned that AVT is elaborated by ependymo-secretion. Moreover, the ependymal cells of the fetal epiphysis are apparently capable of synthesizing AVT de novo, with the pineal progressively losing this ability during ontogenetic development. Interestingly, the adult rat pineal gland retains its ability to synthesize AVT in organ culture, albeit to a limited extent compared with fetal glands (25). Only the apical half of the pineal gland, which they believe contains an ependymal-lined pineal recess, synthesizes AVT whereas the basal part of the gland stores it. These observations and their interpretation, however, are not in accord with the actual neuroanatomical relationship between the rat pineal and the underlying epithalamus. In the rat, the pineal is attached to the brainstem via a rather long stalk in which there is a conspicuous absence of a pineal recess (26,27). Furthermore, the pineal stalk rarely, if ever, remains attached to the pineal on its removal from the brain. Therefore, at least in this species, the synthesis of AVT must occur not in ependymal cells but in pineal parenchymal cells.

Research on the physiological and pharmacological stimuli to AVT synthesis and/or release lags considerably behind that for melatonin. For example, only two reports thus far have addressed the issue of the effects of photoperiod on AVT. Calb et al. (28) documented a diurnal rhythm in the vasotocin content of the rat pineal gland, with AVT reaching its apogee at noon and its nadir at midnight in 12:12 light:dark cycle. Whereas a 24-hour period of exposure to constant light lowers pineal AVT levels, constant darkness causes an increase in glandular content of AVT. Still, other workers (29) have found that long-term light deprivation over a period of 2 months results in decreased pineal AVT levels, perhaps suggesting an increase in vasotocin secretion at the expense of its synthesis.

It is not known whether the effects of darkness on AVT release occur via a β-adrenergic receptor-mediated mechanism. However, there is some pharmacological data to suggest that both adrenergic and cholinergic mechanisms might be involved in the release of AVT in vivo and in vitro respectively (30,31).

Other stimuli for the release of biologically active AVT into the CSF of cats include injections of hypertonic saline, LHRH, thyrotrophin releasing hormone (TRH), somatostatin, and melanocyte inhibiting factor (MIF) (24,32,33). Apparently, these "hypothalamic peptides" are also effective in stimulating the release of neurohypophyseal AVP as well (34). It is important to recall that LHRH, TRH, and somatostatin have been identified in the pineal gland by immunoassay and/or bioassay techniques (35,36). Whether these peptides are synthesized or only stored in the pineal is a matter of conjecture.

Despite these numerous stimuli to AVT release, Pavel (37) has promoted the idea that only melatonin is the physiological releasing factor for vasotocin based primarily on the observation that injections of melatonin into urethane-anesthetized cats causes a decrease in pineal levels and an increase in CSF and plasma levels of AVT (Figure 1). Furthermore,

III VENTRICLE

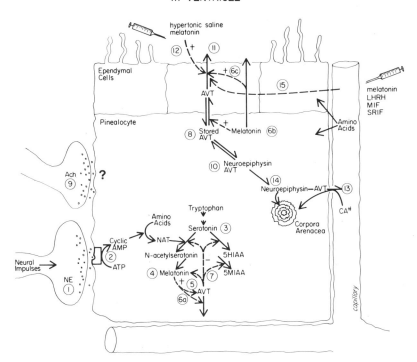

FIGURE 1. Hypotheses concerning the synthesis and regulation of secretion of AVT from the pineal gland. Steps 1 through 4 describe the synthesis of melatonin in response to the stimulation of β-adrenergic receptors by norepinephrine **(NE)** released from postganglionic sympathetic nerve fibers. Melatonin may directly promote the release of AVT into the vascular system of the pineal **(6a)** or, alternatively, may act intracellularly **(6b)** to affect conversion of stored AVT **(8)** to a readily releasable form. The releasable pool of AVT may then be literated into the CSF **(11)** or possibly secreted into the blood in exchange for Ca^{++}. Cholinergic input may also be involved in the release of AVT. Systemic injections of LHRH, TRH, somatostatin, MIF **(15)**, melatonin, and hypertonic saline **(12)** cause the release of AVT into the CSF **(11).** *From Vaughan (42).*

melatonin administered during the dark phase of a photoperiodic cycle is 500-fold more effective in stimulating AVT secretion than when it is injected during the light phase, suggesting a diurnal rhythm of sensitivity to the indole (38). The same demonstration of melatonin's effect on AVT release in unanesthetized animals would certainly strengthen Pavel's hypothesis. Interestingly, melatonin has been shown to stimulate the release of neurohypophyseal AVP as well (39).

In addition to its stimulatory effect on neurohypophyseal AVP, melatonin also enhances the release of LHRH, TRH, and somatostatin from hypothalamic tissue in vitro (40). Therefore, in Pavel's scheme one could easily envisage any or all of these hypothalamic factors being involved in the mechanism of melatonin-induced AVT secretion. This hypothesis gains more credence from the fact that LHRH, TRH, and somatostatin also induce the release of AVP from the neurohypophysis in vitro. As previously proposed (41,42), the actual secretion of AVT from the pineal may involve its dissociation from a hypothetical neurophysin as it is released into the vascular system in exchange for calcium, a process very reminiscent of that which occurs for its evolutionary descendants AVP and OT (Figure 1).

Effects on Reproduction: In Vitro Studies

In vitro studies aimed at elucidating the role of AVT in the regulation of reproductive physiology have been primarily focused on the ability of this compound to alter the release of anterior pituitary hormones. With few exceptions, virtually all such studies have demonstrated a direct progonadotrophic effect of AVT on pituitary hormone secretion rather than its reputed antigonadotrophic activity (6). For example, concentrations of AVT in the microgram range stimulate the secretion of both LH and prolactin (PRL) from rat and hamster anterior pituitary

FIGURE 2. Effects of AVT or PRL release from clonal (2B8) cells into culture medium during 6 hours of incubation. Means ± SEM are indicated. *From Hanew et al. (44).*

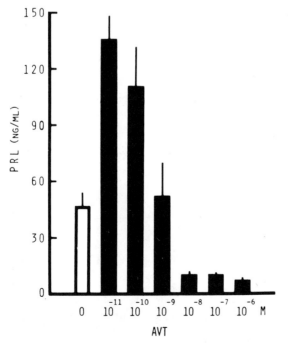

glands in a short-term incubation system (6,43). The effects of AVT on PRL in particular are apparently not pharmacological since concentrations of the neuropeptide in the physiological range (10^{-11} M) cause a marked augmentation of PRL secretion from clonal PRL cells in culture. Conversely, micromolar amounts of AVT have potent PRL-inhibitory effects in this system (44,45) (Figure 2).

Not only is basal LH secretion increased by AVT, but LHRH-stimulated LH release also is augmented by vasotocin (46). However, other laboratories have found AVT either to inhibit LHRH-induced LH secretion (47) or to have no effect on either basal or LHRH-stimulated release (48). These seemingly discordant results might be ascribable to differences in experimental design with respect to the incubation conditions, length of incubation, the use of hemipituitaries versus monolayer cultures, and/or the steroid milieu of the pituitary donor animals. As will be seen, however, both the anti- and progonadotrophic effects of AVT have been corroborated in vivo.

Effects on Reproduction: In Vivo Studies

From experiments in vivo, a great deal of evidence has been marshaled to indicate an antigonadotrophic role for AVT in reproductive processes. This conclusion has been based largely on studies demonstrating AVT's ability to inhibit gonadotrophin-stimulated reproductive organ growth and ovulation in immature animals as well as ovulation in adult species. Additionally, AVT not only increases the length of the estrous cycle by prolonging the diestrous phase, but it also possesses abortifacient activity as well (6,42).

Recent studies centering on the possible mechanisms by which AVT manifests its antireproductive capabilities at the ovarian level have produced some surprising results. For example, whereas AVT effectively inhibits pregnant mare's serum (PMS)-induced ovulation in immature rats, it does so without inhibiting the preovulatory gonadotrophin surge (49). In fact, vasotocin actually potentiates the preovulatory LH surge in this animal model. It was inferred from these findings that AVT might act directly at the ovarian level to inhibit follicular growth by either blocking the action of pituitary hormones or interfering with some steroid-controlled mechanism of follicular growth. Support for the latter hypothesis derives from a recent study showing vasotocin injections to suppress human chorionic gonadotrophin (hCG) cyclic AMP-stimulated ovarian progesterone biosynthesis in immature rats (50). Inasmuch as AVT has no effect on I^{125}-hCG binding to cell membrane preparations, it is apparent that AVT may act at a site in the ovary distal to that of the gonadotrophin-receptor interaction and cyclic AMP formation.

Another plausible explanation for the results of Johnson and coworkers (49) is that the augmentation of the preovulatory LH surge downregulated LH receptors in the ovary, thus suppressing ovulation. As alluded to previously, AVT can act in a progonadotrophic manner by augmenting the response of hemipituitaries to the LH-stimulatory effect

of LHRH in vitro. Similarily, in vivo, a single injection of AVT together
with LHRH significantly augments the circulating levels of LH compared
with animals treated with LHRH alone (51). Hence, a synergism between
AVT and LHRH may occur in the PMS model as well, resulting in higher
levels of circulating LH, which perhaps down-regulate ovarian LH receptors, and causing an inhibition of ovulation.

Pursuant to experiments designed to elucidate a possible neural site
of action of AVT, one group of investigators (52–54) found that the
intraventricular injection of nanogram quantities of AVT inhibited or
delayed the preovulatory surge of LH and subsequent ovulation in freely
moving, unanesthetized rats. Whereas the FSH surge was unaffected,
the proestrous surge of PRL was inhibited by AVT. Inasmuch as AVT
failed to block LH secretion induced with the administration of LHRH,
prostaglandin E_2, or electrochemical stimulation of the medial preoptic
area (mPOA), an antigonadotrophic action of this peptide at a neuroendocrine level lower than the mPOA area seemed unlikely. Contrary to
Cheesman's work, however, other investigators have observed an inhibitory effect of AVT on LHRH-induced LH release in vivo, indicating
that, under certain experimental conditions, vasotocin's antigonadotrophic effect may be exerted at the pituitary level (47,55).

In subsequent experiments (56), we examined the possibility that AVT
inhibits the estrogen-induced gonadotrophin surge in ovariectomized
rats since the preovulatory surge of LH is due to a positive feedback
effect of estrogen presumably on its receptors in the POA. Multiple
injections of AVT were completely effective in suppressing the estrogen-
induced LH surge, but not the FSH surge, suggesting that the POA is
the likely site of action of AVT in blocking the preovulatory LH surge
in adult cycling female rats (Figure 3).

In male rats, we have found that AVT partially suppresses the
postcastration rise in plasma gonadotrophin levels that occurs in response to the elimination of negative steroidal feedback (51). Ostensibly,
this might be due to an inhibition of LHRH release from neurosecretory
neurons in the medial basal hypothalamus (MBH) since the content of
biologically active LHRH of the MBH in these animals is significantly
increased as compared with controls. Alternatively, the increase in LHRH
might simply be the consequence of reduced negative short-loop feedback of circulating LH on LHRH neurons in the MBH.

Some of our more recent studies (57,58) suggest that the endogenous
opiate system is involved in the mechanism of antigonadotrophic action
of AVT. For example, naloxone, an opioid receptor blocker, completely
abrogates the ability of AVT to suppress the postcastration elevation in
LH in male rats. Moreover, naloxone inhibits both the PRL-stimulatory
and inhibitory effects of AVT as well. Since the endogenous opiates
suppress LH and stimulate PRL secretion (59), it is conceivable that AVT
activates opiate neurons that may impinge on LHRH, prolactin inhibiting
factor (PIF), and/or prolactin releasing factor (PRF) neurons.

One frequent criticism of experiments designed to elucidate a physiological role for AVT in the control of reproductive function is that the

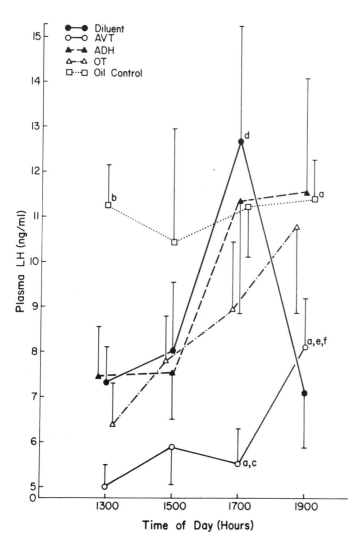

FIGURE 3. Effects of AVT on the surge of plasma LH induced by estradiol benzoate in ovariectomized rats. ADH and OT were administered as control peptides. Vertical lines from means are SEM. *From Blask et al. (56).*

concentrations of the peptide employed usually fall well within a range considered to be pharmacological. The cogency of this argument is further strengthened by the fact that the levels of AVT in the pineal gland are just at the sensitivity of most radioimmunoassays for AVT. However, this criticism may be moot, particularly when one considers the fantastic statement by Pavel and his Roumanian colleagues that AVT "represents the most active hormone so far known." They have based this claim on rather compelling evidence that as little as 10^{-7} pg (only 60 molecules) of AVT injected intraventricularly inhibits the release of cortisol in cats (60).

Further substantiating its biological potency with respect to reproductive physiology, these workers have shown that the intraventricular injection of 10^{-4} pg of AVT into urethane-anesthetized rats causes a significant reduction in circulating LH titers with a concomitant elevation in hypothalamic serotonin levels. When parachlorophenylalanine (pCPA), a serotonin (5-HT) synthesis inhibitor, is also administered, the LH-inhibitory and 5-HT stimulatory effects of AVT are abolished. The additional treatment with a 5-HT precursor, 5-hydroxytryptophan (5-HTP), partially reverses the effects of pCPA (61). Subsequently, they reported that AVT completely obviates the pinealectomy-induced increase in LH and FSH release as well as the decrease in hypothalamic 5-HT content (62). In yet another study along similar lines, they found that the PRL-stimulatory effect of 10^{-4} pg of vasotocin in urethane-treated rats was markedly potentiated if the animals were also treated with fluoxitene, a 5-HT reuptake inhibitor (60).

These dramatic findings have prompted Pavel to reaffirm his belief that AVT is in fact the physiologically active pineal principle that exerts its effects on gonadotrophin and PRL output via serotoninergic mechanisms. These studies may be flawed, however, from the standpoint that urethane anesthesia was used. This is an important point inasmuch as urethane has been shown to modify the neuroendocrine responsiveness to LHRH as well as AVT (63,64). In urethane-treated animals, certain biological responses to AVT, even at ultralow concentrations, may actually represent an artifact of a urethane-induced alteration in neuroendocrine sensitivity to vasotocin. Such a change in sensitivity might be brought about by alterations in neurotransmitter synthesis known to occur in certain brain areas of urethane-treated animals (65). Hence, the urethane-anesthetized rat model may not be suitable for demonstrating physiological effects of AVT or any other putative pineal hormone. Whenever possible, experiments of this type must be duplicated in unanesthetized animals before any firm conclusions can be drawn about the physiological significance of AVT.

Until the issue of the presence of AVT in the mammalian pineal gland is unequivocally resolved, it must be assumed that this neuropeptide is still in contention as a potential pineal hormone. A resolution of this problem will require a greater effort by scientists to adopt the most sophisticated and reliable biochemical and analytical techniques in their efforts to measure AVT in the pineal gland and body fluids under a variety of physiological and pharmacological conditions known to stimulate pineal activity. The immediate benefactors of such an approach will be the AVT physiologists who will in turn be better able to design "physiologically meaningful" experiments aimed at the elucidation of AVT's potentially important role in reproductive physiology.

OTHER PINEAL PEPTIDES

Seasonal photoperiodic fluctuations dramatically alter the functional reproductive status and breeding behavior of photosensitive fossorial rodents; the pineal-dependent nature of this response has been reviewed (3,66). Although one pineal indole, namely melatonin, has been strongly implicated as the potential pineal hormone that can convincingly mimic the action of short photoperiod on reproductive competency (3), one contingent of pinealologists has mounted compelling evidence that antigonadotrophic polypeptides and/or proteins from the pineal are responsible in part for its reproductive effects (42).

Evidence for Their Presence in the Pineal

Supporting evidence for the proteinaceous nature of a pineal antigonadotrophin can be gleaned from early 20th-century reports of European investigators (67); however, the presence of indolic compounds in some of these extracts cannot be conclusively excluded. Thieblot et al. (68), strong advocates for the peptidic nature of the pineal antireproductive substance for many years, eliminated melatonin from their extracts by the use of organic solvents. More recently, investigators have employed sophisticated extraction techniques as well as ultrafiltration and gel filtration methods for the separation of indoles from the peptide-containing pineal fractions (69–73). The number of species from which peptide-containing pineal extracts have been isolated has steadily expanded to now include rats (74), sheep (69,75), cattle (72,76,77), pigs (78), and man (79).

The amino acid sequence of two reputed antireproductive peptides of pineal origin (AVT and threonylseryllysine) are known, although the gland seemingly contains additional unidentified presumptive polypeptides (18,70,80,81) as well as an immunoreactive LHRH-like substance (36,82–84). The pineal literature is replete with references concerning this sizable number of unidentified polypeptides and/or proteins found in crude or partially purified extracts that affect the mammalian reproductive system. A partial listing of this subset of peptides includes: anestrine (85), anovulin (86), epithalmin (87), A_1 and A_3 fractions (88,89), pineal antigonadotrophin (PAG) (70), sheep UM-05R fraction (90), and E_5 (18). Recent progress on at least three of these peptides (sheep UM-05R, PAG, and E_5) provide a hope that these elusive small peptides will be fully characterized and sequenced in the coming decade.

Reproductive Effects

THREONYLSERYLLYSINE (TSL)

The newest of the potential pineal hormones to be characterized culminated several years of research for Orts and his colleagues (73, 91–93). The antireproductive tripeptide, TSL, was one of three antigonadotrophic fractions isolated from bovine pineal glands. Both the naturally occurring (73,93,94) and synthetic (95) peptide inhibit compensatory ovarian hypertrophy (COH) following unilateral ovariectomy (UO) in mice; this observation spurred these investigators to speculate that the synthesis and/or release of follicle stimulating hormone (FSH) was affected by the tripeptide. Additional studies by Orts and colleagues (73) demonstrated significantly reduced FSH levels in UO mice 24 hours after surgery and tripeptide administration. Similarly, TSL significantly delayed the FSH surge in urethane-anesthetized 60-day-old male rats treated with LHRH; these data lent support to the original hypothesis that TSL inhibited or modified FSH secretion. Corroborating evidence, however, was not forthcoming in studies by Vaughan and collaborators (93) who attempted to block the FSH rise attendant on castration in adult male rats. In these studies, subcutaneous injections of 10 or 100 μg TSL every 3 hours for 48 hours failed to affect the elevated levels of FSH or LH observed in orchidectomized rats. The reason for this discrepancy is not obvious at the present time; further testing in other model systems that are dependent on an FSH surge may provide the answer to this curious dilemma.

Since pituitary and plasma levels of prolactin are depressed by short photoperiod or blinding and partially or fully restored by pinealectomy in the male hamster, this adenohypophyseal hormone has become the focal point for many studies involving potential pineal hormones. Intravenous injections of TSL acutely lower pituitary levels of prolactin in a dose-dependent manner in estrogen-progesterone primed, urethane-anesthetized adult male rats (Figure 4); plasma levels of prolactin, however, were unaffected. When various doses of TSL are incubated with a prolactin-secreting clonal cell line (2B8), secretion of the pituitary lactogen was increased (45). Thus the results of these two experiments

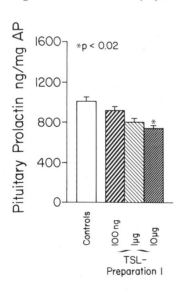

FIGURE 4. Pituitary levels of PRL [ng/mg anterior pituitary (AP)] in adult male rats after intravenous administration of 100 ng, 1 μg, or 10 μg of the tripeptide TSL. Means ± SEM are indicated.

suggest that one site of action of TSL on prolactin secretion is directly at the level of the pituitary to enhance its release from the lactotrophs.

Perturbations in gonadal and accessory organ weight following daily injections of TSL vary with the species, duration of treatment, and dose. Male mice receiving subcutaneous injections of 1 μg TSL for 15 days had significantly lower testicular, ventral prostate, and accessory organ weights than did vehicle-treated controls (95); curiously, similar treatment of another group with 10 μg TSL daily was not as effective as the 1 μg dose. In general, where statistically significant results have been obtained in intact female rodents, an augmentation of ovarian or uterine weight was evident (95). These preliminary results are fragmentary, and variables (e.g., time of day of injection and photoperiod length) known to be critical in obtaining positive data with other pineal substances have not been fully explored.

PINEAL ANTIGONADOTROPHIN (PAG)

A collaborative venture among Drs. Benson, Ebels, and their colleagues has narrowed down the active fraction of a sheep pineal extract to a small substance named PAG. The bioassay method used as the tracer for the antigonadotrophic substance through the complex purification process was the conpensatory hypertrophy in ovarian weight obtained after UO in female mice. The residue obtained after filtration of one active fraction through a UM-05 Diaflo membrane contained a substance(s) that inhibited COH, retarded vaginal opening time in immature mice, and reduced mouse ventral prostate weight (70,80,96). Gel filtration on Sephadex G-10 column separated the active fraction from the indoles, melatonin, 5-methoxytryptophol, and 5-hydroxytryptophol (97). AVT has been categorically ruled out as a possible trace contaminant of PAG (98).

Injection of PAG over a 10-day period reduced fertility in female mice, and single iv injections at various times during the estrous cycle inhibited ovulation in female rats (70). This substance, however, was ineffective in reducing the action of exogenously administered gonadotrophin in immature female mice; interestingly, this bioassay model is used to trace the active component of fractionation methods by most other pinealologists. More recently, further characterization of the active Sephadex G-15 fraction has been attempted using ion-exchange chromatography on DEAE-Sephadex A-25. A major ninhydrin-positive component of the PAG fraction obtained after this chromatography step is oxidized glutathione (79). The sulfur containing amino acid taurine is also intimately associated with the COH-inhibiting activity, but neither synthetic taurine nor oxidized glutatione appreciably inhibit COH.

E_5 PEPTIDE OF NEASCU

Since the preliminary description of the isolation and amino acid analysis of an antigonadotrophic peptide from bovine pineal glands by Neascu

(18), virtually nothing has been done to further characterize the sequence or the action of the substance referred to as E_5. The peptide, as originally described, has 14 amino acids and has many of the biological properties of the nonapeptide previously discussed, AVT.

Initial experiments implied that E_5 had an inhibitory action on LH rather than on FSH; however, one obvious shortcoming of these studies was that only organ weights were measured with no estimates of hormone levels (18). Recently, a small amount of this peptide was made available to us by Drs. Neascu and Pévet. When administered to intact male rats every 12 hours for five injections, E_5 significantly depressed plasma LH and pituitary weight (99); however, no effect was observed on the castration-induced rise in plasma LH and FSH. More importantly, though, are the effects that E_5 had on PRL secretion using the same protocol as described previously. Both castrated and intact male rats had significantly lower pituitary levels of PRL after treatment with E_5 (Figure 5). Further studies utilizing the prolactin secreting 2B8 clonal cell line demonstrated that E_5 had a biphasic response on prolactin secretion: a high dose (100 ng) was stimulatory whereas a low dose (1 fg) was inhibitory (unpublished observations). Unfortunately, the availability of extracted compounds such as E_5 are so limited that long-term injection

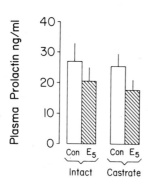

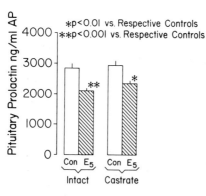

FIGURE 5. Plasma (ng/ml) and pituitary [ng/ml anterior pituitary **(AP)**] levels of PRL in intact or castrated male rats that had received five subcutaneous injections of the partially purified peptide E_5. Means ± SEM are indicated.

studies (as commonly used to demonstrate the effects of melatonin in the hamster) are impossible until the unidentified peptide is fully characterized and synthesized.

BOVINE PINEAL EXTRACT OF MILCU AND COLLEAGUES

In 1963, Milcu and co-workers (7) prepared an extract of bovine pineal glands by boiling acetonic pineal powder with Na_2Co_3; the resulting supernatant was subjected to successive precipitations with HCl and NaOH. The extract is purportedly melatonin-free (100) but may contain AVT (101).

Studies that demonstrate the antireproductive potential of this pineal extract include the inhibition of the hCG-induced hypertrophy of the uterus in mice (72) and decreased serum and testicular testosterone levels in rats (102). Daily injections of 2 ml of extract (30 mg/ml) to adult male rats for 3 days significantly inhibited serum levels of LH and FSH (45% and 36%, respectively); ventral prostate weights were also significantly ($p < 0.001$) decreased (103). Further characterization of the extract by gel filtration and ultrafiltration has revealed two groups of antigonadotrophic substances: $F_1 > 10,000$ and $F_2 < 10,000$ molecular weight (MW) (72).

OTHER PEPTIDES AND/OR PROTEINS THAT AFFECT
GONADOTROPHIN-INDUCED OVULATION

One biological test model that provides a quick and reliable assessment of the antiovulatory potential of a substance is the gonadotrophin (usually, PMS and hCG) induced ovulation or hypertrophy of the ovaries and uterus in mice or rats. This screening process has been employed to "locate" the fraction containing the antigonadotrophic substance(s) in pineal gland extracts by a number of investigators (76–78,86,104–106).

Hipkin (104) observed that a protein-free extract of bovine pineal glands prepared by the trichloroacetic acid method significantly blocked the hCG-induced hypertrophy of the mouse uterus. That same year, Russian scientists (86) prepared an extract from acetonic pineal powder that inhibited PMS + LH induced ovulation in rats; the active fraction, apparently an albumino-peptide, was appropriately named anovulin. Of the five fractions obtained after Sephadex G-50 gel chromatography, Chazov and colleagues observed that the potential for inhibiting ovulation weakened as the MW decreased. Curiously, the exact opposite relationship between MW and antiovulatory capacity was observed recently by Sorensen and Hacker (77). Four fractions of their bovine pineal glands contained antigonadotrophic substances, but, contrary to the results of Chazov and coworkers (86), the proportion on animals ovulating increased as the MW of the fraction increased. Thus these seemingly disparate reports suggest that at least two and perhaps more antigonadotrophins of considerably different MW exist within pineal extracts. Support for this hypothesis has been provided by the F_1 ($> 10,000$ MW) and F_2 (< 10,000 MW) fractions mentioned earlier (72) and also by Ota and colleagues (106). The Japanese investigators extracted acetone-defatted bovine pineal powder with a borate buffer; this procedure was similar to that used previously by this same group for extraction of gonadotrophin-inhibiting substance in urine. The antiovulatory activity of their pineal extract was concentrated in two fractions: one large (MW > 10,000) thermostable fraction and one small (MW < 10,000) melatonin and AVT-free thermolabile substance located in the UM-2 filtrate. Further corroboration of a large ($\cong$ 100,000 MW) antigonadotrophic globular protein was provided by Cheesman and Forsham (76).

Slama-Scemama and coworkers (107) presented some evidence that two of their active fractions (XM-100R and PM-30R) had "complexes" that could be destroyed by chemical manipulation. This observation, along with the previously mentioned evidence that the pineal contains various "sizes" of peptide and/or protein molecules, could be the signal for a disconcerting problem. The pineal may contain large molecular weight storage or prohormone forms of the proteinaceous antigonadotrophin, which, under normal circumstances in situ may be broken down, packaged, and secreted in smaller MW forms. Extraction procedures used by many investigators may damage or inactivate the peptide or may inadvertently cleave portions of the large molecule; the resultant "antigonadotrophic or progonadotrophic" peptide and/or proteins fragments may or, more likely, may not be true representatives of the normally secreted product.

IMMUNOREACTIVE PINEAL LHRH

Over the past 6 years, sporadic reports have appeared in the literature alluding to the presence of an immunoreactive LHRH-like substance in bovine, ovine, and porcine pineal glands (36,82–84,108–110); one negative report is also found (111). Characterization of the molecule from ovine pineal glands revealed an immunoreactive and biologically active molecule that varied considerably in size from a maximum of 60,000 in May/June to 2,000 in January/February (110). Treatment of the 60,000 MW immunoreactive species with trypsin enhanced LHRH activity but reduced the MW to about 12,000. Biological activity was assessed by means of the ability of the extract to release LH and FSH from dispersed pituitary cells in vitro. It is uncertain if the gland synthesizes this immunoreactive form of LHRH; however, other investigators have shown that the pineal can sequester synthetic LHRH (112,113).

UNIDENTIFIED PINEAL FRACTIONS WITH PROLACTIN RELEASING AND INHIBITING ACTIVITY

Light deprivation, early afternoon melatonin injections, or blinding results in pineal-mediated atrophy of the gonads and diminished plasma and pituitary levels of PRL in the hamster (3). A modulatory role of the pineal gland on the complex hypothalamic control of this hormone has previously been proposed (114). Besides melatonin, AVT, and TSL, which were discussed earlier, other unidentified pineal PRF and PIF factors influence the synthesis and/or release of this hormone by pituitary lactotrophs.

Crude, neutralized extracts of bovine, rat, and human pineal glands provoked the release of PRL from normal male rat hemipituitaries in vitro (89); two purified fractions of bovine pineal glands, A_1 and A_3, inhibited release in the same experiment. Similarly, Chang and coworkers (115) found evidence for both a PRF (MW < 10,000) and several PIF-like substances (UM-2 residue, MW > 1,000; UM-05 filtrate, MW < 500; UM-05 residue, MW > 500 and < 1,000). Trypsin inactivation suggested that one PIF may be a peptide or contain a peptide moiety indispensable for its biological activity. Demoulin and colleagues (116) observed PIF activity from extracts of defatted ovine pineal powder on both the basal and TRH-stimulated secretion of pituitary monolayer cultures.

Further support for both PRF and PIF activity in rat pituitaries was provided by Zryakov (117). In his experiment, male rats exposed to a light:dark environment of 9:15 were killed at various times during the photoperiod to determine the PRF and/or PIF activity of their pineal glands. The glands were homogenized in 0.5 ml 4% formic acid in n-butanol. The acidic organic phase was dried, redissolved, and subjected to thin-layer chromatography. The biologically active fractions were determined after incubation with isolated hemipituitaries derived from ovariectomized, estrogen-progesterone primed female rats. PRF activity was maximal in pineal glands derived from rats at 9 A.M. and 9 P.M. and at a minimum at 4 A.M.; conversely, PIF activity was maximal at 2 A.M. Unfortunately, this investigator does not indicate the time of lights on and lights off and the photoperiodic schedule of his animal room (light:dark cycles of 9:15) is also an uncommon one. Thus, at this point, it is impossible to speculate how his data correlate with the known peak period of PRL secretion in rats maintained under 12:12 or 14:10 or with other known pineal phenomena such as the N-acetyltransferase and melatonin rhythms.

CONCLUDING REMARKS

The definitive characterization as well as the specific localization of active pineal polypeptides has been a slow and tedious process. Although for a number of years AVT had gained some favor as a potential pineal hormone, enthusiasm has waned recently because of the inability of several groups of workers to identify the nonapeptide within the gland. TSL and Neascu's E_5 fraction are presently receiving increased attention but, again, the fact that they are not commercially available retards the physiological studies. The bulk of the other alleged inhibitory factors continue to be investigated, but progress, although steady, has been slow. Their chemical structure has thus far remained elusive and, furthermore, there is no proof that any of them are normally produced within and secreted from the pineal gland. There are probably many organs that contain compounds capable of influencing the neuroendocrine-reproductive axis; but if they are never discharged into the circulation, they may be inconsequential in terms of reproductive function.

Physiologically, the action of the peptides that have been studied are complex and, in some cases, variable. It required years to identify the effective mode of administration of melatonin; possibly the proper experimental approaches for testing the gonadally active pineal peptides have escaped detection.

It appears that these areas of investigation will continue to receive attention, but a major breakthrough will be required to make them flourish. Perhaps this advance is just over the horizon.

REFERENCES

1. Relkin R. The Pineal. Eden, Montreal, 1976.
2. Reiter R J. The Pineal, vol 5. Eden, Montreal, 1980.
3. Reiter R J. The pineal and its hormones in the control of reproduction in mammals. Endocrinol Rev 1:109–130, 1980.
4. Wiener H. External chemical messengers. IV. Pineal gland. NY State J Med 68:912–938, 1968.
5. Vliegenthart J F G, Versteeg D H G. Evolution of the vertebrate neurohypophysial hormones. Gen Comp Endocrinol 5:712, 1965.
6. Vaughan M K, Blask D E. Arginine vasotocin—a search for its function in mammals. In The Pineal and Reproduction, ed R J Reiter. Karger, Basel, 1978, pp 90–115.
7. Milcu S M, Pavel S, Neascu C. Biological and chromatographic characterization of a polypeptide with pressor and oxytocic activities isolated from bovine pineal gland. Endocrinology 72:563–566, 1963.
8. Pavel S. Evidence for the presence of lysine vasotocin in the pig pineal gland. Endocrinology 77:812–817, 1965.
9. Cheesman DW. Structural elucidation of a gonadotrophin-inhibiting substance from the bovine pineal gland. Biochim Biophys Acta 207:247–253, 1970.
10. Bowie E P, Herbert D C. Immunocytochemical evidence for the presence of arginine vasotocin in the rat pineal gland. Nature 261:5555, 1976.
11. Rosenbloom A A, Fisher D A. Radioimmunoassay of arginine vasotocin. Endocrinology 95:1726–1732, 1974.
12. Legros J J, Louis F, Demoulin A, Franchimont P. Immunoreactive neurophysins and vasotocin in human foetal pineal glands. J Endocrinol 69:289–290, 1976.
13. Negro-Vilar A, Sanchez-Franco F, Kwiatkowski M, Samson W K. Failure to detect radioimmunoassayable arginine vasotocin in mammalian pineals. Brain Res Bull 4:784–792, 1979.
14. Pévet P, Dogterom J, Buijs R M, Ebels I, Swabb D F, Arimura A. Presence of α-MSH, AVT-, and LHRH-like compounds in the mammalian pineal and subcommissural organ and their relationship with the UMO5R pineal fraction. Xth Conf Europ Comp Endocr Sorrento, 1979, p. 21.
15. Dogterom J, Snijdewint F G M, Pevet P, Buijs R M. On the presence of neuropeptides in the mammalian pineal gland and subcommissural organ. In The Pineal Gland of Vertebrates Including Man, eds J Ariëns-Kappers, P Pévet. Elsevier North-Holland, Amsterdam, 1979, pp 465–470.
16. Biujs R M, Pévet P. Vasopressin- and oxytocin-containing fibers in the pineal gland and subcommissural organ of the rat. Cell Tissue Res 205:11–17, 1980.

17. Pévet P, Ebels I, Swaab D F, Mud M T, Arimura A. Presence of AVT-, α-MSH-, LHRH-, and somatostatin-like compounds in the rat pineal gland and their relationship with UMO5R pineal fraction. Cell Tissue Res 206:341–353, 1980.

18. Neascu C. The mechanism of antigonadotropic activity of a polypeptide extracted from a bovine pineal gland. Rev Roum Physiol 9:161–169, 1972.

19. Fernstrom J D, Fisher L A, Cusack B M, Gillis M A. Radioimmunologic detection and measurement of nonapeptides in the pineal gland. Endocrinology 106:243–251, 1980.

20. Fisher L A, Fernstrom J D. Measurement of nonapeptides in pineal and pituitary using reversed-phase, ion-pair liquid chromatography with post-column detection by radioimmunoassay. Life Sci 28:1471–1481, 1981.

21. Gharib C L, Geelen G, Allevard-Burguburu A M. Radioimmunoassay of AVP, OT and AVT-like material in human pineal gland. 2nd Colloquium of the European Pineal Study Group, EPSG Newsl Suppl 3:30–31, 1981.

22. Pavel S. Arginine vasotocin as a pineal hormone. J Neural Transm Suppl 3:135–155, 1978.

23. Pavel S. Evidence for the ependymal origin of arginine vasotocin in the bovine pineal gland. Endocrinology 89:613–614, 1971.

24. Pavel S, Goldstein R, Gheorghui C, Calb M. Pineal vasotocin: release into cat cerebrospinal fluid by melanocyte-stimulating hormone release-inhibiting factor. Science 197:179–180, 1977.

25. Pavel S, Goldstein R, Ghinea E, Calb M. Chromatographic evidence for vasotocin biosynthesis by cultured pineal ependymal cells from rat fetuses. Endocrinology 100:205–208, 1978.

26. Gregorek J C, Seibel H R, Reiter R J. The pineal complex and its relationship to other epithalamic structures. Acta Anat 99:425–434, 1977.

27. Boeckmann D. Morphological investigation of the deep pineal of the rat. Cell Tissue Res 210:283–294, 1980.

28. Calb M, Goldstein R, Pavel S. Diurnal rhythm of vasotocin in the pineal of the male rat. Acta Endocrinol 84:523–526, 1977.

29. Sartin J, Bruot B, Orts R J. Blinding induced alterations in pineal gland arginine vasotocin and pituitary and plasma LH, FSH and prolactin. Fed Proc 37:437, 1978.

30. Cusack B M, Fisher L A, Fernstrom J D. Increase in plasma vasotocin levels following norepinephrine injection. Fed Proc 37:437, 1978.

31. Sartin J L, Bruot B C, Orts R J. Neurotransmitter regulation of arginine vasotocin release from rat pineal glands in vitro. Acta Endocrinol 91:571–576, 1979.

32. Goldstein R, Pavel S. Vasotocin release into the cerebrospinal fluid of rats induced by luteinizing hormone releasing hormone, thyrotrophin releasing hormone and growth hormone releasing-inhibiting hormone. J Endocrinol 75:175–176, 1977.

33. Pavel S, Coculescu M. Arginine vasotocin-like activity of cerebrospinal fluid induced by injection of hypertonic fluid into the third cerebral ventricle of cats. Endocrinology 91:825–827, 1972.

34. Skowsky E, Swan L. Effects of hypothalamic releasing hormones on neurohypophyseal arginine vasopressin (AVP) secretion. Vth Int Cong Endocrinol, Hamburg, p 197, 1976

35. Pelletier G, Leclerc R, Dube D, Labrie F, Buviani R, Arimura A, Schally A V. Localization of growth hormone release-inhibiting hormone (somatostatin) in the rat brain. Am J Anat 142:397–400, 1975.

36. White W F, Hedlund M T, Weber G F, Rippel R H, Johnson E S, Wilber J F. The pineal gland: a supplemental source of hypothalamic-releasing hormones. Endocrinology 94:1422–1426, 1974.

37. Pavel S. Arginine vasotocin release into cerebrospinal fluid of cats induced by melatonin. Nature 154:183–184, 1973.

38. Pavel S, Goldstein R. Further evidence that melatonin represents the releasing hormone for pineal vasotocin. J Endocrinol 82:1–6, 1979.

39. Leway A, Brouillette A, Denizeau F, Lavoie M. Melatonin- and serotonin-stimulated release of vasopressin from rat neurohypophysis perifused *in vitro*. Progr 61st Ann Mtg Endocrinol Soc, St. Louis, Mo., 1979, p 161.

40. Hollander C S, Prasad R, Richardson S, Horrooka Y, Suzuki S. Melatonin modulates hormonal release from organ cultures of rat hypothalamus. J Neural Transm Suppl 13:369, 1978.

41. Lukaszyk A, Reiter R J. Histophysiological evidence for the secretion of polypeptides by the pineal gland. Am J Anat 143:451–464, 1975.

42. Vaughan M K. Arginine vasotocin in vertebrate reproduction. *In* The Pinea Gland, vol 2, Reproductive Effects, ed R J Reiter. CRC Press, Boca Raton, Florida, 1982, pp 125–164.

43. Blask D E, Vaughan M K, Reiter R J. Arginine vasotocin alters hamster pituitary LH and prolactin secretin *in vitro*. Comp Biochem Physiol in press.

44. Hanew K, Shiino M, Rennels E G. Effect of indoles, AVT, oxytocin, AVP on prolactin secretion in rat pituitary clonal (2B8) cells. Proc Soc Exp Biol Med 164:257–261, 1980.

45. Vaughan M K, McGill J R, Richardson B A, Johnson L Y, Pévet P, Neascu C, Reiter R J. Responsiveness of a prolactin-secreting clonal cell line (2B8) or male rat hemipituitaries to incubation with arginine vasotocin, threonylseryllysine (TSL) or a partially purified peptide (E$_5$) from bovine pineal glands. Neuroendocrinol Lett 3:189–194, 1981.

46. Vaughan M K, Vaughan G M, Blask D E, Barnett M P, Reiter R J. Arginine vasotocin: structure activity relationships and influence on gonadal growth and function. Am Zool 16:25–34, 1976.

47. Bruot B C, Sartin J L, Orts R J. The effect of arginine vasotocin on luteinizing releasing hormone stimulated luteinizing hormone release *in vivo* and *in vitro*. Physiologist 21:14, 1978.

48. Demoulin A, Hudson D, Franchimont P, Legros J J. Arginine vasotocin does not affect gonadotrophin secretion *in vivo*. J Endocrinol 27:105–106, 1977.

49. Johnson L Y, Vaughan M K, Reiter R J, Blask D E, Rudeen, P K. The effects of arginine vasotocin on pregnant mare's serum-induced ovulation in the immature female rat. Acta Endocrinol 87:367–376, 1978.

50. Kahn J K, Menon K M J. Evidence that arginine vasotocin inhibits human chorionic gonadotropin and cyclic adenosine 3′,5′-monophosphate stimulated ovarian steroidogenesis. Biochem Biophys Res Commun 100:100–104, 1981.

51. Vaughan M K, Trakulrungsi C, Petterborg L J, Johnson L Y, Blask D E, Trakulrungsi W, Reiter R J. Interaction of luteinizing hormone-releasing hormone, cyproterone acetate and arginine vasotocin on plasma levels of luteinizing hormone in intact and castrated adult male rats. Mol Cell Endocrinol 14:59–71, 1979.

52. Cheesman D W, Osland R B, Forsham P H. Effects of 8-arginine vasotocin on plasma prolactin and follicle-stimulating hormone surges in the proestrous rat. Proc Soc Exp Biol Med 156:369–372, 1977.

53. Cheesman D W, Osland R B, Forsham P H. Suppression of the preovulatory surge of luteinizing hormone and subsequent ovulation in the rat by arginine vasotocin. Endocrinology 101:1194–1202, 1977.

54. Osland R B, Cheesman D W, Forsham P H. Studies on the mechanism of the suppression of the preovulatory surge of luteinizing hormone in the rat by arginine vasotocin. Endocrinology 101:1203–1209, 1977.

55. Yamashita K, Mieno M, Yamashita Er. Suppression of the luteinizing hormone releasing effect of luteinizing hormone releasing hormone by arginine-vasotocin. J Endocrinol 81:103–108, 1979.

56. Blask D E, Vaughan M K, Reiter R J, Johnson L Y. Influence of arginine vasotocin on the estrogen-induced surge of LH and FSH in adult ovariectomized rats. Life Sci 23:1035–1040, 1978.

57. Blask D E, Vaughan M K. Naloxone inhibits arginine vasotocin (AVT)-induced prolactin release in urethane-anesthetized male rats *in vivo*. Neurosci Lett 18:181–184, 1980.

58. Vaughan M K, Johnson L Y, Dinh D T, Blask D E, Guerra J C, De los Santos R, Reiter R J. Effect of arginine vasotocin and/or naloxone treatment on plasma prolactin, LH and FSH secretion in unanesthetized adult male rats. Anat Rec 196:195A, 1980.

59. Meites J, Bruni JF, Van Vugt DA. Effects of endogenous opiate peptides on release of anterior pituitary hormones. In Central Nervous System Effects of Hypothalamic Hormones and Other Peptides, ed R Y Collu. Raven Press, New York, 1979, pp 122–128.

60. Pavel S. The mechanism of action of vasotocin in the mammalian brain. In The Pineal of Vertebrates Including Man, eds J Ariëns-Kappers, P Pévet. Elsevier North-Holland, Amsterdam, 1979, pp 445–458.

61. Pavel S, Luca N, Calb M, Goldstein R. Inhibition of release of luteinizing hormone in male rat by extremely small amounts of arginine vasotocin: further evidence for the involvement of 5-hydroxy tryptamine-containing neurons in the mechanism of action of arginine vasotocin. Endocrinology 104:517–524, 1979.

62. Pavel S, Luca N, Calb M, Goldstein R. Reversal by arginine vasotocin of pinealectomy effects on hypothalamic 5-hydroxytryptamine content and plasma luteinizing and follicle-stimulating hormone levels in immature male rats. J Endocrinol 84:159–162, 1980.

63. Carter D A, Dyer R G. Inhibition by pentobarbitone and urethane on the in vitro response of the adenohypophysis to luteinizing hormone releasing hormone in male rats. Br J Pharmacol 67:277–281, 1979.

64. Johnson L Y, Vaughan M K, Reiter R J, Petterborg L J, Chen H J. Acute effects of arginine vasotocin on plasma and pituitary levels of prolactin in the male rat: influence of urethane anesthesia. Horm Res 13:109–120, 1980.

65. Findell P R, Larsen B R, Benson B, Blask D E. Mechanism of the effect of urethane on the secretion of prolactin in the male rat. Life Sci in press.

66. Reiter R J. Circannual reproductive rhythm in mammals related to photoperiod and pineal function: a review. Chronobiologia 1:365–395, 1974.

67. Kitay J I, Altschule M D. The Pineal Gland. Harvard University Press, Cambridge, Massachusetts, 1954.

68. Thieblot L, Alassimone L, Blaise S. Etude chromatographique et électrophorétique du facteur antigonadotrope de la glande pinéale. Ann Endocrinol 24:861–866, 1966.

69. Ebels I, Citharel A, Moszkowska A. Separation of pineal extracts by gelfilgration III. Sheep pineal factors acting either on the hypothalamus, or on the anterior hypophysis of mice and rats in in vitro experiments. J Neural Transm 36:281–302, 1975.

70. Benson B. Current status of pineal peptides. Neuroendocrinology 24:241–248, 1977.

71. Rosenblum I Y, Benson B, Bria C F, McDonnell D, Hruby V J. Localization and chemical characterization of a partially purified bovine pineal antigonadotropin. J Neural Transm 44:197–220, 1979.

72. Damian E, Ianas O, Badescu I. Studies on the purification of the antigonadotropic melatonin-free pineal extract. Rev Roum Med Endocr 17:163–169, 1979.

73. Orts R J, Liao T H, Sartin J L, Bruot B C. Isolation, purification and amino acid sequence of a tripeptide from bovine pineal tissue displaying antigonadotropic properties. Biochim Biophys Acta 628:201–208, 1980.

74. Orts R J, Benson B, Cook B F. Some antigonadotropic effects of a melatonin-free bovine pineal extracts in rats. Acta Endocrinol 76:438–448, 1974.

75. Ebels I. Pineal factors other than melatonin. Gen Comp Endocrinol 25:189–198, 1975.

76. Cheesman D W, Forsham P H. Inhibition of induced ovulation by a highly purified extract of the bovine pineal gland. Proc Soc Exp Biol Med 146:722–724, 1974.

77. Sorensen M T, Hacker R R. Inhibition of ovulation induced with PMSG and HCG in prepuberal mice by bovine pineal glands extracts of different molecular weights. Can J Anim Sci 59:375–380, 1979.

78. Ntunde B N, Hacker R R, Brown R G. Aqueous porcine pineal extract: inhibition of ovulation induced with PMSG and HCG in immature mice. J Anim Sci 48:1422–1428, 1979.

79. Matthews M J, Benson B, Rodin A E. Antigonadotropic activity in a melatonin-free extract of human pineal glands. Life Sci 10:1375–1379, 1971.

80. Ebels I, Benson B, Bria CR, McDonnell D, Chang SY, Hruby VJ. Location by paper chromatography of compensatory ovarian hypertrophy (COH) inhibiting activity in acetic acid extracts from bovine pineals. J Neural Transm 42:275–292, 1978.

81. Thieblot L, Grizard G, Dastugue B, Gachon A M, Thieblot P. Purification du facteur antigonadotrope de la glande pinéale. Ann Endocrinol 40:519–529, 1979.

82. Duraiswami P, Franchimont D, Boucher M, Thieblot M. Immunoreactive luteinizing hormone-releasing hormone (LH-RH) in the bovine pineal gland. Horm Metab Res 8:232–233, 1976.

83. Millar R P, Aehnelt C, Rossier G. Higher molecular weight immunoreactive species of luteinizing hormone releasing hormone: possible precursors of the hormone. Biochem Biophys Res Comm 74:720–731, 1977.

84. Wheaton J E. Immunoreactive luteinizing hormone-releasing hormone (LHRH) in ovine pineal glands. Horm Metab Res 12:314–317, 1980.

85. Bianchini P, Osima B. Studi su di un probabile ormone della pineale: L'anestrina. Boll Soc Ital Biol Sper 36:1674–1677, 1960.

86. Chazov Y I, Isachenkov V A, Krivosheyev O G, Veselova S N, Zhivoderova G V. A factor from the pineal body inhibiting the ovulation induced by luteinizing hormones. Dokl Akad Nauk SSSR 27:246–248 (in Russian), 1972.

87. Anisimov V N, Khavinson V K, Morozov V G, Dilman V M. Lowering of the threshold of sensitivity of the hypothalamo-hypophysial system to the action of estrogens under the effect of an epiphysis extract in old female rats. Dokl Akad Nauk SSSR 213:483–485 (in Russian), 1973.

88. Vaughan M K, Reiter R J, McKinney T, Vaughan G M. Inhibition of growth of gonadal dependent structures by arginine vasotocin and purified bovine pineal fractions in immature mice and hamsters. Int J Fertil 19:103–106, 1974.

89. Blask D E, Vaughan M K, Reiter R J, Johnson L Y, Vaughan G M. Prolactin-releasing and release-inhibiting factor activities in the bovine, rat and human pineal. Endocrinology 99:152–161, 1976.

90. Ebels I, Benson B, Matthews M J. Localization of a sheep pineal antigonadotrophin. Anal Biochem 56:546–565, 1973.

91. Orts R J, Benson B, Cook B F. LH inhibitory properties of aqueous extracts of rat pineal glands. Life Sci 14:1501–1510, 1974.

92. Orts R J, Poe R W, Liao T H. Studies on the characteristics of a partially purified antigonadotrophin from bovine pineal glands. Life Sci 24:985–992, 1979.

93. Orts R J, Bruot B C, Sartin J L. Inhibitory properties of a bovine pineal tripeptide, threonylseryllysine, on serum follicle-stimulating hormone. Neuroendocrinology 31:92–95, 1980.

94. Orts R J, Liao T H, Sartin J L, Bruot B. Purification of a tripeptide with anti-reproductive properties isolated from bovine pineal glands. Physiologist 21:87, 1978.

95. Vaughan M K, Johnson L Y, Blask D E, Brainard G C, Dinh D T, Petterborg L J, Reiter R J. Effect of synthetic threonylseryllysine (TSL), a proposed pineal peptide, on reproductive organ weights and plasma and pituitary levels of LH, FSH and prolactin in intact and castrated immature and mature adult male rodents. Neuroendocrinol Lett 2:235–240, 1980.

96. Ebels I, Benson B, Bria C F, Richardson D, Larsen B R, Hruby V J. Location by paper chromatography of compensatory ovarian hypertrophy (COH) inhibiting activity in isobutanol extracts of bovine pineals. J Neural Transm 45:43–61, 1979.

97. Ebels I, Horwitz-Bresser A E M. Separation of pineal extracts by gel filtration IV. Isolation, location, and identification from sheep pineals of three indoles, identical with 5-hydroxytryptophol, 5-methoxytryptophol and melatonin. J Neural Transm 38:31–41, 1976.

98. Benson B, Matthews M J, Hadley M E, Powers S, Hruby V J. Differential localization of antigonadotrophic and vasotocic activities in bovine and rat pineal. Life Sci 19:747–754, 1976.

99. Vaughan M K, Johnson L Y, Dinh D T, Petterborg L J, Brainard G C, Reiter R J. Effect of synthetic threonine-serine-lysine (TSL), a new pineal peptide, on several reproductive model systems in mice, hamsters, and rats. In Pineal Function, eds C D Matthews, R F Seamark. Elsevier North-Holland, Amsterdam, 1981, pp 165–172.

100. Damian E, Ianas O. The control of melatonin presence in pineal extracts. Stud Cercet Endocrinol 22:449–453, 1971.

101. Coculescu M, Zaoral M, Matulevicius V. Tentative identification of arginine vasotocin in the bovine pineal extract prepared by the Milcu-Nanu method. Rev Roum Med Endocrinol 15:27–33, 1977.

102. Milcu S M, Damian E, Ianas O, Badescu I, Oprescu M. Decrease in serum and testicular testosterone after administration of pineal polypeptides to rats. Endocrinol Exp 9:259–262, 1975.

103. Damian E, Ianas O, Badescu I, Oprescu M. Anti-LH and FSH activity of melatonin-free pineal extract. Neuroendocrinology 26:325–332, 1978.

104. Hipkin L J. Gonadotrophin inhibitory properties of pineal extracts. Nature 228:1202, 1972.

105. Ota M, Horiuchi S, Obara K. Inhibition of ovulation induced with PMS and HCG by a melatonin-free extract of bovine pineal powder. Neuroendocrinology 18:311–321, 1975.

106. Ota M, Shimizu E, Obara K. Separation of non-melatonin anti-ovulatory substances from bovine pineal powder by ultrafiltration. Mol Cell Endocrinol 9:21–31, 1977.

107. Slama-Scemama A, l'Heritier A, Moszkowska A, van der Horst C J G, Noteborn H P J M, de Morée A, Ebels I. Effects of sheep pineal fractions on the activity of male rat hypothalami in vitro. J Neural Transm 46:47–58, 1979.

108. Kozlowski C P, Zimmerman E A. Localization of gonadotropin-releasing hormone (Gn-RH) in sheep and mouse brain. Anat Rec 178:396, 1974.

109. Wheaton J E, Harsdorf S E. Biological and immunological LH-RH activity in ovine pineal glands. Fed Proc 36:279, 1977.

110. Kotaras P J, McIntosh J E A, Seamark R F. Seasonal and protease influences of ovine pineal GnRH activity. In Pineal Function, eds C D Matthews, R F Seamark. Elsevier North-Holland, Amsterdam, 1981, pp 148–154.

111. Carson R S, Matthews C D, Findlay J K, Symons R G, Burger H C. Biological and immunological luteinizing hormone-releasing hormone (LH-RH) activity of the ovine pineal. Neuroendocrinology 24:221–225, 1977.

112. Redding T W, Schally A V. The distribution, half-life and excretion of tritiated luteinizing hormone-releasing hormone (LH-RH) in rats. Life Sci 12:23–32, 1973.

113. Amundson B C, Wheaton J E. Effects of chronic LHRH treatment on brain LHRH content, pituitary and plasma LH, and ovarian follicular activity in the anestrous ewe. Biol Reprod 20:633–638, 1979.

114. Blask D E, Reiter R J. The pineal gland of the blind-anosmic female rat: its influence on medial basal hypothalamic LRH, PIF and/or PRF activity in vivo. Neuroendocrinology 17:362–374, 1975.

115. Chang N, Ebels I, Benson B. Preliminary characterization of bovine pineal prolactin releasing (PPRF) and releasing-inhibiting factor (PPIF) activity. J Neural Transm 46:139–151, 1979.

116. Demoulin A, Hudson D, Legros J J, Franchimont P. Influence d'un extrait de glandes pineales ovines sur la liberation de prolactine in vitro. C R Soc Biol 171:1134–1140, 1977.

117. Zryakov O N. Circadian changes in prolactostatin and prolactoliberin activity in the rat epiphysis. Sechenov Physiol J USSR 9:1324–1328 (in Russian), 1979.

The following three chapters are dedicated

to Elizabeth and Douglas

RICHARD RELKIN, M.D.

PINEAL-HORMONAL INTERACTIONS

This chapter deals with interrelationships between the pineal and other endocrine glands or systems. As the pineal-hypothalamic-pituitary-gonadal axis has already been discussed at length in preceding chapters, it will not be detailed here.

ADRENALS

Adrenal weight has been decreased and compensatory adrenal hypertrophy diminished as a result of the administration of melatonin and other indoles to mice (1), the administration of pineal extracts to rats, increasing pineal activity by blinding or exposing rats to continuous darkness (2), as well as by the administration of arginine vasotocin to mice (3). These effects, measured either grossly or histologically, could be negated by pinealectomy (2,4). In addition, adrenal hypertrophy has been produced in mice (1), and histologic changes compatible with marked adrenal hypertrophy have been produced in rats by pinealectomy without prior treatment (5). Thus it would appear that the overall effect of the pineal is one of adrenocortical inhibition.

From Easton Hospital, Easton, Pennsylvania 18042, and Hahnemann Medical College and Hospital, Philadelphia, Pennsylvania 19102

Aldosterone

Despite early postulation of zona glomerulosa stimulation by a pineal substance dubbed "glomerulotropin" (6) and the apparent finding of increased aldosterone secretion following the administration of melatonin to rats (7), subsequent investigation (8) elicited inhibition of aldosterone secretion by ubiquinone, a component of pineal lipid. Later studies (9,10) were also interpreted as indicating an inhibitory effect of the pineal on aldosterone secretion. More evidence for an inhibitory role of the pineal in aldosterone secretion was adduced when it was shown that aldosterone secretion was elevated 1 and 3 months following pinealectomy (11). Using a factor-isolate of pineal tissue, other workers were later able to produce hyperkalemia in rats (12). Because hyperkalemia is found in only a few situations, such as renal insufficiency, tissue damage, acidosis, hypoaldosteronism, certain diuretic usage, and a few other rarities, this last study provided inferential evidence of a suppressive effect of the pineal on the glomerular zone of the adrenal cortex. Thus, despite some earlier evidence to the contrary, the prevailing view would be that the pineal is inhibitory to aldosterone secretion.

Corticosterone

Melatonin has been reported to lower plasma corticosterone levels in rats (13), and pinealectomy in rat neonates to elevate the levels of this hormone (14). Subsequent work (15) also indicated that melatonin could reduce the rate of corticosterone secretion. However, in another study (16), the intraperitoneal administration to rats of an acid extract of pineal tissue resulted in elevated blood corticosterone levels only in females, whereas a pineal alkaline extract produced the same effect only in males. This last study is difficult to interpret because the sexes responded differently to the extracts. Interestingly, a later study (17), which also used a crude pineal extract, demonstrated decreased production of corticosterone in vitro using a heterogeneous population of adrenal cortex cells. This work also indicated that the pineal and adrenocorticotropin (ACTH) may influence the adrenal cortex via different receptor sites.

Recently, using intact female rats, pinealectomy has been demonstrated to increase plasma corticosterone, corticosterone production, and total adrenal steroidogenesis and, thus, was hypothesized to enhance ACTH secretion in the presence of estrogen (18). Focusing attention more specifically on ACTH, it has been shown that sensory deprivation via blinding and removal of the olfactory bulbs in male rats resulted in a marked augmentation of postadrenalectomy ACTH levels following pinealectomy (19). Neither the sensory deprivation nor pinealectomy alone achieved this effect. It was concluded that an intact pineal, and an intact sensory system, cam dampen the ACTH response to inadequate corticosteroid feedback. In this and the preceding study, there is significant evidence for the necessity of having intact gonadal secretion for the pineal to exert an inhibitory effect on ACTH and, thus, on adrenal steroidogenesis. This implication becomes more obvious when it is recalled that blind, anosmic male rats have lower testicular, seminal vesicle, and ventral prostate weights, as well as depressed levels of serum testosterone.

All the preceding does not settle the question of the site of pineal inhibition of steroid synthesis in the adrenals. Further investigation (20) has shown that melatonin given in vivo stimulates adrenal 5α-reductase, with corresponding enhancement in the secretion of the 5α-reduced metabolites of corticosterone—dihydrocorticosterone and tetrahydrocorticosterone—and a proportionate decrease in corticosterone secretion; this result was obtained even in the absence of the pituitary. This effect on adrenal 5α-reductase was confirmed in a later study (21) by the same authors in which melatonin was used in vitro. In addition, using in vitro preparations of bovine adrenal cortex, melatonin was demonstrated to inhibit corticosteroid biosynthesis, specifically the 17- and 21-hydroxylases (22). These studies would suggest that melatonin's effect on the adrenal cortex is direct, rather than via the hypothalamus and/or pituitary.

The performance of pineal stalk section in rabbits followed by exposure of the animals to cold resulted in earlier and greater elevations in plasma cortisol and corticosterone than that seen in controls (23). This suggested that the pineal normally increases the latency of onset and decreases the amplitude of the corticosteroid response to stress.

Investigation of possible effects the pineal may have on circadian rhythms of adrenocortical activity in rats has revealed, in one study (24), that there was little evidence to implicate the pineal either in the maintenance of normal circadian periodicity or in the shift in circadian rhythm that occurs with blinding. However, another experiment (25) in rats revealed that blinding elevated morning corticosterone levels; pinealectomy partially reversed; and immunization against melatonin and N-acetylserotonin (NAS) completely reversed these elevations. Pinealectomy alone did not affect morning corticosterone levels, but did lower evening levels. In addition, antimelatonin-anti-NAS immunization significantly lowered corticosterone levels during the 24-hour cycle. Unlike the preceding study, this one appears to show that melatonin and/or NAS may be involved in regulating basal diurnal corticosteroid secretion.

Taking all available evidence into account, it would appear that the pineal is mainly inhibitory to adrenal corticosteroid synthesis and secretion, the latter decrease partly the result of accelerated degradation. This inhibition would seem to have two sites of action: the hypothalamus and/or pituitary and the adrenal cortex. These inhibitory effects would liken pineal action to that of prolactin, which has been demonstrated to have a direct effect on luteinizing-hormone releasing factor (LRH) as well as on gonadal steroidogenesis.

Examining the effect of the adrenals on the pineal, one group of investigators found that bilateral adrenalectomy in female rats resulted in an alteration in the amount of contact area between pinealocyte processes and glial processes, respectively, and the perivascular space (26).

Normally, 40% of the contact area was occupied by pinealocyte processes and 60% by glial processes; following bilateral adrenalectomy, this proportion was reversed. To determine whether the histologic changes represented an increase in pineal activity, the authors measured hydroxyindole-O-methyltransferase (HIOMT) activity. Following bilateral adrenalectomy, HIOMT activity was found to be significantly increased.

Catecholamines

Pinealectomy has been observed to result in hypertrophy of adrenomedullary cells, with accumulation of secretory granules (27). When pineal extract was given, however, only slight changes were observed in these cells.

Dopamine-β-hydroxylase (DBH) is the enzyme responsible for the conversion of dopamine to norepinephrine. As DBH has been observed to have a 24-hour periodicity, a study (28) was devised to ascertain whether the pineal exerts any control over DBH in rats. Within 1 hour after the onset of darkness, the DBH activity increased approximately sixfold; this rise did not occur when the lights were kept on or when prior pinealectomy had been performed.

In quantitating the number of large granular vesicles (LGV) and small clear vesicles (SCV) in the nerves ending on norepinephrine-containing cells of the adrenal medulla, it was found that the SCV peaked at the middle of the light and dark phases of a 12:12-hour light-dark cycle (29). The LGV peaked at the onset and middle of the dark phase. Pinealectomy resulted in loss of the SCV peak in the dark phase and of the LGV peak at the onset of the dark phase. As prior work (30) on synaptic vesicles in nerves ending on epinephrine-containing adrenomedullary cells had shown rhythmic patterns and quantitative results differing from those just mentioned, it was concluded that epinephrine and norepinephrine adrenomedullary cells are subject to different neuroendocrine and preganglionic regulatory mechanisms.

It appears that rat pineal serotonin-N-acetyltransferase (NAT) activity can be stimulated either by norepinephrine released from postganglionic sympathetic nerve endings in the pineal acting on β-receptors or by circulating adrenomedullary catecholamines (31). The increases in pineal NAT and melatonin generated by the stress of immobilization were observed, in this study, to be prevented by bilateral adrenalectomy, but not by surgical or chemical (6-hydroxydopamine) pineal denervation. In addition, α-adrenergic blockade with phenoxybenzamine potentiated the pineal response to stress, as judged by increased NAT activity; β-adrenergic blockade with propranolol had previously been shown to block this increase in NAT activity (32). The mechanism by which phenoxybenzamine increased pineal NAT activity was unclear. However, it was postulated that either the pineal contained both α- and β-adrenergic receptors, a block of the α-receptors presumably releasing unopposed β activity, or that phenoxybenzamine had acted presynaptically to increase norepinephrine release (33). In any event, the sum and substance of the study appears to be that the increased pineal melatonin synthesis seen with immobilization stress is probably mediated by adrenomedullary catecholamines.

PANCREAS

Insulin

The pineal appears to antagonize the effects of insulin. Melatonin decreased insulin secretion in rat pancreas organ cultures, inhibited glucose-stimulated insulin secretion (34), and increased blood glucose levels in monkeys (35). Blinding rats resulted in depressed insulinlike activity and elevated blood glucose levels (36). Conversely, pinealectomy increased insulin levels after glucose administration in rats (37), reduced blood sugar levels in rats (38), and enhanced the incorporation of tyrosine in the islets of Langerhans (39). When pineal peptides were administered to pinealectomized animals, the enhanced glucose tolerance was reversed (40). More recently, rats made alloxan-diabetic 10 days after either pinealectomy, sham-pinealectomy, or anesthesia without surgery were found to have significantly less hyperglycemia as a result of sham-pinealectomy than that resulting from pinealectomy or no operation at all; the latter two groups did not differ significantly (41). These unusual results were interpreted as signifying a pineal-independent, partially protective effect of sham surgery. Although the explanation for these results seems elusive, the authors postulated a beneficial effect of intracranial surgery per se on glucose homeostasis in these diabetic animals.

PARATHYROIDS

Pinealectomy in rats has been reported to depress parathyroid activity (42) as well as causing hyperplasia of parafollicular cells in the thyroid (43). As the parafollicular cells secrete calcitonin, these effects of pinealectomy would appear to result in a dual mechanism for lowering serum calcium. Nevertheless, previous studies in rats had reported parathyroid hyperactivity with hypercalcemia as a result of pinealectomy (44) and decreased parathyroid function with lowered serum calcium levels following administration of pineal extract (45). Seemingly confirmatory of these latter findings was the observation that hypocalcemia could be produced in rats by administration of pineal 5-methoxytryptamine (5-MeO-T) (46). However, as neither 5-methoxytryptophol (5-MTP) nor melatonin duplicated the effect of 5-MeO-T, and as the latter substance affected both parathyroidectomized and thyroidectomized animals, the observed hypocalcemia must have been produced via a mechanism that did not involve either of these glands. One possibility is that, like calcitonin, 5-MeO-T directly inhibits bone resorption.

Rather than resolving the question of the role of the pineal in parathyroid activity, other work up to the present appears only to have raised more questions. One study (47) reported the advent of muscle spasms and death in pinealectomized, thyroparathyroidectomized rats. It was felt that it was the absence of parathyroid tissue, not the thyroid, that resulted in seizures when combined with pinealectomy (48). Further investigation (49) revealed that seizures in parathyroidectomized, pinealectomized rats apparently involved not only the voluntary nervous system but the autonomic as well. Indeed, pargyline, a monoamine oxidase (MAO) inhibitor, prevented seizures in parathyroidectomized rats which otherwise convulsed following pinealectomy (50). Pargyline resulted in increased concentrations of norepinephrine and dopamine in the telencephalon, and of norepinephrine in the brainstem. Those rats that did not receive pargyline and convulsed were found to have only lowered norepinephrine levels in the telecephalon and brainstem. Investigating four different strains of rats having undergone parathyroidectomy plus pinealectomy, it was found that, while telencephalic norepinephrine was depressed in one strain of rats, it was serotonin (5-hydroxytryptamine, 5-HT) that was lowered in the telencephalon of a different strain; convulsions occurred in 70–75% of these latter two strains (51). Seizures, characterized by wild running, tonic-clonic movements, and, on occasion, death, have been produced in gerbils by pinealectomy alone (52). These seizures totally resembled those in pinealectomized, parathyroidectomized rats, except for a shorter latency to onset. When melatonin was administered to gerbils prior to pinealectomy, these animals manifested fewer seizures than did pinealectomized gerbils that did not receive melatonin (53). These results indicated that melatonin has a suppressive effect on pinealectomy-induced seizures in gerbils; an effect not unlike that reported for pineal extract in electrically induced seizures in cats (54). Just how pinealectomy induces seizures, and how melatonin suppresses them, is still an enigma. To compound the difficulty in unraveling these complexities was a recent report (55) of protection of mice from rapid-shaking-induced convulsions by pinealectomy. This protection was 100% for 23 days following pinealectomy, following which the degree of protection dropped to 70% at 60 days postpinealectomy; however, the latter figure was still greater than the less-than-10% protection rate for sham-operated animals at 60 days.

PINEAL

Hypothalamic Peptides

Various hypothalamic peptides have been found in the pineal. LRH has been found in bovine (56), sheep (57), and rat (58) pineals. Oxytocin and vasopressin have been reported as contents of the bovine pineal (59). Somatostatin has been detected in the pineal of guinea pigs (60) and rats (61), and thyrotropin-releasing hormone (TRH) in bovine, ovine (62,63), and porcine (62) pineals. In the latter instances (62), the amounts of TRH detected in the pineals were similar to previously reported values for the hypothalami of the same species. Whether all these peptides are synthesized in the pineal or transported there via blood or cerebrospinal fluid (CSF) is, at present, unsettled.

Melatonin

Aside from being synthesized primarily in the pineal, secreted, and resulting in various central and peripheral effects outside the pineal, melatonin also appears to have direct effects on the pineal itself. When administered to rats, melatonin resulted in an increase in HIOMT and NAT activities (64). It also increased the number of annulate lamellae, Golgi apparatus, microtubules, procentrioles, and ribosomes. All these alterations would indicate enhanced pineal activity. Some confirmation of this work was found when hamsters were exposed to short photoperiods (1L:23D) and given melatonin (65). The testicular regression that normally occurs with this lighting was prevented by melatonin. A smaller-than-average diameter of pinealocyte nuclei, with the latter having more heterochromatin, less polymorphism, a reduction of hypertrophic smooth endoplasmic reticulum and lipid droplets, all appeared to indicate that melatonin was inhibiting the pineal and, thus, reversing the testicular regression brought about by exposure to short photoperiods. The number of pinealocyte dense-cored secretory vesicles, membrane whorls, and large mitochondria increased, however, implying increased pineal activity.

When ferrets were given melatonin, the circadian rhythm of pineal 5-HT changed to that characteristic of animals exposed to short photoperiods (66). It was suggested that the rhythm of pineal 5-HT might be indicative of the pineal mechanism that controls hypothalamic LRH under different environmental lighting conditions.

Among its many reported effects, melatonin has also been deemed to be the releasing hormone for pineal arginine vasotocin (AVT) (67,68).

Vasotocin

The presence of the arginine form of vasotocin, first purported to be present in bovine pineal extracts (69), was subsequently confirmed to be present in the mammalian pineal (70–73). In the pig, vasotocin was present as the lysine form (74). Other work (75) identified AVT in the CSF of cats, such activity being induced either by injection of hypertonic saline into the third ventricle or by injection of melatonin (67). In addition, in studying bovine pineals, evidence was adduced for an ependymal origin of AVT (76,77); the same finding applied in rats (77) and rabbits (78).

When AVT was injected into the third ventricle of mice, it prevented the increase in pituitary prolactin that had been observed to follow pinealectomy (79) (see Pituitary, Prolactin following).

PITUITARY

As a result of exposure of rats to constant light or removal of the pineal, pituitary MAO activity increases; constant darkness or the addition of melatonin in vitro reduces MAO activity (80). In addition, pinealectomy results in a significant increase in the mitotic rate of cells of the rat pituitary (81).

Conversely, hypophysectomy results in decreased pineal weight in mature as well as immature rats, with the latter manifesting diminished HIOMT activity (82). Ultrastructural examination of the rat pineal following pituitary ablation has revealed alterations compatible with atrophy in the endoplasmic reticulum and ribosomes (83,84).

Thus it would appear that the pineal may exert a generalized inhibitory effect on the pituitary. Indeed, as the pituitary is under hypothalamic control, the finding of a higher affinity binding of melatonin in bovine medial basal hypothalamus (85,86) versus other brain areas tested (i.e., occipital cortex, cerebellar cortex, amygdala, corpus striatum, and pons) would indicate at least one mechanism by which the pineal could modify pituitary function. Furthermore, it would also appear that a normal pituitary is necessary for the development and continued functioning of the pineal.

Growth Hormone

When rats were blinded, the result was a lower pituitary growth hormone (GH) content than that found in blinded-pinealectomized animals or controls; adding anosmia to blinding caused even lower pituitary GH levels as compared to anosmic-blind-pinealectomized rats or controls (87,88). In a study by the author (89), constant darkness significantly lowered rat pituitary and plasma GH levels; these effects were reversed by pinealectomy. It was hypothesized that enhanced pineal activity depressed both the synthesis and secretion of GH. This effect could have been due to an inhibition of α-adrenergic or dopaminergic hypothalamic stimuli or to a direct inhibitory action on the pituitary somatotrophs.

Findings inferred to be the result of removal of pineal inhibition of GH secretion were presented in another study (90) in which the incorporation of ^{35}S-methionine into protein and the amount of liver protein were found to be increased following pinealectomy.

The foregoing would implicate the pineal as being capable of inhibiting GH production and release. However, a recent study (91) expressed the opinion that the results of preceding investigations may have been influenced by stress and/or anesthesia, both of which have been reported to inhibit GH release in the rat (92,93). As a result, this study (91) utilized frequent blood sampling for GH from freely moving, cannulated, purportedly nonstressed rats. It was found that there was a diurnal pattern of GH release in which GH was released less at night. Within this pattern, pinealectomy, versus sham-operated controls, significantly reduced GH release during the day, but there was no further reduction at night. Examination of the methodology in this experiment raises the question as to whether these animals were truly without stress. In any event, if this work can be confirmed, it would necessitate a change in the current concepts of pineal influence on GH secretion.

Melanocyte-Stimulating Hormone

It is of historical interest to note some early observations on the relationship of melanocyte-stimulating hormone (MSH) to the pineal. As early as 1917, it was noted that bovine pineal extract could cause a blanching of tadpole skin (94). Results of reinvestigation of this phenomenon, published 41 years later, revealed that it was melatonin that had produced melanocyte-pigment-granule contraction, the latter leading to skin blanching (95). This latter study also found that melatonin could produce the blanching effect in a concentration of 10^{-12} gm/ml of medium.

Exploring possible treatments for canine melanosis, it was demonstrated that melatonin was effective in decreasing pigmentation (96). However, a subsequent study (97) in mice noted no effect of melatonin on dermal melanocytes.

In the rat, however, a temporary elevation of pituitary MSH resulted from pinealectomy (98). After this initial increment, an apparent compensatory adjustment took place; this was postulated to be the result of an overriding effect of MSH-inhibiting factor (MIF). However, when rats were exposed to constant light, the result was a more prolonged elevation of pituitary MSH (99).

Melanocyte-lightening activity (MLA), defined as the ability to lighten frogs' skin previously made melanotic by hypothalamic destruction, has been noted to be increased in the plasma of hypophysectomized rats (100). Destruction of the hypothalamus in these animals resulted in decreased MLA, as did pinealectomy. In addition, the plasma of the hypophysectomized rats was found to contain increased amounts of MIF and melatonin; MIF enhanced the skin-lightening effect of melatonin. These results would appear to point to the existence of an inhibitory feedback on MIF and melatonin by MSH. Evidence that might indicate an influence of the hypothalamus itself on the pineal was presented in a study (101) using ^{14}C-leucine or ^{3}H-proline MIF (H-Pro-Leu-Gly-NH$_2$) injected iv into rats. The labeled materal was found to accumulate in greatest concentration in the pineal and pituitary. As the intermediate lobe of the pituitary is the main site of action of MIF, its high concentration there is not unexpected. However, in the pineal the labeled MIF was present unchanged and the tissue to plasma ratio increased.

Studying the diurnal rhythm of pituitary MSH, it was found that this rhythm bore no direct relationship to the light-dark cycle, nor was it regulated by melatonin or any other known pineal product (102).

As melatonin has been shown to have an effect on melanocytes, and as the synthesis of melatonin is dependent on activation of NAT, ordinarily via norepinephrine released from postganglionic nerve terminals acting on β-adrenergic receptors on pinealocytes, an experiment (103) was devised to ascertain whether there was any interaction between α-MSH and the pineal β-adrenergic system. This in vitro study demonstrated that, whereas norepinephrine produced hyperpolarization of rat pinealocytes, the addition of α-MSH resulted in significant depolarization and considerably reduced the cyclic-adenosine monophosphate (cyclic-AMP) accumulation that ordinarily follows incubation with norepinephrine. Cyclic-AMP is known to be the second messenger involved in the induction of NAT (104,105). These findings (103) are consonant with the hypothesis offered previously (100) regarding feedback inhibition by MSH on pineal melatonin.

Prolactin

Dissimilar in the nature of its control from other pituitary hormones, with the possible exception of MSH in subhuman mammals, prolactin is tonically held in check by prolactin-inhibiting factor (PIF) (106). The substance currently considered to be a prime candidate for PIF is dopamine (107); however, other substances have been implicated (108).

In studies by the author (109,110), pituitary prolactin concentrations in male rats were significantly greater and plasma prolactin concentrations significantly less than in controls as a result of pinealectomy. Results comparable to those seen with pinealectomy were observed following exposure to constant light. Depressed concentrations of pituitary prolactin with elevated concentrations of plasma prolactin were noted when rats were exposed to constant darkness; these effects were negated by pinealectomy. Blinding, as well as constant darkness, has also been noted to lower the content of pituitary prolactin in rats (111). Electron microscopic study (112) of lactotrophs under various lighting conditions revealed diminished numbers of cytoplasmic granules in sham-pinealectomized male rats exposed to constant darkness, whereas there were numerous granules in similarly operated animals exposed to constant light. The preceding studies would indicate that PIF activity is interfered with by pineal overactivity, eventuating in increased pituitary secretion of prolactin. The result is a diminished content of pituitary prolactin in conjunction with elevated levels of plasma prolactin; constant light or pinealectomy causes the reverse. Previous work (113) in rats had also demonstrated an increased pituitary secretion of prolactin resulting from melatonin.

Another investigation (114) of lactotroph ultrastructural changes, produced in immature female rats using pineal extract, revealed evidence compatible with both enhanced synthesis and release of prolactin.

Lower pituitary prolactin levels occurred in blinded-anosmic, 3-week-old male rats; this decrement was reversed by pinealectomy. In addition, the reduction in pituitary prolactin levels lasted only until age 125 days, at which time these levels had returned to normal (115). Although no hypothesis was offered, a similar compensatory adjustment with the passage of time had been observed previously when elevated pituitary prolactin levels were found following pinealectomy (109). When extracts from the medial basal hypothalamus of blind-anosmic female rats (animals with lowered pituitary and elevated plasma prolactin levels) were injected into ovariectomized, estrogen-progesterone treated rats, plasma prolactin levels fell, whereas when similar extracts from blind-anosmic-pinealectomized rats were used, an increase in plasma prolactin resulted (116). These results appeared to reflect the effect of PIF in the blind-anosmic rats and the effect of a prolactin-releasing factor (5-HT, TRH, vasoactive intestinal polypeptide?) in similarly operated but also pinealectomized animals; this study remains an enigma.

Other workers found, however, that blind-anosmic-castrated, as well as blind-anosmic-noncastrated, male rats had depressed serum prolactin levels and that pinealectomy did not alter the result (117). As these investigators pointed out, one would have expected elevated serum prolactin levels to result from increased pineal activity. They proposed that sightlessness and anosmia reduced the stress of anesthesia and blood sampling, resulting in depressed serum prolactin levels. That stress does not seem to be the entire problem was made evident in another report (118) in which anosmic male rats manifested depressed serum prolactin levels in response to exogenous melatonin. This effect was not seen in anosmic-pinealectomized animals or in intact animals. It was suggested that anosmia sensitizes the site at which melatonin acts to inhibit prolactin levels. This experiment was cited as being confirmatory of previous work by one of the investigators (119). The findings here, like those in the previously cited study (117), are difficult to reconcile with much of what has already been presented. However, other recent work appears consonant with what has preceded. Examining the effects of melatonin in ovariectomized, superior-cervical ganglionectomized or pinealectomized adult female rats primed with estrogen and progesterone, it was found that serum prolactin concentrations were significantly depressed by ganglionectomy. In addition, melatonin produced an elevation of serum prolactin in the controls, but not in the ganglionectomized rats. Pinealectomy blocked the release of prolactin produced by melatonin (120). The effects here demonstrate that exogenous melatonin requires an intact pineal to increase serum prolactin levels.

In another recent study (121), not only did melatonin, injected into the lateral cerebral ventricle, cause a significant increase in plasma prolactin, but so did 5-HT and one of its metabolites, 5-hydroxykynurenamine. The finding of a prolactin-releasing effect of 5-HT had been reported previously (113).

As previously mentioned (see Pineal, Vasotocin), injection of AVT into the third ventricle of mice has been demonstrated to inhibit the increase in pituitary prolactin that occurs following pinealectomy (79). However, when AVT was injected into the anterior pituitary of pinealectomized mice, it was without effect on pituitary prolactin. It was postulated that the intraventricular site of injection enabled AVT to inhibit the synthesis or release of PIF. Indeed, an earlier study (122) had described the presence of modified ependymal cells found around the base of the infundibular and optic recesses of the third ventricle of vervet monkeys. These cells, termed tanycytes, possessed elongated basal processes that extended into the hypothalamic neural tissue beneath them. It was hypothesized that these tanycytes can absorb substances that have been secreted into the CSF, thereby enabling such substances (e.g., indoleamines, peptides) to exert a significant influence over hypothalamic function. These anatomic findings fit nicely with the experiment using AVT, cited earlier.

When a possible relationship of the pineal to the diurnal rhythm of plasma prolactin was explored in rats, the initial conclusion was that the pineal exerted no influence on this rhythm (123). Subsequently, however, another study (124) in rats reported pinealectomy to prevent the rise in serum prolactin normally seen early in the morning. Recent investigation of the association between the pineal and prolactin rhythms has revealed that the circaannual rhythm of prolactin secretion in ewes is primarily determined by the length of the photoperiod in any given season, with the pineal being an essential mediator of this effect (125). Plasma prolactin concentrations were consistently low during the short photoperiods of the winter months and elevated during the summer months. In pinealectomized ewes, prolactin levels were generally raised throughout the year. As regards the diurnal rhythm of prolactin, there was a positive effect of long (i.e., 16L:8D) photoperiods on plasma prolactin in castrated sheep having intact pineals; this effect did not obtain in pinealectomized animals (126). Interestingly, pinealectomy did not abolish the rise in prolactin occurring at dusk. In another study (127), an early morning prolactin peak was observed in male rats, as mentioned earlier. Mean concentrations of prolactin were higher during dark periods, and pinealectomy resulted in prominent peaks during the light periods. In this experiment, the total period for measurement of secretory patterns was 6 hours.

PROSTAGLANDINS

An in vitro study (128), utilizing bovine pineals, demonstrated the release of prostaglandin E- and F-like substances. The release of this material was more than doubled by the addition of norepinephrine to the medium. The presence of high-affinity binding of prostaglandin E_2 and prostaglandin $F_{2\alpha}$ by pineal tissue was established. The significance of these findings requires further elucidation.

THYROID

The overall effect of the pineal on thyroid function would appear to be inhibitory. Pineal extract has been reported to produce a decreased radioactive iodine uptake (RAIU) in mice (129). Melatonin administered to rats decreased RAIU and thyroid weight (130). The secretory rate of thyroxine (T_4) in rats has been shown to be increased by pinealectomy (131) and decreased by melatonin administration (132,133). Not only enhanced T_4 secretory rate, but thyroid hypertrophy as well, has been produced by pinealectomy (134,135). The finding of increased thyroid weight and elevated blood thyrotropin (TSH), as a result of administration of melatonin to rats (136), was interpreted as a direct suppressant effect of melatonin on the thyroid itself, producing findings similar to those produced by goitrogens (137). In keeping with the results of pinealectomy on thyroid activity, another study (138) found enhanced RAIU in rats as a result of using p-chlorophenylalanine, an inhibitor of indoleamine synthesis.

Constant darkness had been reported to increase RAIU in mice, the opposite applying with exposure to constant light (139). A more recent study (140) in rats revealed consonant findings: melatonin, 5-HT, and constant darkness brought about an increase in thyroidal cyclic-AMP, and 5-hydroxytryptophol, 5-MTP, and 5-HT produced an increase in serum T_4 levels, whereas 5-HT and melatonin decreased intrathyroidal T_4 content. The data were interpreted as reflecting a stimulatory effect of pineal indoles on thyroid hormone secretion. Other work (141) in rats has also shown a stimulatory effect of 5-HT, this compound enhancing the incorporation of iodine into follicular cells of the thyroid; however, melatonin inhibited such incorporation. Because melatonin and 5-HT were presented as antagonists in this investigation, it is difficult to understand why they should have worked in concert in the prior study (140), as regards cyclic-AMP. In the case of 5-HT, the decreased intrathyroidal T_4 found could have been the result of enhanced secretion of T_4 because, unlike melatonin, 5-HT elevated serum T_4 levels, whereas the effect of melatonin in decreasing intrathyroidal T_4 could have been due to a block in T_4 synthesis. Indeed, in addition to the studies (132,133) already cited, in which T_4 secretory rate was depressed by melatonin, subsequent work (142,143) in hamsters has shown a depression of plasma T_4 as a result of melatonin administration.

The two studies just mentioned (142,143), as well as one other (144), also demonstrated that blinding hamsters resulted in lowered levels of plasma T_4. The author had previously demonstrated that 21-day-old intact rats, subsequently exposed to 3 days of continuous darkness, manifested depressed levels of plasma and pituitary TSH, as well as plasma protein-bound iodine (PBI). Constant light or pinealectomy resulted in depressed pituitary TSH and elevated plasma TSH and PBI levels; this indicated enhanced secretion of TSH (145). Unlike previous work (136,137) that had hypothesized a direct suppressant effect of melatonin on the thyroid, this work appeared to indicate an effect of the pineal at a central level. A subsequent study (146) by the author demonstrated that, in the same-aged rats treated with saline, constant light, pinealectomy, and constant darkness produced the same effects as previously detailed (except that T_4 levels replaced PBI measurements). However, following intraperitoneal TRH, all rats showed elevated plasma TSH levels as compared to saline-treated controls. Another part of this investigation entailed either no treatment, giving cerebral intraventricular saline or melatonin, or giving intraventricular melatonin plus intraperitoneal TRH to 25-day-old rats reared in diurnal lighting. Melatonin decreased plasma TSH levels compared to nontreated and saline-treated animals; the concurrent administration of TRH with melatonin obviated the effect of melatonin, increasing plasma TSH above control levels. These results would indicate that the inhibitory effect of the pineal on TSH secretion is exerted at the level of hypothalamic secretion of TRH.

Recent work (147) on plasma levels of T_4, triiodothyronine (T_3), and TSH in the developing rat revealed TSH to peak on day 13 of life, T_4 on day 16, and T_3 on day 20. Rats reared in constant darkness from birth, however, manifested significantly reduced T_3 levels on day 20, as compared to controls. Although the authors also spoke of depressed T_4 and elevated TSH levels in the dark-reared versus control animals, they failed to demonstrate any statistically significant differences between these groups for the respective parameters.

Pinealectomy has been demonstrated to increase plasma TSH levels and alter the diurnal rhythm of TSH in rats exposed to 1L:23D (148). Antimelatonin and anti-NAS immunization also resulted in elevated plasma TSH levels in animals exposed to 1L:23D. It was concluded that melatonin and/or NAS may be involved in the maintenance of basal TSH levels and that the pineal may play a role in entraining TSH rhythm to environmental lighting.

Testing both a low- and high-molecular weight fraction of rat pineals on hypophyseal function, it was found that the low-molecular weight fraction stimulated the release of TSH, the response being similar to that seen with TRH (149).

Contrary to current concepts about pineal-hypothalamic-pituitary-thyroid interactions, a recent study (150) found no evidence for any significant effect of the pineal on thyroid function.

Not only does the great bulk of evidence to date indicate an effect of the pineal on the hypothalamic-pituitary-thyroid axis, but apparently the converse is also true. An in vitro study (151) demonstrated that norepinephrine-stimulated accumulation of cyclic-AMP in rat pineal tissue was inhibited by TRH. In another in vitro study (152), the effect of TSH, T_4, and T_3 on basal and norepinephrine-stimulated indoleamine metabolism was examined. TSH was found to be without effect on pineal tryptophan metabolism, irrespective of the presence or absence of norepinephrine in the culture medium. T_4 increased melatonin concentration and, when norepinephrine was also present, increased NAS. T_3, when used in a low dose, increased melatonin and, when used at a higher dose, increased the concentrations of melatonin, 5-HT, NAS, 5-hydroxytryptophol and 5-hydroxyindoleacetic acid, as well as enhancing norepinephrine-stimulated NAS. The investigators interpreted the results as indicating a direct positive feedback of the thyroid on the pineal.

REFERENCES

1. Vaughan M K, Vaughan G M, Reiter R J, Benson B. Effect of melatonin and other pineal indoles on adrenal enlargement produced in male and female mice by pinealectomy, uni-lateral adrenalectomy, castration and cold stress. Neuroendocrinology 10:139–154, 1972.

2. Dickson K L, Hasty D L. Effects of the pineal gland in unilaterally adrenalectomized rats. Acta Endocrinol (Kbh) 70:438–444, 1972.

3. Pavel S, Matrescu L, Pretrescu M. Central corticotrophin inhibition by arginine vasotocin in the mouse. Neuroendocrinology 12:371–375, 1973.

4. Ziegels J, Devecerski V, Duchesne P Y. Étude histochimique de la cortico-surrénale du rat après épiphysectomie. C R Soc Biol 170:206–211, 1976.

5. Losada J. Efectos de la pinealectomia experimental. An Anat 26:133–153, 1977.

6. Kennedy A, Kilshaw D, Reid N C, Taylor W H. Pineal enlargement: with hypernatremia, hypokalaemic alkalosis, and thyrotoxicosis. Br Med J 2:641–644, 1962.

7. Gromova E A, Kraus M, Krecek J. Effect of melatonin and 5-hydroxytryptamine on aldosterone and corticosterone production by adrenal glands of normal and hypophysectomized rats. J Endocrinol 39:345–350, 1967.

8. Fabre L F Jr, Banks R C, McIsaac W M, Farrell G. Effects of ubiquinone and related substances on secretion of aldosterone and cortisol. Am J Physiol 208:1275–1280, 1965.

9. Kinson G A, Singer B. Effect of pinealectomy on adrenocortical secretion in normal rats and in rats with experimental renal hypertension. J Endocrinol 37:37–38, 1967.

10. Kinson G A, Wahid A K, Singer B. Effect of chronic pinealectomy on adreno-cortical hormone secretion rates in normal and hypertensive rats. Gen Comp Endocrinol 8:445–454, 1967.

11. Kinson G A, Singer B, Grant L. Adrenocortical hormone secretion at various time intervals after pinealectomy in the rat. Gen Comp Endocrinol 10:447–449, 1968.

12. Chazov E I, Isachenkov V A, Krivosheev O G, Tuzhilin V D. A hyperkalemic factor from the pineal gland. Bull Exp Biol Med 74:1475–1477, 1973.

13. Motta M, Fraschini F, Piva F, Martini L. Hypothalamic and extra-hypothalamic mechanisms controlling adrenocorticotropin secretion. In Memoirs of the Society for Endocrinology, vol 17. Cambridge University Press, 1968, pp 3–18.

14. Henzl M R, Spaur C L, Magoun R E, Kincl F A. A note on endocrine functions of neonatally pinealectomized rats. Endocrinol Exp (Bratisl) 4:77–81, 1970.

15. Golikov P P, Fominykh E S. Melatonin action on the rate of aldosterone and corticosterone secretion in intact, pseudoepiphyse- and epiphysectomized rats. Farmakol Toksikol 37:696–698, 1974.

16. Golikov P P, Konyushko S D. The effect of the extracts of the epiphysis on the content of 11-OCS in the peripheral blood of rats. Probl Endokrinol (Mosk) 20:81–85, 1974.

17. Heiman M L, Porter J R. Inhibitory effects of a pineal extract on adrenal cortex. Lack of competition with ACTH. Horm Res 12:104–112, 1980.

18. Ogle T F, Kitay J I. Effects of pinealectomy on adrenal function in vivo and in vitro in female rats. Endocrinology 98:20–24, 1976.

19. Vaughan G M, Allen J P, Vaughan M K, Siler-Khodr T M. Influence of pinealectomy on corticotropin (ACTH). Experientia 36:364–365, 1980.

20. Ogle T F, Kitay J I. Effects of melatonin and an aqueous pineal extract on adrenal secretion of reduced steroid metabolites in female rats. Neuroendocrinology 23:113–120, 1977.

21. Ogle T F, Kitay J I. In vitro effects of melatonin and serotonin on adrenal steroidogenesis. Proc Soc Exp Biol Med 157:103–105, 1978.

22. Mehdi A Z, Sandor T. The effect of melatonin on the biosynthesis of corticosteroids in beef adrenal preparations in vitro. J Steroid Biochem 8:821–823, 1977.

23. Rivest R W, Roberts K D, Lepore F. The pineal gland and stress: effect of pineal stalk section on the plasma corticosteroid response to cold in rabbits. Psychol Rep 44:883–890, 1979.

24. Takahashi K, Inoue K, Takahashi Y. No effect of pinealectomy on the parallel shift in circadian rhythms of adrenocortical activity and food intake in blinded rats. Endocrinol Jap 23:417–421, 1976.

25. Niles L P, Brown G M, Grota L J. Endocrine effects of the pineal gland and neutralization of circulating melatonin and N-acetylserotonin. Can J Physiol Pharmacol 55:537–544, 1977.

26. Deussen-Schmitter M, Garweg G, Schwabedal P E, Wartenberg H. Simultaneous changes of the perivascular contact area and HIMOT activity in the pineal organ after bilateral adrenalectomy in the rat. Anat Embryol 149:297–305, 1976.

27. Petrescu C, Simionescu N. Experimental studies on the relation between the pineal body and the adrenal medulla in the albino rat. Stud Cercet Endocrinol 21:339–343, 1970.

28. Banerji P K, Quay W B. Adrenal dopamine-β-hydroxylase activity: 24-hour rhythmicity and evidence for pineal control. Experientia 32:253–255, 1976.

29. Kachi T, Banerji T K, Quay W B. Circadian and ultradian changes in synaptic vesicle numbers in nerve endings on adrenomedullary noradrenaline cells, and their modifications by pinealectomy and sham operations. Neuroendocrinology 30:291–299, 1980.

30. Kachi T, Banerji T K, Quay W B. Daily rhythmic changes in synaptic vesicle contents of nerve endings on adrenomedullary adrenaline cells, and their modification by pinealectomy and sham operations. Neuroendocrinology 28:201–211, 1979.

31. Lynch H J, Ho M, Wurtman R J. The adrenal medulla may mediate the increase in pineal melatonin synthesis induced by stress, but not that caused by exposure to darkness. J Neural Transm 40:87–97, 1977.

32. Lynch H J, Eng J P, Wurtman R J. Control of pineal indole biosynthesis by changes in sympathetic tone caused by factors other than environmental lighting. Proc Nat Acad Sci USA 70:1704–1707, 1973.

33. Enero M A, Langer S Z, Rothlin R P, Stefano F J E. Role of the α-adrenoceptor in regulating noradrenaline overflow by nerve stimulation. Br J Pharmacol 44:672–688, 1972.

34. Bailey C J, Atkins T W, Matty A J. Melatonin inhibition of insulin secretion in the rat and mouse. Horm Res 5:21–28, 1974.

35. Burns J K. Serum sodium and potassium and blood glucose levels in cynamolgus monkeys after administration of melatonin. J Physiol (Lond) 232:84–85P, 1973.

36. Benson B, Miller C W, Sorrentino S. Effects of blinding on blood glucose and serum insulin-like activity in rats. Tex Rep Biol Med 29:513–525, 1971.

37. Milcou S M, Nanu-Ionescu L, Milcou I. The effect of pinealectomy on plasma insulin in rats. In The Pineal Gland, ed G E W Wolstenholme, J Knight. Churchill, Livingstone, London & Edinburgh, 1971, pp 345–357.

38. Csaba G, Baráth P. Are Langerhans' islets influenced by the pineal body? Experientia 27:962, 1971.

39. Csaba G, Nagy U. The regulatory role of the pineal gland on the thyroid gland, adrenal medulla and islets of Langerhans. Acta Biol Med Ger 31:617–619, 1973.

40. Nanu L, Marcean R, Ionescu V, Milcou I. Correlations between pineal body and pyruvemia levels. Rev Roum Endocrinol 6:141–147, 1969.

41. Gorray K C, Quay W B. Effects of pinealectomy and of sham-pinealectomy on blood glucose levels in the alloxan-diabetic rat. Horm Metab Res 10:389–392, 1978.

42. Kiss J, Banhegyi D, Csaba G. Endocrine regulation of blood calcium level. II. Relationship between the pineal body and the parathyroid glands. Acta Med Acad Sci Hung 26:363–370, 1969.

43. Miline R, Scepovic M, Krstic R. Influence de l'epiphysectomie sur les cellules parafolliculaires de la glande thyroid. C R Assoc Anat 139:893–898, 1968.

44. Krstic R. Über Veränderungen der Epithelkörperchen nach Epiphysektomie. Z Zellforsch Mikrosk Anat 77:8–24, 1967.

45. Krstic R. Über die Wirkung von Epiphysenextrakt auf die Struktur der Epithelkörperchen der Ratte. Z Zellforsch Mikrosk Anat 89:73–79, 1968.

46. Choe J-Y, Peng T-Ch. Effect of 5-methyoxytryptamine on serum calcium and phosphate in rats. J Pharmacol Exp Ther 189:593–602, 1974.

47. Reiter R J, Sorrentino S Jr, Hoffman R A. Muscular spasms and death in thyroparathyroidectomized rats subjected to pinealectomy. Life Sci 12:123–133, 1972.

48. Reiter R J, Morgan W W. Attempts to characterize the convulsive response of parathyroidectomized rats to pineal gland removal. Physiol Behav 9:203–208, 1972.

49. Reiter R J, Blask D E, Talbot J A, Barnett M P. Nature and the time course of seizures associated with surgical removal of the pineal gland from parathyroidectomized rats. Exp Neurol 38:386–397, 1973.

50. Herrera H H, Morgan W W, Reiter R J. Brain norepinephrine levels in parathyroidectomized rats induced to convulse by pinealectomy. Exp Neurol 48:595–600, 1975.

51. Philo R, Reiter R J. Brain amines and convulsions in four strains of parathyroidectomized, pinealectomized rat. Epilepsia 19:133–137, 1978.

52. Philo R, Reiter R J. Characterization of pinealectomy induced convulsions in the mongolian gerbil (Meriones unguiculatus). Epilepsia 19:485–492, 1978.

53. Rudeen P K, Philo R C, Symmes S K. Antiepileptic effects of melatonin in the pinealectomized mongolian gerbil. Epilepsia 21:149–154, 1980.

54. Roldan E, Anton-Tay F. EEG and convulsive threshold changes produced by pineal extract administration. Brain Res 11:238–245, 1968.

55. Hata T, Kita T. A newly designed method for removal of the pineal body, and depression of convulsions and enhancement of exploratory movements by pinealectomy in mice. Endocrinol Jap 25:407–413, 1978.

56. Duraiswami S, Franchimont P, Boucher D, Thiebolt M. Immunoreactive luteinizing hormone-releasing hormone (LH-RH) in the bovine pineal gland. Horm Metab Res 8:232–233, 1976.

57. Kotaras P, McIntosh J E A, Seamark R F. Gonadotropin releasing hormone activity of the sheep pineal gland. J Neural Transm (Suppl) 13:374, 1978 (Abstract)

58. Pevet R, Ebels I, Swaab D F, Mud M T, Arimura A. Presence of AVT- α-MSH- LHRH- and somatostatin-like compounds in the rat pineal gland and their relationship with the UM05R pineal fraction. Cell Tissue Res 206:341–353, 1980.

59. Fisher L A, Spindel E R, Fernstrom J D. Nonapeptide content of the bovine pineal gland. Endocrine Soc Abstr, p 103, 1980.

60. Dube D, LeClerc R, Pelletier G. Immunohistochemical detection of growth hormone inhibiting hormone (SRIF) in guinea pig brain. Cell Tissue Res 161:385–392, 1975.

61. Pelletier G, LeClerc R, Dube D, Labrie F, Puviani R, Arimura A, Schally A V. Localization of growth hormone-releasing-inhibiting hormone (somatostatin) in the rat brain. Am J Anat 142:397–401, 1975.

62. White W F, Hedlund M T, Weber G F, Rippel R H, Johnson E S, Wilber J F. The pineal gland: a supplemental source of hypothalamic-releasing hormones. Endocrinology 94:1422–1426, 1974.

63. Youngblood W W, Humm J, Kizer J S. TRH-like immunoreactivity in rat pancreas and eye, bovine and sheep pineals, and human placenta: non-identity with synthetic Pyroglu-His-Pro-NH₂ (TRH). Brain Res 163:101–110, 1979.

64. Freire F, Cardinali D P. Effects of melatonin treatment and environmental lighting on the ultrastructural appearance, melatonin synthesis, norepinephrine turnover and microtubule protein content of the rat pineal gland. J Neural Transm 37:237–257, 1975.

65. Barratt G F, Nadakavukaren M J, Frehn J L. Effect of melatonin implants on gonadal weights and pineal gland fine structure of the golden hamster. Tissue Cell 9:335–345, 1977.

66. Yates C A, Herbert J. Differential circadian rhythms in pineal and hypothalamic 5-HT induced by artificial photoperiods or melatonin. Nature 262:219–220, 1976.

67. Pavel S. Arginine vasotocin release into cerebrospinal fluid of cats induced by melatonin. Nature 246:183–184, 1973.

68. Pavel S, Goldstein R. Further evidence that melatonin represents the releasing hormone for pineal vasotocin. J Endocrinol 82:1–6, 1979.

69. Milcu S M, Pavel S, Neascu C. Biological and chromatographic characterization of a polypeptide with pressor and oxytocic activities isolated from bovine pineal gland. Endocrinology 72:563–566, 1963.

70. Pavel S. Endocrine functions of arginine vasotocin from mammalian pineal gland. Gen Comp Endocrinol 9:481–485, 1967.

71. Cheesman D W. Structure elucidation of a gonadotropin inhibiting substance from the bovine pineal gland. Biochim Biophys Acta 207:247–253, 1970.

72. Pavel S. Vasotocin content in the pineal gland of fetal, newborn and adult male rats. J Endocrinol 66:283–284, 1975.

73. Rosenbloom A A, Fisher D A. Radioimmunoassayable AVT and AVP in adult mammalian brain tissue: comparison of normal and Brattleboro rats. Neuroendocrinology 17:354–361, 1975.

74. Pavel S. Evidence for the presence of lysine vasotocin in the pig pineal. Endocrinology 77:812–817, 1965.

75. Pavel S, Coculescu M. Arginine vasotocin-like activity of cerebrospinal fluid induced by hypertonic saline injected into the third cerebral ventricle of cats. Endocrinology 91:825–827, 1972.

76. Pavel S. Evidence for the ependymal origin of arginine vasotocin in the bovine pineal gland. Endocrinology 89:613–614, 1971.

77. Benson B, Matthews M J, Hadley M E, Powers S, Hruby V J. Differential localization of antigonadotropic and vasotocic activities in bovine and rat pineal. Life Sci 19:747–754, 1976.

78. Rosenbloom A A, Fisher D A. Arginine vasotocin in the rabbit subcommissural organ. Endocrinology 96:1038–1039, 1975.

79. Pavel S, Calb M, Georgescu M. Reversal of the effects of pinealectomy on the pituitary prolactin content in mice by very low concentrations of vasotocin injected into the third cerebral ventricle. J Endocrinol 66:289–290, 1975.

80. Urry, R L, Ellis L C. Monoamine oxidase activity of the hypothalamus and pituitary: alterations after pinealectomy, changes in photoperiod or addition of melatonin *in vitro*. Experientia 31:891–892, 1975.

81. Bindoni M, Raffaele R. Mitotic activity in the adenohypophysis of rats after pinealectomy. J Endocrinol 41:451–452, 1968.

82. Urry R L, Barfuss D W, Ellis L C. HIOMT activity of male rat pineal glands following hypophysectomy and HCG treatment. Biol Reprod 6:238–243, 1972.

83. Lupulescu A. Ultrastructure of the pineal gland after hypophysectomy. Experientia 24:482–484, 1968.

84. Karasek M. Ultrastructure of the epiphysis in white rats under normal conditions and after hypophysectomy. Endokrynol Pol 22:13–26, 1971.

85. Cardinali D P, Vacas M I, Boyer E E. High affinity binding of melatonin in bovine medial basal hypothalamus. J Int Res Commun 6:357, 1978.

86. Cardinali D P, Vacas M I, Boyer E E. Specific binding of melatonin in bovine brain. Endocrinology 105:437–441, 1979.

87. Sorrentino S Jr, Reiter R J, Schalch D S. Pineal regulation of growth hormone synthesis and release in blinded and blinded-anosmic male rats. Neuroendocrinology 7:210–218, 1971.

88. Sorrentino S Jr, Reiter R J, Schalch D S, Donofrio R J. Role of the pineal gland in growth restraint of adult male rats by light and smell deprivation. Neuroendocrinology 8:116–124, 1971.

89. Relkin R. Effects of pinealectomy, constant light and darkness on growth hormone in the pituitary and plasma of the rat. *J Endocrinol* 53:289–293, 1972.

90. Gasanov S G, Akhmedova N A. Effect of the pineal body on regulation of protein metabolism. Bull Exp Biol Med 73:49–51, 1972.

91. Rønnelkeiv O K, McCann S M. Growth hormone release in conscious pinealectomized and sham-operated male rats. Endocrinology 102:1694–1701, 1978.

92. Schalch D S, Reichlin S. Plasma growth hormone concentration in the rat determined by radioimmunoassay: influence of sex, pregnancy, lactation, anesthesia, hypophysectomy and extrasellar pituitary transplant. Endocrinology 79:275–280, 1966.

93. Krulich L, Hefco E, Illner P, Read C B. The effects of acute stress on secretion of LH, FSH, prolactin and GH in the normal male rat, with comments on their statistical evaluation. Neuroendocrinology 16:293–311, 1974.

94. McCord C P, Allen F P. Evidences associating pineal gland function with alterations in pigmentation. J Exp Zool 23:207–224, 1917.

95. Lerner A B, Case J D, Takahashi Y, Lee T H, Mori W. Isolation of melatonin, the pineal gland factor that lightens melanocytes. J Am Chem Soc 80:2587, 1958.

96. Rickards D A. The therapeutic effect of melatonin on canine melanosis. J Invest Dermatol 44:13–16, 1965.

97. Reams W M Jr, Shervette R E, Dorman W H. Refractoriness of mouse dermal melanocytes to hormones. J Invest Dermatol 50:338–339, 1968.

98. Kastin A J, Redding T W, Schally A V. MSH activity in rat pituitaries after pinealectomy. Proc Soc Exp Biol Med 124:1275–1277, 1967.

99. Kastin A J, Schally A V, Viosca S, Barrett L, Redding T W. MSH activity in the pituitaries of rats exposed to constant illumination. Neuroendocrinology 2:257–262, 1967.

100. Kastin A J, Viosca S, Nair R M G, Schally A V, Miller M C. Interactions between pineal hypothalamus and pituitary involving melatonin, MSH release-inhibiting factor and MSH. Endocrinology 91:1323–1328, 1972.

101. Redding T W, Kastin A J, Nair R M G, Schally A V. Distribution, half-life, and excretion of ^{14}C- and ^{3}H-labeled L-prolyl-L-leucyl-glycinamide in the rat. Neuroendocrinology 11:92–100, 1973.

102. Tilders F J H, Smelik P G. A diurnal rhythm in melanocyte-stimulating hormone content of the rat pituitary gland and its independence from the pineal gland. Neuroendocrinology 12:296–308, 1975.

103. Sakai K K, Schneider D, Felt B, Marks B H. The effect of αMSH on β-adrenergic receptor mechanisms in the rat pineal. Life Sci 19:1145–1150, 1976.

104. Deguchi T. Role of the beta-adrenergic receptor in the elevation of adenosine cyclic 3′,5′-monophosphate and induction of serotonin N-acetyltransferase in rat pineal glands. Mol Pharmacol 9:184–190, 1973.

105. Klein D C, Weller J L. Adrenergic-adenosine 3′,5′-monophosphate regulation of serotonin N-acetyltransferase activity and the temporal relationship of serotonin N-acetyltransferase activity to the synthesis of ^{3}H-N-acetylserotonin and ^{3}H-melatonin in the cultured rat pineal gland. J Pharmacol Exp Ther 186:516–527, 1973.

106. Schally A V, Meites J, Bowers C Y, Ratner A. Identity of prolactin-inhibiting factor (PIF) and luteinizing hormone-releasing factor (LRF). Proc Soc Exp Biol Med 117:252–254, 1964.

107. Gibbs D M, Neill J D. Dopamine levels in hypophyseal stalk blood in the rat are sufficient to inhibit prolactin secretion in vivo. Endocrinology 102:1895–1900, 1973.

108. Chang N, Ebels I, Benson B. Preliminary characterization of bovine pineal prolactin releasing (PPRF) and release-inhibiting factor (PPIF) activity. J Neural Transm 46:139–151, 1979.

109. Relkin R. Rat pituitary and plasma prolactin levels after pinealectomy. J Endocrinol 53:179–180, 1972.

110. Relkin R. Effects of variations in environmental lighting on pituitary and plasma prolactin levels in the rat. Neuroendocrinology 9:278–284, 1972.

111. Donofrio R J, Reiter R J. Depressed pituitary prolactin levels in blinded anosmic female rats: role of the pineal gland. J Reprod Fertil 31:159–162, 1972.

112. Relkin R., Adachi M, Kahan S A. Effects of pinealectomy and constant light and darkness on prolactin levels in the pituitary and plasma and on pituitary ultrastructure of the rat. J Endocrinol 54:263–268, 1972.

113. Kamberi I A, Mical R S, Porter J C. Effects of melatonin and serotonin on the release of FSH and prolactin. Endocrinology 88:1288–1293, 1971.

114. Kozyritsky V G, Zryakov O N, Gordienko V M. Changes in lactotropocytes upon administration of the epiphyseal factor stimulating prolactin secretion. Tsitologiya 22:405–408, 1980.

115. Reiter R J. Pituitary and plasma prolactin levels in male rats as influenced by the pineal gland. Endocrinol Res Commun 1:169–180, 1974.

116. Blask D E, Reiter R J. The pineal gland of the blind-anosmic female rat; its influence on medial basal hypothalamic LRH, PIF and/or PRF activity in vivo. Neuroendocrinology 17:362–374, 1975.

117. Rønnekleiv O K, McCann S M. Effects of pinealectomy, anosmia and blinding on serum and pituitary prolactin in intact and castrated male rats. Neuroendocrinology 17:340–353, 1975.

118. Blask D E, Nodelman J L. An interaction between the pineal gland and olfactory deprivation in potentiating the effects of melatonin on gonads, accessory sex organs, and prolactin in male rats. J Neurosci Res 5:129–136, 1980.

119. Blask D E, Vaughan M K, Reiter R J, Johnson L Y, Vaughan G M. Prolactin-releasing and release-inhibiting factor activities in the bovine, rat and human pineal gland: in vitro and in vivo studies. Endocrinology 99:152–162, 1976.

120. Cardinali D P, Faigon M R, Scacchi P, Moguilevsky J. Failure of melatonin to increase serum prolactin levels in ovariectomized rats subjected to superior cervical ganglionectomy or pinealectomy. J Endocrinol 82:315–319, 1979.

121. Iwasaki Y, Kato Y, Ohgo S, Abe H, Imura H, Hirata F, Senoh S, Tokuyama T, Hayaishi O. Effects of indoleamines and their newly identified metabolites on prolactin release in rats. Endocrinology 103:254–258, 1978.

122. Knight B K, Hayes M M M, Symington R B. An anatomical study of the pineal body of the vervet monkey (Cercopithecus aethiops). S Afr J Med Sci 39:133–141, 1974.

123. Kizer J S, Zivin J A, Jacobowitz D M, Kopin I J. The nyctohemeral rhythm of plasma prolactin: effects of ganglionectomy, pinealectomy, constant light, constant darkness or 6-OH-dopamine administration. Endocrinology 96:1230–1240, 1975.

124. Rønnekleiv O K, Kurlich L, McCann S M. An early morning surge of prolactin in the male rat and its abolition by pinealectomy. Endocrinology 92:1339–1342, 1973.

125. Munro C J, McNatty K P, Renshaw L. Circa-annual rhythms of prolactin secretion in ewes and the effect of pinealectomy. J Endocrinol 84:83–89, 1980.

126. Brown W B, Forbes J M. Diurnal variations of plasma prolactin in growing sheep under two lighting regimes and the effect of pinealectomy. J Endocrinol 84:91–99, 1980.

127. Willoughby J O. Pinealectomy mildly disturbs the secretory patterns of prolactin and growth hormone in the unstressed rat. J Endocrinol 86:101–107, 1980.

128. Cardinali D P, Ritta M N, Speziale N S, Gimeno M F. Release and specific binding of prostaglandins in bovine pineal gland. Prostaglandins 18:577–589, 1979.

129. Anton-Tay F, Anton S, Tover-Zamora E. Inhibicien de la function-tiroridea producido par la administracion de extracto pineal. Rev Invest Clin 15:367–375, 1963.

130. Baschieri L, De Luca F, Cramarossa L, De Martino C, Oliverio A, Negri M. Modifications of thyroid activity by melatonin. Experientia 19:15–17, 1963.

131. Ishibashi T, Hahn D W, Srivastava L, Kumaresan P, Turner C W. Effect of pinealectomy on feed consumption and thyroid hormone secretion rate. Proc Soc Exp Biol Med 122:644–647, 1966.

132. Singh D V. Effect of various hormones upon thyroxine secretion rate in experimental animals. Diss Abstr 28:3043, 1968.

133. Singh D V, Narang G D, Turner C W. Effect of melatonin and its withdrawal on thyroid hormone secretion rate of female rats. J Endocrinol 43:489–490, 1969.

134. Houssay A B, Pazo J H. Role of the pituitary in the thyroid hypertrophy of pinealectomized rats. Experientia 24:813–814, 1968.

135. De Fronzo R A, Roth W D. Evidence for the existence of a pineal-adrenal and a pineal-thyroid axis. Acta Endocrinol (Kbh) 70:35–42, 1972.

136. Panda J N, Turner C W. The role of melatonin in the regulation of thyrotropin secretion. Acta Endocrinol (Kbh) 57:363–373, 1968.

137. Panda J N. Neural control of thyrotropin (TSH) secretion. Diss Abstr 28:3042, 1968.

138. De Prospo N, Melgar M. Effects of p-chlorophenylalanine on pineal serotonin and ^{131}I uptake by the thyroid glands of rats. J Endocrinol 66:295–296, 1975.

139. Puntriano G, Meites J. The effects of continuous light or darkness on thyroid function in mice. Endocrinology 48:217–224, 1951.

140. Nir I, Hirschmann N, Puder M, Petrank J. Changes in rodent thyroid hormones and cyclic-AMP following treatment with pineal indolic compounds. Arch Int Physiol Biochim 86:353–362, 1978.

141. Csaba G, Richter T. Collaboration of serotonin and melatonin in the control of thyroid function. Acta Biol Med Ger 34:1097–1100, 1975.

142. Vriend J, Reiter R J. Free thyroxin index in normal, melatonin-treated and blind hamsters. Horm Metab Res 9:231–234, 1977.

143. Vriend J, Reiter R J, Anderson G R. Effects of the pineal and melatonin on thyroid activity of male golden hamsters. Gen Comp Endocrinol 38:189–195, 1979.

144. Vriend J, Sackman J W, Reiter R J. Effects of blinding, pinealectomy and superior cervical ganglionectomy on free thyroxine index of male golden hamsters. Acta Endocrinol (Kbh) 86:758–762, 1977.

145. Relkin R. Effects of pinealectomy and constant light and darkness on thyrotropin levels in the pituitary and plasma of the rat. Neuroendocrinology 10:46–52, 1972.

146. Relkin R. Use of melatonin and synthetic TRH to determine site of pineal inhibition of TSH secretion. Neuroendocrinology 25:310–318, 1978.

147. Ooka-Souda S, Draves D J, Timiras P S. Developmental patterns of plasma TSH, T_4 and T_3 in rats deprived of light from birth. Mech Ageing Dev 6:287–291, 1977.

148. Niles L P, Brown G M, Grota L J. Role of the pineal gland in diurnal endocrine secretion and rhythm regulation. Neuroendocrinology 29:14–21, 1979.

149. Demoulin A. Influence de la glande pinéale sur la fonction hypophysaire du rat *in vitro*. Arch Int Physiol Biochim 87:119–153, 1979.

150. Brammer G L, Morley J E, Geller E, Yuwiler A, Hershman J M. Hypothalamus-pituitary-thyroid axis interactions with pineal gland in the rat. Am J Physiol 236:E416–E420, 1979.

151. Tsang D, Martin J B. Effect of hypothalamic hormones on the concentration of adenosine 3′, 5′-monophosphate in incubated rat pineal glands. Life Sci 19:911–918, 1976.

152. Nir I, Hirschmann N. The effect of thyroid hormones on rat pineal indoleamine metabolism *in vitro*. J Neural Transm 42:117–126, 1978.

RICHARD RELKIN, M.D.

MISCELLANEOUS EFFECTS
OF THE PINEAL

As can be seen from what follows, the pineal apparently exerts its influence in many diversified areas in addition to those already described in preceding chapters. The significance and pathophysiology in many of these instances has yet to be clarified.

AGING

The treatment of rats with a pineal extract polypeptide in doses of 0.1 or 0.5 mg for 20 months resulted in a lifespan that was increased by 10 and 25% respectively (1). Comparing ultrastructural changes in the pineals of 1-month-old and 28-month-old rats, it was found that increasing age was accompanied by increased capsule thickness, increased collagen infiltration, increased amounts of granular deposits between cells, greater variability in the number of light pinealocytes, increased numbers of pinealocytes with nuclear invaginations and nuclear inclusions, increased numbers of cytoplasmic dense bodies in pinealocytes and gliocytes, increased maximum diameter of lipid droplets in pinealocytes, no

From Easton Hospital, Easton, Pennsylvania 18042, and Hahnemann Medical College and Hospital, Philadelphia, Pennsylvania 19102.

change in granular endoplasmic reticulum, and occasional cells with reticulated mitochondria; some cell processes had an appearance allied to that of neuroaxonal dystrophy (2).

BEHAVIOR

Activity

Treadwheel recordings taken 12 weeks after pinealectomizing rats revealed greater activity than that seen in controls; treadwheel activity was reduced following administration of pineal extract (3). In this study, the number of rats used was small and some were female. As it has long been known that female-rat activity increases during estrus (4), further investigation was necessary. When rats were deprived of food and then given melatonin, their treadwheel activity decreased; however, this depressant effect abated after 5 days of treatment (5). Other work (6) revealed that pinealectomy had no effect on the activity cycle of rats exposed to diurnal or constant lighting. Subsequently, the effect of prepubertal and postpubertal pinealectomy on treadwheel activity of male rats was investigated by the author (7). Animals were either pinealectomized or sham-pinealectomized at age 2–4 days or 93–98 days of age. Commencing at age 42–45 days, both groups were tested in bright light and constant darkness. The rats operated on at age 93–98 days were rerun on the treadwheel at age 108–113 days. It was found that neither mean revolutions per hour in darkness and light nor dark versus light comparisons differed significantly for any of the groups.

Increased exploratory activity has been observed in female rats pinealectomized at 2–3 days of age and tested in an open field at age 80 days; treatment with pineal extract decreased this activity in both pinealectomized and control groups, melatonin having no effect (8). However, a subsequent study (9), though confirming the absence of an effect of melatonin on exploratory activity in rats, also found no effect from pinealectomy. Comparing adult hypoactive to adult hyperactive rats, it was found that the former group demonstrated increased exploratory behavior following pinealectomy, whereas the latter group manifested no behavioral change (10). In another report (11), blinded-anosmic female rats showed increased locomotor activity in open-field running; weekly melatonin implants or pinealectomy reversed this effect. This study was based on the prior findings that blinding results in hyperactivity in rats (12), as does anosmia (13). In addition, chronic melatonin administration apparently vitiates the effects of the pineal (14), resulting in a functional pinealectomy (15).

A recent experiment (16) has demonstrated that the running activity of pinealectomized female hamsters could be reentrained to photoperiod reversal in 5.1 days as compared to 7.3 days for control animals.

When the effects of prepubertal and postpubertal pinealectomy on maze performance were examined in male rats, it was discovered that this learning activity was not affected by the operation (17).

Aggression

As a result of 15-minute pairing of sham-pinealectomized, sham-pine-alectomized plus pinealectomized, or pinealectomized adult wild-derived male rats, it was observed that the mean latency to initiation of fighting doubled and the duration of fighting decreased by 35–41% in pairs in which one or both members were pinealectomized [18]. This work was subsequently confirmed by other investigators who found that, in addition to pinealectomy, melanocyte-stimulating hormone (MSH) also lowered aggression levels [19]; however, the effects of MSH and pinealectomy were not additive.

Ethanol Preference

Rats with intact pineals, but congenitally blind or exposed to continuous darkness, manifest a preference for ethanol versus water [20,21]. In congenitally blind, pinealectomized rats, as well as in intact animals with normal vision, exposed to diurnal lighting, the preference was for water, not ethanol [22]. These results imply that pineal hyperactivity dictates a preference for ethanol. Other workers, however, found that rats preferred 4% ethanol to water, irrespective of lighting conditions [23]. Nevertheless, environmental lighting did affect the amount of ethanol consumption, the latter being increased by continuous darkness, as well as by melatonin. Ethanol intake was not affected by pinealectomy under any lighting condition. These results were interpreted as indicating that the pineal is not involved in ethanol preference or amount consumed. This interpretation, however, still leaves the explanation of some of the findings unanswered.

Passive Avoidance

The effect of MSH and melatonin on the acquisition and extinction of a passive avoidance response was tested in rats [24]. It was found that MSH delayed extinction of the passive avoidance response, whereas melatonin enhanced its extinction. MSH also increased and maintained high defecation rates during both acquisition and extinction phases of the passive avoidance response, whereas melatonin did not cause a significant increase in defecation during acquisition and had no influence on defecation during extinction. These results suggest a positive effect of MSH on long-term memory and emotionality and an inhibitory effect by melatonin on these parameters.

As the effects of MSH and pinealectomy were similar in an experiment mentioned previously (see Aggression), it is not surprising to find MSH and melatonin having opposite effects here.

Saccharin Neophobia

Based in large part on findings such as those just mentioned, an experiment [25] was designed to determine whether melatonin would alter the usual neophobic response of rats to a novel taste. This phobic response is usually accompanied by emotional responses such as biting or rattling the drinking tube that delivers the new substance. Melatonin caused a significant increase in the consumption of saccharin solution, once again demonstrating this indoleamine's ability to inhibit emotional responses.

Salt Preference

It had previously been demonstrated that sexually mature female rats drink more saline than do males in a situation in which there is a free choice between water and 3% saline (26). These results also applied in the instance of ovariectomy at age 20 days. However, saline intake could be decreased to that seen in intact adult males by testosterone propionate administration to females at age 2 days (27). In a follow-up study (28), it was found that increased saline intake by female rats could be accelerated by neonatal pinealectomy, the increased intake occurring only in sexually immature females, however. Neonatal "masculinization" of female rats, using testosterone propionate, reversed the increased saline intake in adult females, as well as reversing the accelerated appearance of enhanced saline intake in pinealectomized, immature females. When male rats were subjected to neonatal gonadectomy, increased saline intake was observed in adult-aged rats, but not in young animals. However, if neonatal pinealectomy was added to gonadectomy, increased saline intake also occurred in the young rats (29). As the male hypothalamus can be "feminized" by neonatal gonadectomy (30), the female hypothalamus "masculinized" by neonatal androgen administration (31), and maturation of gonadal function accelerated by pinealectomy (32), it would appear that the degree of saline versus water intake in rats is sex-dependent.

Social Isolation

Social isolation of the immature rat has been observed to induce pineal hypertrophy (33).

Stress

Stress has been reported to result in increased synthesis and release of melatonin in rats (34). Subjecting rats to acute psychic stress was observed to result in an enhanced pineal uptake of tryptophan, precursor of melatonin (35).

BRAIN

Melatonin controls dispersion and aggregation of melanin granules (36), and the antimitotic agent colchicine causes disruption of the movement of melanocyte pigment granules (37). Prior work (38,39) had shown that granule movement follows microtubular alignment. It had also been shown that melatonin antagonizes the antimitotic effect of colchicine (40), melatonin apparently displacing colchicine from tubulin, the assembly of which latter subunits comprise microtubules. Nevertheless, melatonin does not, itself, result in mitotic arrest. However, an in vitro study (41) of bovine brain microtubules subsequently revealed that melatonin had no effect on their assembly.

Alterations in levels of tryptophan, 5-hydroxytryptamine (serotonin, 5-HT), 5-hydroxyindoleacetic acid (5-HIAA), dopamine, and norepinephrine were sought in various brain regions of the rat following pinealectomy (42). The results revealed no change in brain tryptophan in either sex. For pinealectomized females versus controls, 5-HT levels were higher in the striatum, midbrain, and cortex; 5-HIAA levels were lower in the cerebellum and hypothalamus; dopamine levels were not significantly different for any area measured; and norepinephrine levels were higher in the cortex. For pinealectomized versus control males, 5-HT levels did not differ significantly for any area measured; 5-HIAA levels were lower in the hypothalamus, midbrain, and hippocampus; and levels of dopamine and norepinephrine were lower in the cortex. The data were interpreted as providing confirmation for the brain being a site of action of pineal hormones.

Cerebellum

Investigating the amount of N-acetylserotonin (NAS) in the granular layer of rat cerebella, it was found that following treatment with p-chlorophenylalanine there was an increase in NAS (43). Parachlorophenylalanine is an inhibitor of indoleamine synthesis, blocking tryptophan-5-hydroxylase, an essential enzyme for the synthesis of 5-HT from tryptophan. The significance of the findings in this study, as they relate to the pineal, is unclear.

Cerebrospinal Fluid

Following injection of melatonin into the cisterna magna of rabbits, the cerebrospinal fluid (CSF) concentration of 3',5' cyclic guanosine monophosphate (c-GMP) was observed to rise (44). Acetylcholine also caused a CSF rise of c-GMP; however, melatonin was 1000 times more potent than acetylcholine in producing this effect. Nevertheless, the minimal effective dose of melatonin (i.e., 1 μg) may have been pharmacologic, as it represented approximately 25 times the amount present in rabbit pineals. As the discussion of this study points out, the hypothalamic areas beneath the third ventricle are some of the prime candidates for sites of action of pineal hormones; the latter, if normally secreted by the pineal into the CSF, would be secreted into the third ventricle. Yet, in this study, intracisternally injected melatonin would have bathed the surfaces of the cerebral cortex, cerebellum, and spinal cord, with only a fraction of the original dose reaching the proposed melatonin action sites neighboring the third ventricle. It was concluded that before c-GMP is deemed a mediator of melatonin's central nervous system (CNS) actions, melatonin must be injected into the CSF at sites other than the one chosen for this investigation.

Hypothalamus

Blinding or exposing male rats to constant light, commencing at age 21 days, resulted in a higher rate of oxygen consumption in the hypothalamus in the former group and a lower rate in the latter group, as compared to controls, when these rates were measured 48 days later (45). No change in oxygen consumption was found in either the amygdala or hippocampus. This work suggests that the alterations in hypothalamic oxygen consumption may be related to changes in gonadotropin secretion, as blinding depresses gonadotropin secretion and continuous lighting enhances it.

Unlike the study mentioned earlier (41), in which whole brains were measured, melatonin administered to rats was observed to decrease microtubule protein by 44% in the arcuate-median eminence region of the hypothalamus and by 19% in the remainder of the hypothalamus; no effect was seen in the cerebral cortex (46).

In an in vitro experiment (47), in which synaptosome-rich rat hypothalamic homogenates were preincubated with melatonin, it was found that there were significant decreases in hypothalamic uptake of dopamine, glutamate, norepinephrine, and 5-HT. It was suggested that exogenous melatonin may affect neurotransmitter accumulation and release in the hypothalamus by modifying the mechanism of transmitter uptake rather than by competition with the transmitter for its uptake.

Another in vitro study (48) revealed that the indole derivatives 5-hydroxytryptophol and 6-methoxytetrahydroharman were competitive inhibitors of 5-HT uptake by the rat hypothalamus. Neither these indole derivatives nor other compounds tested (i.e., melatonin, 6-hydroxy-melatonin, 5-methoxytryptophol, 6-hydroxytetrahydroharman) affected hypothalamic norepinephrine uptake. The results were cited as supportive evidence for a role for pineal indole metabolites in modulating aminergic mechanisms in the hypothalamus.

Myelination

In several studies (49,50), the author and coworkers demonstrated that neonatal pinealectomy in the rat resulted in a delay in brain maturation, seen at first by a decrease in brain lipids and then by observing a decrease in myelin itself. Subsequent work (51) in rats has revealed alterations in the levels of a number of the long-chain fatty acids of myelin following neonatal pinealectomy.

There are diseases of dysmyelination in humans, such as phenylketonuria, maple syrup urine disease, oasthouse urine disease, and some cases of adrenoleukodystrophy. In addition, Tay-Sachs' disease is associated not only with brain accumulation of GM_2 ganglioside but with brain dysmyelination as well (52,53). It is, thus, of interest to note that, in the first ultrastructural study of the pineal in Tay-Sachs' disease, striking abnormalities were noted (54). Although this association does not necessarily imply a cause-and-effect relationship between the pineal and dysmyelination, if it can be shown that other dysmyelinating diseases are also associated with pineal abnormalities, the findings in rats reported herein may assume considerable significance.

Pituitary

Constant darkness or melatonin in vitro were observed to reduce rat pituitary monoamine oxidase (MAO) activity; continuous lighting or pinealectomy produced the opposite effect (55). A similar pattern of MAO activity was found in the hypothalamus, but to a lesser extent. It was hypothesized that MAO might be a target enzyme for melatonin.

In an in vitro study (56) in rats, a dose-dependent increase in pituitary cell incorporation of leucine and thymidine was produced by pineal extract. This effect was postulated to be related either to stimulation of nucleic acid and protein synthesis or to an inhibition of newly synthesized protein secretion.

Sleep

Sleep has been induced in cats by intrahypothalamic administration of melatonin (57). In addition, arginine vasotocin (AVT) injected into the third ventricle of unanesthetized cats suppressed rapid-eye-movement (REM) sleep while inducing non-REM sleep (58). AVT also resulted in a rise of 5-HT and a decrease in 5-HIAA. Fluoxetine, an inhibitor of 5-HT uptake, enhanced the non-REM sleep induced by AVT, whereas metergoline, a 5-HT-receptor blocking agent, prevented this effect of AVT. Neither arginine vasopressin nor oxytocin had any effect on brain indole levels or on sleep. It was suggested that the effect of AVT on sleep is secondary to an interference with 5-HT release at postsynaptic receptor sites.

Prior work (59) on the effects of pinealectomy on paradoxical and slow-wave sleep in rats had revealed that, though there were no changes in the total amount of paradoxical and slow-wave sleep in a 24-hour period, paradoxical sleep increased during dark exposure and decreased during light exposure. Circadian periodicity and diurnal variations of slow-wave sleep remained as they had been under control conditions; but the circadian periodicity of paradoxical sleep virtually disappeared. It appears that the pineal is important to the diurnal and circadian rhythmicity of paradoxical sleep.

CARTILAGE

A study (60) in rats has demonstrated hypoplasia of growing metaphyseal cartilage as a result of the effect of pineal extract. This effect was documented histologically and hypothesized to be related to pineal influence on the adenyl cyclase system.

DRUG EFFECTS

Depressed electrophysiologic reactions of the female-rat brain and heart to lethal doses of pentobarbitone have been found to result from pinealectomy (61). As regards the diurnal rhythm of drug metabolism in general, however, pinealectomy has been reported to have no effect (62).

The acute administration of various antidepressants, such as desmethylimipramine, imipramine, clomipramine, maprotiline, pargyline, and L-5-hydroxytryptophan was observed to result in elevated plasma and pineal melatonin levels (63). However, chronic treatment with clomipramine reduced these elevations. The acutely increased levels of melatonin were probably the result of a β-adrenergic agonistic action common to all these antidepressants. As an example, it has been demonstrated that desmethylimipramine causes an increased conversion of tryptophan to melatonin (64), as well as increasing serotonin-N-acetyltransferase (NAT) activity (65). The reduced levels of melatonin following chronic administration of an antidepressant were most likely secondary to reduced β-adrenergic sensitivity that occurs with such prolonged drug usage.

EYE

The production of experimental allergic uveitis in the guinea pig, by injecting an extract of homologous retina homogenate, prompted a study (66) to ascertain whether antibody to this homogenate would react with pineal tissue. This idea arose from the established structural and functional relationship between the retina and pineal in submammalian vertebrates (67). Specific immunofluorescence was demonstrated in the cytoplasm of pinealocytes of guinea pigs using homologous serum from guinea pigs sensitized to the retinal homogenate. The same investigators then proceeded to demonstrate that, during the induction of experimental allergic uveitis, the pineal is also involved (68). Lymphocytic infiltration was seen in the pineal, and, at times, such infiltrate was seen before the appearance of ocular disease.

When pigmented guinea pigs were treated with melatonin, pigmented cells in the retinal pigment layer and choroid of the eye were aggregated (69). This resulted in a lightening effect on the eye pigmentation, which in turn could be expected to enhance the diffusion of light in the visual layer and/or to enhance the reflection of light from the choroid. The effect of melatonin here would correspond to the observation that guinea pig eye pigments aggregate during darkness and disperse during light exposure (70). As melatonin and NAS have been found in the retinae of rats and chickens (71), and as hydroxyindole-0-methyltransferase has also been found in the vertebrate retina (72), these findings would suggest de novo synthesis of melatonin in the retina (71). Thus it would appear that both locally synthesized retinal melatonin, as well as melatonin secreted by the pineal, may regulate eye pigmentation in vertebrates.

In addition to the findings just presented, although no active uptake of melatonin could be demonstrated in the retinal neurons of rabbits, uptake was shown for 5-HT (73). It was suggested that 5-HT is a neurotransmitter in special retinal neurons.

GASTROINTESTINAL TRACT

Destroying the apparently nonsecretory pineals of 15–17-day-old rat fetuses resulted in significant alterations in the epithelial cells of the lower ileum (74). However, when pinealectomy was performed in prenatal rats after pineal secretion was judged to have commenced, no ileal changes were observed (75).

Melatonin has been reported to suppress the duodenal motility in rats that ordinarily follows administration of 5-HT (76).

GLUCOSE METABOLISM

The disrupted process of gluconeogenesis that occurs in animals with chronic hepatitis has been reported to undergo improvement as a result of the use of pineal polypeptides (77).

Melatonin has been demonstrated to decrease glucose oxidation, glucose incorporation into glyceride-glycerol fractions, and fatty acid synthesis in rabbit perirenal fat (78).

HYPERTENSION

In early work (79) on this subject, it was suggested that a previously observed hypotensive effect of pineal extract may have been due to the histamine content of pineal mast cells. Subsequently, it was noted that systolic hypertension developed 15 days following pinealectomy in rats (80). This hypertension was still present 1 month after operation and resulted in hypertensive changes in the renal vasculature. In another study (81), a mild hypertension of 20 mm Hg was produced by pineal electrocoagulation in rats. The two preceding investigations resulted in the postulate that the hypertension was secondary to overactivity of the renin-angiotensin-aldosterone system. It was then demonstrated in rats that pinealectomy-induced hypertension, and accompanying hypokalemia, could be offset by spironolactone (82). The finding of elevated plasma renin activity in such hypertensive rats prompted the suggestion that sympathetic activity was increased (83,84). It was also postulated that melatonin or other pineal indoleamines may act as antihypertensives, possibly via stimulation of central inhibitory adrenergic pathways. In a subsequent study (85), when melatonin was administered via drinking water to pinealectomized rats, commencing in the immediate postoperative period, it prevented the appearance of hypertension. Furthermore, melatonin actually depressed the blood pressure of these pinealectomized rats below that of the controls. Administration of melatonin to those rats that had been allowed to become hypertensive produced a decline in blood pressure to below control levels after 2 weeks of treatment.

The hypertension produced by pinealectomy has been demonstrated to persist beyond the 1-month period mentioned earlier, the effect being observed for 60 days, with total remission by 90 days (86). Histologic examination of the kidneys of the pinealectomized, hypertensive rats revealed a patchy distribution of arteriolar-wall thickening, adventitial fibrosis, and hypernucleated or sclerosed glomeruli.

In another approach to this problem, pinealectomy was performed in both prepubertal (43-day-old) and postpubertal (55-day-old) male rats (87). When the sole source of fluid was 1% saline, administered from day 96 to day 123, hypertension was found in prepubertally, but not postpubertally pinealectomized rats. In addition, the hypertensive animals consumed more saline than did sham-pinealectomized controls. The investigators suggested that prepubertal pinealectomy may predispose to hypertension, the latter becoming overt when salt intake is increased.

The vascular reactivity of the mesenteric arterial vessels of pinealectomized rats was observed following injections of 50 and 100 ng of angiotensin and of norepinephrine, 0.5 and 1.0 μg of 5-HT, and 1.5 and 3.0 mg of potassium (88). Vascular responsiveness to both concentrations of 5-HT and norepinephrine were greater in pinealectomized animals, as was also true with the higher concentration of angiotensin; potassium caused no significant change in either dose. Injection of melatonin in vivo 3 hours prior to dissection, or subsequent in vitro perfusion of melatonin, either reduced vasoconstrictor responses or reversed vasoconstrictor responses, respectively, in the pinealectomized rats, but had little effect in controls. It was hypothesized that the increased vascular responsiveness of pinealectomized rats may be specific for agents that stimulate the release of calcium from intracellular stores, such as angiotensin and norepinephrine, rather than those that cause calcium influx from extracellular fluid, such as potassium; the mechanism of vascular responsiveness to 5-HT is unknown. It was further suggested that melatonin deficiency may underlie the alterations in vascular responsiveness observed in this study.

Using varying combinations of pinealectomy, sham-pinealectomy, no operation, 1% saline or water for drinking, unilateral nephrectomy, and pressor response to cadmium chloride, a recent study (89) concluded that pinealectomy does not always cause hypertension and that cardiovascular instability may occur in pinealectomized rats. The investigators expressed doubt about the existence of true hypertension following pinealectomy in these animals.

Hypertension that is spontaneous, rather than postpinealectomy, may also occur in rats. Beta-adrenergic blocking agents have been demonstrated to delay the onset of this type of hypertension. Thus it was proposed that there might be an alteration in β-adrenergic receptors in this condition (90). To test this theory, isoproterenol was given to normal and spontaneously hypertensive rats, and NAT induction in the pineal was measured (as mentioned previously, NAT activation is known to be controlled by β-adrenergic stimulation). The activity of pineal NAT in spontaneously hypertensive male rats was double that found in normal males; the respective value in female rats was a 1.5-fold elevation. As the hypertensive rats apparently had an inherited propensity for increased induction of pineal NAT, the hypertension was postulated to be secondary to either a greater number or an enhanced catecholamine sensitivity of β receptors, or both.

Another type of hypertension found in rats is that occurring following adrenal enucleation; so-called adrenal-regeneration hypertension. This has been attributed to mineralocorticoid hypersecretion, the compounds incriminated not including aldosterone but, rather, desoxycorticosterone or 18-hydroxydesoxycorticosterone (91). Exploring the effect of pinealectomy on this type of hypertension, it was discovered that pinealectomy reduced blood pressure only in rats having had hypertension induced prior to puberty (92). The investigators, invoking salt balance in this type of hypertension, proposed that their findings could be explained by loss of a salt-regulating function of the pineal, such loss occurring with sexual maturation.

IMMUNITY

The immune capacity of rats previously pinealectomized as neonates has been observed to remain intact, whereas pinealectomy performed at 6 weeks of age resulted in a partial, transient dysfunction of the immune response (93). In another study (94), antibody-mediated and cellular immune responses were examined in adult rats that had been thymectomized and/or pinealectomized within 36 hours after birth. Skin graft rejection, hemolytic plaque formation, hemagglutinating antibody formation in response to sheep red cells, and phytohemagglutinin stimulation of splenic lymphoid cells were measured. Pinealectomy alone had no significant effect on the immune competence of adult rats. However, hemagglutinating antibody response was found to be less depressed in thymectomized-pinealectomized rats than in rats having undergone thymectomy alone. It was suggested that this latter finding might have been due to a shortening of the immunodepressed state, resulting from an accelerated proliferation of immunocompetent cells in pinealectomized animals. In another investigation (95), however, hemagglutinating antibody response of mice to sheep red cells was seen to increase in response to pineal (and thymic) extracts. Thus it would appear that: (1) pinealectomy performed in the rat neonate does not alter the animal's immune status; (2) there may be a limited offsetting effect of pineal removal on the immunodepressed state resulting from thymectomy; (3) with the administration of thymic or pineal constituents, there is enhancement of some aspects of the immune response of mice. However, why pinealectomy and pineal extract should both enhance certain antibody responses remains enigmatic (see Nerve Growth Factor below).

KIDNEY

Pineal extract administered to nephrectomized rats has been reported to reduce the level of blood urea following amino acid infusion; the converse applied following pinealectomy (96,97).

LIVER

Nine-week-old rats, which were previously pinealectomized at age 21 days, manifested greater growth and weight gain than did controls, despite an initial period of weight deceleration (98). It was found that these pinealectomized rats had poorer glyine absorption than did controls; however, their eventual superior growth was thought to be the result of enhanced hepatic protein synthesis.

Developing an enzyme-inhibition assay for melatonin in rats produced the in vitro finding of inhibition of liver N-acetyltransferase by both NAS and melatonin (99).

MALARIA

Apparently, the mouse pineal may exert control over the growth, division synchrony, vascular entrapment, and release of late growth forms of malarial parasites (100). Furthermore, the normally enhanced growth and division synchrony of plasmodia, which results from photoperiod rhythmicity, was found to be abolished by pinealectomy in mice (101,102).

NERVE GROWTH FACTOR

Pinealectomy as well as a long-acting melatonin preparation were both observed to produce a reduction in nerve growth factor in the mouse submaxillary gland (103). As noted by the investigators, these seemingly contradictory results may have been, in part, a function of the chronicity with which melatonin was released. In addition, melatonin apparently does not totally disappear from the circulation after pinealectomy, other sources of production having been demonstrated (71).

PELAGE

Acceleration of hair waves in mice has been observed to follow pinealectomy, whereas melatonin slows the progression of hair waves in pinealectomized and intact animals (104,105).

In a study of the annual pelage color change in the Siberian (Djungarian) hamster, tyrosinase activity of hair-follicle homogenates was found to peak at both the spring and autumn molts, despite the fact that only the spring molt was associated with the production of pigmented hair (106). The melanin content of hair-follicle homogenates was high in the summer and low in the winter, however. It was opined that a factor must exist that prevents the elevated tyrosinase levels of the autumn molt from being translated into melanogenesis. Attention was focused on the pineal as being the unknown factor because pinealectomy has been demonstrated to prevent the change to white winter pelage that normally occurs in this hamster when exposed to less daylight (107) and melatonin can prevent the appearance of a pigmented pelage at the time of molting of this animal when it is exposed to long photoperiods (108).

PERIPHERAL NERVE

Intraocular administration of melatonin has been observed to impair fast axonal transport in the optic pathway of rabbits (46). It has been suggested that this effect may be related to alterations in microtubules (see the earlier section on Brain). In a subsequent experiment (109), melatonin, tryptamine, 5-HT, NAS, 5-methoxytryptamine, 5-HIAA, and 5-methoxyindoleacetic acid were all tested for their ability to impair fast axonal transport by their injection in close proximity to the sciatic nerve of rats. Axonal transport was measured by using [^{3}H] leucine injected intraganglionically. Melatonin was more potent than all its analogues in impairing axonal transport; however, all the analogues did cause such impairment. A similar effect has been observed in frog sciatic nerve using tryptamine (110).

PHENYLKETONURIA

Prior work (111,112) had shown that melatonin either attenuated or prevented learning defects in rats artifically made phenylketonuric. The explanation for these findings probably lies with the observations that decreased 5-HT metabolism has been demonstrated in human phenylketonurics (113,114), decreased cerebral 5-HT has been shown to produce behavioral abnormalities (115,116), and melatonin has been observed to raise levels of 5-HT in the brain (117). However, in a recent study (118), melatonin failed to improve maze-learning impairment in rats made phenylketonuric on days 1–8 of life. No significant learning impairment was evident from phenylketonuria that was induced on days 9–16 or 17–24 of life. The investigators, in comparing their results with previous reports, attributed the discrepancies to methodologic differences.

POLYAMINES

The polyamines, consisting of putrescine, spermidine, and spermine, participate in protein and nucleic acid synthesis and stabilize nucleic acid and ribosome structure, protecting the latter from denaturation (119). Synthesis of polyamines takes place in four stages, in the first of which ornithine is converted to putrescine by the enzyme L-ornithine decarboxylase (ODC). In adult male rats, killed at seven-day intervals up to 6 weeks postpinealectomy, ODC activity was found to be decreased in the thymus and testes, whereas enzyme activity was increased in the hypothalamus, pituitary, and prostate. In both the kidneys and liver,

ODC activity decreased 1-week postpinealectomy, only to increase in the third and fourth weeks, respectively (120). As tissue levels of polyamines have been found to be positively correlated with tissue growth (121), it would appear that the pineal can exert a significant control over growth that may be separate and distinct from its effect on growth hormone (see Chapter 6, Pituitary, Growth Hormone).

PORPHYRINS

Unlike the situation existing in mice (122), rabbits (123), and rats (124), gross ultrastructural differences exist between the Harderian glands of male and female hamsters (125–127). In addition, as a result of castration, the Harderian gland of the male hamster can be made "female" in type, which includes morphologic changes as well as increased porphyrin content (128,129). In a recent investigation (130), when Δ-aminolevulinic acid (ALA) was added to incubated Harderian glands of young adult golden hamsters, increases in tissue and media porphyrin concentrations resulted. However, the addition to the incubation media of estradiol, gonadotropins, melatonin, and testosterone, respectively, along with ALA, had no effect on porphyrin concentrations. It was concluded that male-hamster Harderian tissue is deficient in ALA and that ALA induces synthesis and release of porphyrins from both male and female Harderian glands.

In another study (131), the exposure of male rats to continuous darkness resulted in an increase in Harderian-gland porphyrin content, whereas MSH decreased such porphyrin content.

PREGNANCY

Based on the secretory capability apparently possessed by the fetal rat pineal in the third trimester of pregnancy, one experiment (132), in which the fetal pineal was destroyed, revealed changes indicating massive fetal absorption of amniotic fluid proteins.

THERMOREGULATION

When bats were subjected to auditory stimuli during hibernation, changes reflecting involution were observed in the pineal (133). These same investigators later found that exposure of rats to cold produced progressive structural changes compatible with enhanced activity in the pineal (134). It was postulated that the pineal may be an integrated component of a cold-adaptation system in the rat. Further evidence implicating the pineal as a temperature transducer was put forth when it was noted that alterations occurred in the pineals of heat-exposed rats (135).

Daily subcutaneous administration of melatonin has been observed to increase the incidence and duration of hibernation in the ground squirrel, C. lateralis (136). An in vitro part of this experiment revealed a depressed duration of electrical activity of isolated hearts from both hibernating and nonhibernating animals when melatonin was added to the bathing solution.

Measuring the core temperature of female rats revealed the existence of bimodal 24-hour rhythm (137). Under conditions of 14L:10D, the main peak in temperature occurred during darkness, with a lesser peak occurring 3–4 hours after the onset of light exposure. Although, by altering the phase of the photoperiod or the total proportion of light, the core temperature rhythm was seen to be light-entrained, the two peaks were governed by different mechanisms. By exposing the rats to a 20-hour photoperiod, constant light or constant darkness, it was concluded that the rhythm of the main peak was endogenous, being entrained only by circadian photoperiods, whereas that of the lesser peak was exogenous, requiring circadian light-dark cycles. It was of interest to note that, with constant darkness, not only did the secondary peak disappear but the primary peak occurred with precision every 24 hours. With exposure to continuous light, however, although the secondary peak was also absent, the core temperature rhythm appeared to be free-running, having a periodicity of 25.8 hours. Pinealectomy reduced the mean core temperature along the spectrum from constant darkness to constant light. The investigators interpreted the data to indicate that the pineal is not essential to controlling body temperature rhythm in the rat, nor is the gland a transducer for the entrainment of core temperature rhythm by photic information. Rather, the pineal was postulated to be a modulator of the set point around which the circadian core-temperature rhythm oscillates.

Mice maintained on short photoperiods of 9L:15D and exposed to cold of 13°C were observed to become torpid nine times more frequently than did animals exposed to 16L:8D (138). In addition, chronic melatonin administration resulted in a 2.5-fold increase in daily torpor incidence as compared to sham-treated mice. A gradual increase in daily torpor has been reported in mice exposed progressively to photoperiods of 13L:11D to 12L:12D and 10L:14D to 9L:15D (139). Pinealectomy prevented the extent of torpor seen in sham-operated controls when all animals were kept on a 9L:15D photoperiod.

The influence of short (9L:15D) and long (15L:9D) daily photoperiods on basal metabolic rate, rectal temperature, and norepinephrine-induced nonshivering thermogenesis was investigated in rats (140). Short-day plus cold exposure (8 ± 2°C) resulted in a positive response to norepinephrine, resulting in nonshivering thermogenesis with an elevation of the metabolic rate by 23% above the basal level and elevation of the mean daily lowest rectal temperature to above that found with warm-acclimated (21 ± 2°C) rats exposed to 9L:15D. As compared to warm-exposed controls, melatonin administration lowered the mean daily lowest rectal temperature in warm-acclimated animals exposed to both short and long photoperiods and elevated the mean daily lowest rectal temperature of rats exposed to cold and both short and long photoperiods (apparently overriding the latter's effect) when the respective cold and warm groups were compared with each other. Melatonin also enhanced the combination of short photoperiods plus cold in causing an increase in mean pineal weight as compared to cold-, long-photoperiod-exposed rats treated with melatonin. These results were interpreted as indicating the importance of short photoperiods in preparing and eliciting metabolic responses that enable adaptation to the cold. The participation of the pineal, ostensibly via melatonin, in this process of adaptation could be inferred from the increased mean rectal temperatures of both the 9L:15D and 15L:9D animals exposed to cold and treated with melatonin as compared to the depressed mean rectal temperatures observed with melatonin in warm-exposed rats subjected to both short and long photoperiods. However, as the effect of melatonin in cold-exposed, 9L:15D-exposed rats was no greater than the effect of cold plus short photoperiod alone, it was suggested that melatonin's function here may be that of a set-point adjuster. The depressant effect on mean rectal temperatures seen with melatonin in warm-acclimated animals exposed to both types of photoperiods was ascribed to the hormone's sedative effects on metabolism (141).

THYMUS

Thymic weight was found to be unaffected by pineal extract given to intact rats; however, when the animals underwent unilateral gonadectomy, pineal extract significantly increased the weight of the thymus (142). Inexplicably, melatonin was without effect in either instance. Thymic atrophy (143) and structural disorganization (144) were observed following pinealectomy in the rat. The latter findings would imply a stimulatory effect of the pineal on the thymus. For the role of the thymus in immune responses, see the earlier section on Immunity. For the relation of the thymus to oncogenesis see the section that immediately follows.

TUMOR GROWTH

An early report (145) on this subject described the absence of pineal tumors 3–21 months following implantation of a carcinogen into fetal or newborn rat pineals. Other studies (146,147) found that pinealectomized hamsters developed larger melanomas and more extensive metastases than did nonpinealectomized animals. Pinealectomy also resulted in greater tumor volume in rats with Walker 256 carcinosarcoma, as compared to control animals (148), as well as producing an increase in number and size of melanomas induced in hamsters by the administration of 9,10-dimethyl-1,2-benzanthracene (149). Using this same carcinogen to induce fibrosarcomas in rats, it was found that pineal weights did not differ in affected rats versus controls. However, the pinealocytes and their nuclei were larger and contained more lipid in tumor-bearing rats as compared to control animals (150). These findings were interpreted as signifying increased metabolic activity in the pineals of the fibrosarcoma-bearing animals. In another investigation (151), one-half hour following injection of either melatonin or a control vehicle to BALB/

c mice, transplantable leukemia (LSTRA) cells were injected. Injections of melatonin or the vehicle were then continued for 14 days, when the animals were killed. The melatonin-treated mice had developed fewer tumors and had lower mean tumor weight than did the controls. Subsequently, a partially purified substance was isolated from sheep pineal glands that inhibited the in vitro multiplication of three different cell strains (152). The unidentified antimitotic substance was shown to have different effects from such antineoplastic drugs as daunorubicin and methotrexate, as the pineal substance produced rapid (i.e., 3–6 hour) shrinkage of cytoplasm and nucleus of these cell lines, whereas the antineoplastic drugs produced a slower (i.e., 1–3 day) and less-pronounced effect.

The inoculation with Yoshida sarcoma of 10–12-week-old rats, which had been pinealectomized and/or thymectomized within 24 hours of birth, resulted in reduced survival of the operated animals as compared with inoculated-unoperated controls (153). The inoculated-unoperated controls survived a mean of 55.5 days as compared with 29.2 days in pinealectomized-inoculated rats, 21.5 days in thymectomized (i.e., immunodepressed; see the earlier section on Immunity) inoculated rats, and 17.3 days in pinealectomized-thymectomized-inoculated rats. The same investigator then studied the effect of polyoma virus injection into neonate rats immediately following pinealectomy and/or thymectomy (154). Approximately two-thirds of the thymectomized rats and one-third of the pinealectomized-thymectomized rats died of renal tumors 3–5 months following inoculation. Controls and pinealectomized rats, however, survived tumor-free until killed at age 10–12 months. It was concluded that, unlike the situation with certain other tumors, pinealectomy did not have an enhancing effect on the ability of the polyoma virus to produce noeplasm. Almost identical findings were reported in another paper (155).

Because reserpine has been reported to exert a suppressive effect on immune competence (156), an experiment (157) was performed in which the effect of reserpine on the incidence of 9,10-dimethyl-1,2-benzanthracene-induced tumors in neonatally pinealectomized and/or thymectomized rats was studied. Following reserpine treatment, the incidence of these tumors was found to be greater in pinealectomized and pinealectomized-thymectomized rats than in intact or thymectomized animals. These findings were construed as indicating that: (1) neonatal pinealectomy alone does not enhance oncogenesis from 9,10-dimethyl-1,2-benzanthracine; (2) the immunocompromised state resulting from neonatal thymectomy alone does not enhance the susceptibility of the animal to the oncogenic effects of this chemical; (3) reserpine does not enhance the chemical's ability to produce tumor as long as the pineal remains intact, but when reserpine is added to the effect of neonatal pinealectomy, tumor growth is stimulated. It was hypothesized that neonatal pinealectomy results in latent neuroendocrine changes, the latter becoming manifest after the exhibition of reserpine, a CNS catecholamine and 5-HT depletor. The relationship between this hypothesis and tumor growth was based on prior work (158) in which it was reported that lesions in the hypothalamus and amygdala can influence the development of carcinogen-induced mammary tumors in rats. Such mammary tumors, as well as ear-duct tumors, both of which occurred in the experiment under discussion (157), are hormone-dependent. Thus the pineal may influence tumor growth via pineal-hypothalamic-pituitary hormone interplay. Unexplained by this work is the absence of tumor enhancement by neonatal thymectomy. This contrasts with the decreased survival of neonatally thymectomized rats with Yoshida sarcoma (153) and with polyoma-virus-induced renal tumors (154), mentioned earlier.

In another report (159), melatonin was found to prolong the survival of pinealectomized female rats with Yoshida sarcoma. In addition, in this experiment, several sheep pineal fractions were studied; fraction UM-2R reduced the survival time of intact rats with this sarcoma, and fraction UM-05R prolonged survival in intact animals. Using Lewis lung carcinoma cells in intact DBF1 male mice, the pineal fraction UM-05F prolonged survival slightly, whereas melatonin reduced survival. With methylcholanthrene-induced sarcoma in DBF1 female mice, melatonin delayed the increased incidence of tumor seen with the passage of time, whereas fraction UM-2R even further delayed the incidence of sarcomas. The investigators noted that, in prior in vitro experiments (160), (1) the pineal fraction UM-2R had shown an inhibition of hypothalamic-stimulatory influence on the pituitary of the male rat; (2) the fraction UM-05R could stimulate the hypothalamus; and (3) the UM-05F fraction could diminish the gonadotropic activity of the male-rat anterior pituitary. In vivo, in mice the UM-05R fraction exerted an inhibitory effect on the compensatory ovarian hypertrophy that follows unilateral ovariectomy. Thus, of the various fractions tested previously in vitro and in vivo, and where information for the same sex could be obtained, fraction UM-05R prolonged survival of female animals with Yoshida sarcoma and exerted a gonadotropin-inhibitory effect, whereas fraction UM-05F slightly prolonged survival of male animals with Lewis lung carcinoma and had antigonadotropic activity. In the latter instance, the effect of melatonin on survival ran counter to the effect of UM-05F. Judging from some of these slender clues, it would appear that, at least in certain instances, the effect of the pineal on tumor growth may be via the hypothalamus and pituitary, as suggested earlier. Further evidence for this line of reasoning was supplied in work (161) on female rats in which 7,12-dimethyl-1,2-benzanthracene was used to induce mammary tumors. In this instance, the carcinogen itself was found to alter pituitary levels of 5-HT, particularly in the intermediate lobe. In addition, melatonin administered to hamsters having melanoma reversed the enhanced tumor growth associated with pinealectomy; however, melatonin administered to intact animals had no effect on melanoma growth (162). It was concluded that melatonin has no effect on tumor growth and that the effect of pinealectomy on tumor growth is secondary to melantonin deficiency. Citing previously reported effects of the pineal on the hypothalamus and midbrain, it was suggested that these same effects may explain the enhanced growth of tumor seen with melatonin deficiency following pinealectomy.

Seeking to unravel further the chain of events by which the pineal may affect tumor growth, a recent study (163) suggested several possible modes of action: (1) the effect of the pineal on immunocompetence; (2) the inhibitory effect of the pineal on growth hormone secretion (see Chapter 6, Pituitary, Growth Hormone); (3) a peripheral inhibitory action of the pineal on somatomedin (164); (4) pineal inhibition of adrenocortical secretions (see Chapter 6, Adrenals, Corticosterone); and, (5) the effect of the pineal on catecholamine synthesis and secretion (see Chapter 6, Adrenals, Catecholamines). In addition, the investigators invoked phase alterations in various circadian rhythms as mediating pineal effects on tumor growth. Some of those aspects specifically alluded to were the circadian rhythm of rat blood glucose (165), in relation to the relatively increased level of aerobic glycolysis of neoplasms, and the fact that the susceptibility of tumors to chemotherapeutic agents is time-dependent, not only as regards the phase timing of circadian rhythms within the tumor tissue but also in the host's tissues (166).

REFERENCES

1. Dilman V M, Anisimov V N, Ostroumova M N, Khavinson V K, Morozov V G. Increase in lifespan of rats following polypeptide pineal extract treatment. Exp Pathol (Jena) 17:539–545, 1979.

2. Johnson J E Jr. Fine structural alterations in the aging rat pineal gland. Exp Aging Res 6:189–211, 1980.

3. Reiss M, Davis R H, Sideman M B, Plichta E S. Pineal gland and spontaneous activity of rats. J Endocrinol 28:127–128, 1963.

4. Long J A, Evans H N. The oestrus cycle in the rat and its associated phenomena. Memoirs Univ California 6, 1922.

5. Wong R, Whiteside C B C. The effect of melatonin on the wheel-running activity of rats deprived of food. J Endocrinol 40:383–384, 1968.

6. Remley N R, Bryon D M, Wilson F R. The effects of pinealectomy on the activity levels in rats. Psychon Sci 15:175–176, 1969.

7. Relkin R. The influence of prepuberal and postpuberal pinealectomy on treadwheel activity. Physiol Behav 5:341–343, 1970.

8. Sampson P H, Bigelow L. Pineal influence on exploratory behavior of the female rat. Physiol Behav 7:713–715, 1971.

9. Kovacs G L, Gajari I, Telegdy G, Lissak K. Effect of melatonin and pinealectomy on avoidance exploratory activity in the rat. Physiol Behav 13:349–355, 1974.

10. Krapp C H, Der Einfluss der Epiphyse auf die Lokomotionsaktivität bei Ratten. Experientia 33:731–732, 1977.

11. Sackman J W, Reiter R J. Hyperactivity in the blind-anosmic female rat: role of the pineal gland. Physiol Behav 18:321–323, 1977.

12. Klein D, Brown T S. Exploratory behavior and spontaneous alternation in blind and anosmic rats. J Comp Physiol Psychol 68:107–110, 1969.

13. Sieck M H, Baumbach H D. Differential effects of peripheral and central anosmia producing techniques on spontaneous behavior. Physiol Behav 13:407–425, 1974.

14. Reiter R J, Vaughan M K, Blask D E, Johnson L Y. Melatonin: its inhibition of pineal antigonadotropic activity in male hamsters. Science 185:1169–1171, 1974.

15. Reiter R J, Blask D E, Vaughan M K. A counter antigonadotropic effect of melatonin in male rats. Neuroendocrinology 19:72–80, 1975.

16. Finkelstein J S, Baum F R, Campbell C S. Entrainment of the female hamster to reversed photoperiod: role of the pineal. Physiol Behav 21:105–111, 1978.

17. Relkin R. Influence of prepuberal and postpuberal pinealectomy on maze performance. Am J Physiol 218:328–331, 1970.

18. McKinney T D, Vaughan M K, Reiter R J. Pineal influence on intermale aggression in adult house mice. Physiol Behav 15:213–216, 1975.

19. Paterson A T, Rickerby J, Simpson J, Vicker C. Possible interaction of melanocyte-stimulating hormone (MSH) and the pineal in the control of territorial aggression in mice. Physiol Behav 24:843–848, 1980.

20. Geller I. Ethanol preference in the rat as a function of photoperiod. Science 173:456–459, 1971.

21. Reiter R J, Blum K, Wallace J E, Merritt J H. Effect of the pineal gland on alcohol consumption by congenitally blind male rats. Q J Stud Alcohol 34:937–939, 1973.

22. Blum K, Merritt J H, Reiter R J, Wallace J E. A possible relationship between the pineal gland and ethanol preference in the rat. Curr Ther Res 15:25–30, 1973.

23. Burke L P, Kramer S Z. Effects of photoperiod, melatonin and pinealectomy on ethanol consumption in rats. Pharmacol Biochem Behav 2:459–463, 1974.

24. Datta P C, King M G. Effects of melanocyte-stimulating hormone (MSH) and melatonin on passive avoidance and on an emotional response. Pharmacol Biochem Behav 6:449–452, 1977.

25. Golus P, McGee R, King M G. Attenuation of saccharin neophobia by melatonin. Pharmacol Biochem Behav 11:367–369, 1979.

26. Křeček J, Novakova V, Stribral K. Sex differences in taste preference for salt solution. Physiol Behav 8:183–188, 1972.

27. Křeček J. Sex differences in salt taste: the effect of testosterone. Physiol Behav 10:683–688, 1973.

28. Křeček J, Panek M, Salatova J, Zicha J. The pineal gland and the effect of neonatal administration of androgen upon the development of spontaneous salt and water intake in female rats. Neuroendocrinology 18:137–143, 1975.

29. Křeček J. The pineal gland and the development of salt intake patterns in male rats. Dev Psychobiol 9:181–188, 1976.

30. Harris G W. Sex hormones, brain development and brain function. Endocrinology 75:627–648, 1964.

31. Gorski R A. Localisation and sexual differentiation of the nervous structures which regulate ovulation. J Reprod Fertil (Suppl) 1:667–688, 1966.

32. Reiter R J, Sorrentino S Jr. Reproductive effects of the mammalian pineal. Am Zool 10:247–257, 1970.

33. Quay W B, Bennett E L, Rosenzweig M R, Krech D. Effects of isolation and environmental complexity on brain and pineal organ. Physiol Behav 4:489–494, 1969.

34. Lynch H J, Hsuan M, Wurtman R J. Sympathetic neural control of indoleamine metabolism in the rat pineal gland. Adv Exp Med Biol 54:93–114, 1975.

35. Singh P M, Mazumdar S, Prasad G C, Udupa K N. Brain and pineal biogenic amines in response to acute psychic stress. Indian J Exp Biol 17:1071–1073, 1979.

36. Malawista S E, Sato H, Inoue S. Melatonin reversibly augments mitotic spindle birefringence and inhibits the colchicine effect. Biol Bull 129:414, 1965 (Abstract).

37. Malawista S E. The melanocyte model. Colchicine-like effects of other antimitotic agents. J Cell Biol 49:848–855, 1971.

38. Bikle D, Tilney L G, Porter K R. Microtubules and pigment migration in the melanophores of Fundulus heteroclitus L. Protoplasma 61:322–354, 1966.

39. Green L. Mechanisms of movements of granules in melanocytes of *Fundulus hetero-clitus*. Proc Natl Acad Sci USA 59:1179–1186, 1968.

40. Fitzgerald T J, Veal A. Melatonin antagonizes colchicine-induced mitotic arrest. Experienta 32:372–373, 1976.

41. Poffenbarger M, Fuller G M. Is melatonin a microtubule inhibitor? Exp Cell Res 103:135–141, 1976.

42. Sugden D, Morris R D. Changes in regional brain levels of tryptophan, 5-hydroxy-tryptamine, 5-hydroxyindoleacetic acid, dopamine and noradrenaline after pinealectomy in the rat. J Neurochem 32:1593–1595, 1979.

43. Bubenik G A, Brown G M, Grota L J. Immunohistological investigations of N-acetyl-serotonin in the rat cerebellum after parachlorophenylalanine treatment. Experientia 32:579–581, 1976.

44. Rudman D. Injection of melatonin into cisterna magna increases concentration of 3',5' cyclic guanosine monophosphate in cerebrospinal fluid. Neuroendocrinology 20:235–242, 1976.

45. Mas, M, Alonso Solis R. Effects of constant light exposure and blindness on the oxidative metabolism of selected brain areas in male rats. Experientia 33:1390–1391, 1977.

46. Cardinali D P, Freire F. Melatonin effects on brain. Interaction with microtubule protein, inhibition of fast axoplasmic flow and induction of crystaloid and tubular formations in the hypothalamus. Mol Cell Endocrinol 2:317–330, 1975.

47. Cardinali D P, Nagle C A, Freire F, Rosner J M. Effects of melatonin on neurotransmitter uptake and release by synaptosome-rich homogenates of the rat hypothalamus. Neuroendocrinology 18:72–85, 1975.

48. Meyer D C, Quay W B, Yu-Heng M. Comparative inhibition of hypothalamic uptake of 5-hydroxytryptamine and norepinephrine by 5-hydroxy- and 5-methoxy indole derivatives. Gen Pharmacol 285–288, 1975.

49. Relkin R, Fok W Y, Schneck L. Pinealectomy and brain myelination. Endocrinology 92:1426–1428, 1973.

50. Relkin R, Schneck L. Effect of pinealectomy on rat brain myelin. Proc Soc Exp Biol Med 148:337–338, 1975.

51. Kamback D O, Rich R A, Relkin R. Effect of pinealectomy on fatty acid composition of rat brain myelin. Endocrinology 110:907–909, 1982.

52. van Bogaert L. La méthode histopathologique et les problèmes des maladies de la substance blanche. J Belge Neurol Psychiatry 47:82–110, 1947.

53. Thieffry S, Bertrand I, Bargeton E, Edgar G, Arthuis M. Indiotie amaurotique infantile avec alterations graves de la substance blanche. Rev Neurol 102:130–152, 1960.

54. Adachi M, Volk BW, Schneck L, Relkin R. Ultrastructural alterations of endocrine glands in Tay-Sachs disease. Am J Clin Pathol 57:557–561, 1972.

55. Urry R L, Ellis LC. Monoamine oxidase activity of the hypothalamus and pituitary: alterations after pinealectomy, changes in photoperiod, or additions of melatonin *in vitro*. Experientia 31:891–892, 1975.

56. Peress N S, Murthy G G, Balcom R J. Pineal effects upon pituitary protein and nucleic acid synthesis *in vitro*. Neurosci Lett 2:207–210, 1976.

57. Marczynski T J, Yamaguchi N, Ling G M, Grodzinska L. Sleep induced by the administration of melatonin (5-methoxy-N-acetyltryptamine) to the hypothalamus in unrestrained cats. Experientia 20:435–437, 1964.

58. Pavel S. Pineal vasotocin and sleep: involvement of serotonin containing neurons. Brain Res Bull 4:731–734, 1979.

59. Mouret J, Coindet J, Chouvet G. Effect of pinealectomy on sleep stages and rhythms of the male rat. Brain Res 81:97–105, 1974.

60. Scuderi M C, Villari C, Calapso P, Nicotina P A, Giarrizzo S, Sofi A. Modificazioni indotte dall'estratto epifisario sulle cartilagini di accrescimento del ratto albino. Studio isotochimico. Arch Vecchi Anat Patol 62:455–460, 1977.

61. Behroozi K, Assael M, Ivriani I, Nir I. Electrocortical reactions of pinealtomized and intact rats to lethal doses of pentobarbital. Neuropharmacology 9:219–222, 1970.

62. Heikkinen E, Karppanen H, Vapaatalo H, Pelkonen O. Lack of effect of pinealectomy on the diurnal rhythm in drug metabolism. Acta Pharmacol Toxicol (Kbh) 32:157–160, 1973.

63. Wirz-Justice A, Arendt J, Marston A. Antidepressant drugs elevate rat pineal and plasma melatonin. Experientia 36:442–444, 1980.

64. Parfitt A, Klein D C. Increase caused by desmethylimipramine in the production of [³H]melatonin by isolated pineal glands. Biochem Pharmacol 26:904–905, 1977.

65. Parfitt A, Klein D C. Sympathetic nerve endings in the pineal gland protect against acute stress-induced increase in N-acetyltransferase (EC 2.3.1.5.) activity. Endocrinology 99:840–851, 1976.

66. Kalsow C M, Wacker W B. Pineal reactivity of anti-retina sera. Invest Ophthal Vis Sci 16:181–184, 1977.

67. Oksche A. Survey of the development and comparative morphology of the pineal organ. Prog Brain Res 10:3–29, 1965.

68. Kalsow C M, Wacker W B. Pineal gland involvement in retina-induced experimental allergic uveitis. Invest Ophthal Vis Sci 17:774–783, 1978.

69. Pang S F, Yew D T. Pigment aggregation by melatonin in the retinal pigment epithelium and choroid of guinea-pigs, Cavia porcellus. Experientia 35:231–233, 1979.

70. Pang S F, Yew D T, Tsui H W. Photomechanical changes in retina and choroid of guinea pig, Cavia porcellus. Neurosci Lett 10:221–224, 1978.

71. Pang S F, Brown G M, Grota L J, Chambers J W, Rodman R L. Determination of N-acetylserotonin and melatonin activities in the pineal gland, retina, Harderian gland, brain and serum of rats and chickens. Neuroendocrinology 23:1–13, 1977.

72. Quay W B, Retinal and pineal hydroxyindole-0-methyltransferase activity in vertebrates. Life Sci 4:983–991, 1965.

73. Ehinger B, Florén I. Quantitation of the uptake of indoleamines and dopamine in the rabbit retina. Exp Eye Res 26:1–11, 1978.

74. Owman C. Prenatal changes in epithelium of small intestine of rat foetus pinealectomized in utero. Q J Exp Physiol 48:408–422, 1963.

75. Owman C. Further studies on prenatal functional relations between rat pineal gland and epithelium of lower ileum. Acta Endocrinol (Kbh) 47:500–516, 1964.

76. Quastel M R, Rahamimoff R. Effect of melatonin on spontaneous contractions and response to 5-hydroxytryptamine of rat isolated duodenum. Br J Pharmacol Chemother 24:455–461, 1965.

77. Oprescu M, Costiner E. Influenta polipeptidelor pineale asupra procesuliu de gluconeogeneza in ficatul animalelor cu hepatitacronica. Stud Cercet Endocrinol 24:25–29, 1973.

78. Murthy G G, Modesto R R. Effects of melatonin and serotonin on ¹⁴C-glucose metabolism in rabbit adipose tissue. Experientia 31:383–384, 1975.

79. Machado A B M, Faleiro L C M, Da Silva W D. Study of mast cell and histamine contents of the pineal body. Z Zellforsch Mikrosk Anat 65:521–529, 1965.

80. Zanoboni A, Zanoboni-Muciaccia W. Experimental hypertension in pinealectomized rats. Life Sci 6:2327–2331, 1967.

81. Karppanen H, Vapaatalo H, Lahovaara S, Paasonen M K. Studies with pinealectomized rats. Pharmacology 3:76–84, 1970.

82. Karppanen H, Vapaatalo H. Effects of an aldosterone antagonist, spironolactone, on pinealectomized rats. Pharmacology 6:257–264, 1971.

83. Karppanen H, Airaksinen M M, Sarkimaki I. Effects in rats of pinealectomy and oxypertine on spontaneous locomotor activity and blood pressure during various light schedules. Ann Med Exp Biol Fenn 51:93–103, 1973.

84. Karppanen H, Lahovaara S, Mannisto P, Vapaatalo H. Plasma renin activity and *in vitro* synthesis of aldosterone by the adrenal glands of rats with spontaneous, renal, or pinealectomy-induced hypertension. Acta Physiol Scand 94:184–188, 1975.

85. Holmes S W, Sugden D. The effect of melatonin on pinealectomy-induced hypertension in the rat. Br J Pharmacol 55:360P–361P, 1975.

86. Zanoboni A, Forni A, Zanoboni-Muciaccia W, Zanussi C. Effect of pinealectomy on arterial blood pressure and food and water intake in the rat. J Endocrinol Invest 2:125–130, 1978.

87. Vaughan G M, Becker R A, Allen J P, Vaughan M K. Elevated blood pressure after pinealectomy in the rat. J Endocrinol Invest 2:281–284, 1979.

88. Cunnane S C, Manku M S, Oka M, Horrobin D F. Enhanced vascular reactivity to various vasoconstrictor agents following pinealectomy in the rat: role of melatonin. Can J Physiol Pharmacol 5:287–293, 1980.

89. Hall C E, Quay W B. Spontaneous and induced changes in cardiovascular function in pinealectomized rats. Physiol Behav 23:191–195, 1979.

90. Illnerova H, Albrecht I. Isoproterenol induction of pineal serotonin N-acetyltransferase in normotensive and spontaneously hypertensive rats. Experientia 31:95–96, 1975.

91. Relkin R. The pineal, the adrenals and hypertension. *In* The Pineal, Eden Press, Montréal, and Lancaster, England 1976, pp 68–70.

92. Jelinek J, Křeček J. The effect of age and pinealectomy on the hypertension produced by adrenal regeneration. Experientia 24:912–913, 1968.

93. Jankovic B D, Isakovic K, Petrovic S. Effect of pinealectomy on immune reactions in the rat. Immunology 18:1–16, 1970.

94. Rella W, Lapin V. Immunocompetence of pinealectomized and simultaneously pinealectomized and thymectomized rats. Oncology 33:3–6, 1976.

95. Belokrylov G A, Morozov V G, Khavinson V K, Sofronov B N. Effect of low-molecular extracts from heterologous thymus, epiphysis and hypothalamus on the immune response of mice. Biull Eksp Biol Med 81:202–204, 1976.

96. Milcu I, Nanu-Ionescu L, Marcean R, Ionescu V. The influence of the pineal gland on nitrogen metabolism. J Endocrinol 45:175–181, 1969.

97. Nanu-Ionescu L, Marcean R, Ionescu V. Pineal gland and amino acid tolerance in rats. Rev Roum Endocrinol 8:123–129, 1971.

98. Peres G E, Vareilles F. Etude des consequences de la pinealectomie sur l'absorption intestinale de la glycine chez le rat en croissance. C R Soc Biol (Paris) 168:54–58, 1974.

99. Howd R A, Seo K S, Wurtman R J. Rat liver N-acetyltransferase: inhibition by melatonin. Biochem Pharmacol 25:977–978, 1976.

100. Arnold J D, Berger A E, Martin D C. The role of the pineal in mediating photoperiodic control of growth and division synchrony and capillary sequestration of *Plasmodium berghei* in mice. J Parasitol 55:609–616, 1969.

101. Arnold J D, Berger A E, Martin D C. Chemical agents effective in mediating control of growth and division synchrony of *Plasmodium berghei* in pinealectomized mice. J Parasitol 55:617–625, 1969.

102. Arnold J D, Berger A E, Martin D C. Role of the endocrine system in controlling growth and division synchrony of *Plasmodium berghei* in mice. J Parasitol 55:956–962, 1969.

103. Perez-Polo J R, Hall K, Vaughan M K, Reiter R J. Effect of pinealectomy, blinding, castration and melatonin on nerve growth factor levels in the submaxillary glands of mice. Neurosci Lett 10:83–87, 1978.

104. Houssay A B, Pazo J H, Epper C E. Effects of the pineal gland upon the hair cycles in mice. Acta Physiol Lat Am 16:202–205, 1966.

105. Houssay A B, Pazo J H, Epper C E. Effects of the pineal gland upon the hair cycles in mice. J Invest Dermatol 47:230–234, 1966.

106. Logan A, Weatherhead B. Pelage color cycles and hair follicle tyrosinase activity in the Siberian hamster. J Invest Dermatol 71:295–298, 1978.

107. Hoffmann K. Photoperiodic mechanism in hamsters: the participation of the pineal gland. In Environmental Endocrinology, ed J Assenmacher, D S Farner. Springer-Verlag, Berlin, Heidelberg, and New York, 1978, pp 94–102.

108. Hoffmann K. The influence of photoperiod and melatonin on testis size, body weight and pelage color in the Djungarian hamster (Phodopus sungorus). J Comp Physiol 85:267–282, 1973.

109. Prevedello M R, Ritta M N, Cardinali D P. Fast axonal transport in rat sciatic nerve. Inhibition by pineal indoles. Neurosci Lett 13:29–34, 1979.

110. Edström A, Hanson M. The mechanisms of fast axonal transport: a pharmacological approach. Neuropharmacology 14:181–188, 1975.

111. Polidora V J. Behavioral effects of "phenylketonuria" in rats. Proc Natl Acad Sci USA 57:102–106, 1967.

112. Wooley D W, van der Hoeven T. Prevention of mental defect of phenylketonuria with serotonin congeners such as melatonin or hydroxytryptophan. Science 144:1593–1594, 1964.

113. Knox W E. Phenylketonuria. In The Metabolic Basis of Inherited Diseases, ed JB Stanbury, J B Wyngaarden, S Fredrickson, McGraw-Hill, New York, 1972, pp 266–295.

114. Pate C M B, Sandler M, Stacy R S. Decreased 5-hydroxytryptophan decarboxylase activity in phenylketonuria. Lancet 2:1099–1101, 1958.

115. Tennen S S. The effects of p-chlorophenylalanine, a serotonin depletor, on avoidance acquisition, pain sensitivity and related behavior in the rat. Psychopharmacologia 10:204–219, 1967.

116. Vorhees C V, Schaefer G J, Barrett R J. p-chloroamphetamine: behavioral effects of reduced cerebral serotonin in rats. Pharmacol Biochem Behav 3:279–284, 1975.

117. Anton-Tay F, Chou C, Anton S, Wurtman R J. Brain serotonin concentration: elevation following intraperitoneal administration of melatonin. Science 162:277–278, 1968.

118. Butcher R E, Vorhees C V, Kindt C W, Kazmaier-Novak K J, Berry H K. Induced PKU in rats: effects of age and melatonin treatment. Pharmacol Biochem Behav 7:129–133, 1977.

119. Raina A, Jänne J. Physiology of the natural polyamines putrescine, spermidine and spermine. Med Biol 53:121–147, 1975.

120. Fraschini F, Ferioli M E, Nebuloni R, Scalabrino G. Pineal gland and polyamines. J Neural Transm 48:209–221, 1980.

121. Tabor C W, Tabor H. 1,4-diaminobutane (putrescine), spermidine, and spermine. Ann Rev Biochem 45:285–306, 1976.

122. Woodhouse M, Rhodin J. The ultrastructure of the Harderian gland of the mouse with particular reference to the formation of its secretory product. J Ultrastruct Res 9:76–98, 1963.

123. Bjorkman N, Nicander L, Schanz B. On the histology and ultrastructure of the Harderian gland in rabbits. Z Zellforsch Mikrosk Anat 52:93–104, 1960.

124. Kelenyi G, Orban S. Electron microscopy of the Harderian gland of the rat: maturation of the acinar cells and genesis of the secretory droplets. Acta Morphol Acad Sci Hung 13:155–166, 1965.

125. Christensen F, Dam H. A sexual dimorphism of the Harderian gland in hamsters. Acta Physiol Scand 27:333–336, 1953.

126. Paule W, Hayes E, Marks B. The Harderian gland of the Syrian hamster. Anat Rec 121:349–350, 1955.

127. Bucana C, Nadakavukaren M. Fine structure of the hamster Harderian gland. Z Zellforsch Mikrosk Anat 129:178–187, 1972.

128. Hoffman R. Influence of some endocrine glands, hormones and blinding on the histology and porphyrins of the Harderian glands of golden hamsters. Am J Anat 132:463–478, 1971.

129. Clabough J, Norvell J. Effects of castration, blinding and the pineal gland on the Harderian glands of the male golden hamster. Neuroendocrinology 12:344–353, 1973.

130. Jones C W, Hoffman R A. Porphyrin concentration of the hamster (Mesocricetus auratus) Harderian gland: effects of incubation with delta-aminolevulinic acid and various hormones. Int J Biochem 7:135–139, 1976.

131. Joó I, Kahán A. The porphyrin content of Harderian glands in rats and the melatonin-melanocyte stimulating hormone-system. Endokrinologie 65:308–312, 1975.

132. Owman C. On the effects of pinealectomy in the fetal rat. Commun Dept Anat Univ Lund (Sweden) No. 2, 1962.

133. Miline R, Devecerski V, Krstic R. Effects des stimuli auditifs sur la glande pineale de la chauve-souris en hibernation. Acta Anat (Basel) 73 (Suppl) 56:293–300, 1969.

134. Miline R, Devecerski V, Sijacki N, Krstic R. Pineal gland behavior as affected by cold. Hormones 1:321–331, 1970.

135. Nir I, Hirschmann N, Sulman F G. Pineal gland changes of rats exposed to heat. Experientia 28:701–702, 1972.

136. Palmer D L, Riedesel M L. Responses of whole-animal and isolated hearts of ground squirrels, Citellus lateralis to melatonin. Comp Biochem Physiol 53C:69–72, 1976.

137. Spencer F, Shirer H W, Yochim J M. Core temperature in the female rat: effect of pinealectomy or altered lighting. Am J Physiol 231:355–360, 1976.

138. Lynch G R, White S E, Grundel R, Berger M S. Effects of photoperiod, melatonin administration and thyroid block on spontaneous daily torpor and temperature regulation in the white-footed mouse, Peromyscus leucopus. J Comp Physiol 125:157–163, 1978.

139. Lynch G R, Sullivan K, Gendler S L. Temperature regulation in the mouse, Peromyscus leucopus: effects of various photoperiods, pinealectomy and melatonin administration. Int J Biometeorol 24:49–55, 1980.

140. Hagelstein K A, Folk G E Jr. Effects of photoperiod, cold acclimation and melatonin on the white rat. Comp Biochem Physiol 62C:225–229, 1979.

141. Sampson P H. Behavior and pineal functioning. In Frontiers of Pineal Physiology, ed M D Altschule. MIT Press, Cambridge, Mass, 1975, pp 204–222.

142. Casetta R, Osima B, Bianchini P, Barbanti-Silva C. The effects of pineal gland extracts on the thymus of monogonadectomized rats. Biochim Biol Sper 8:173–176, 1969.

143. Baráth P, Csaba G. Histological changes in the lung thymus and adrenal one and a half year after pinealectomy. Acta Biol Acad Sci Hung 25:123–125, 1974.

144. Csaba G, Baráth P. Morphological changes of thymus and the thyroid gland after postnatal extirpation of pineal body. Endocrinol Exp (Bratisl) 9:59–67, 1975.

145. Wragg L E. Refractoriness of rat pineal to chemical carcinogens. Anat Rec 154:496, 1966.

146. Das Gupta T K, Terz J. Influence of pineal gland on the growth and spread of melanoma in the hamster. Cancer Res 27:1306–1311, 1967.

147. Das Gupta T K, Terz J. Influence of pineal body on melanoma of hamsters. Nature 213:1038–1040, 1967.

148. Barone R M, Das Gupta T K. Role of pinealectomy on Walker 256 carcinoma in rats. J Surg Oncol 2:313–322, 1970.

149. Aubert C, Prade M, Bohoun C. Effect of pinealectomy on the melanic tumours of the golden hamster induced by administration (per os) of a single dose of 9,10-dimethyl-1, 2-benzanthracene. C R Acad Sci (D) (Paris) 271:2465–2468, 1970.

150. Tapp E. Pineal gland in rats suffering from malignancy. J Neural Transm 48:131–135, 1980.

151. Buswell R S. The pineal and neoplasia. Lancet 1:34–35, 1975.
152. Bindoni M, Jutisz M, Ribot G. Characterization and partial purification of a substance in the pineal gland which inhibits cell multiplication *in vitro*. Biochim Biophys Acta 437:577–588, 1976.
153. Lapin V. Influence of simultaneous pinealectomy and thymectomy on the growth and formation of metastases of the Yoshida sarcoma in rats. Exp Pathol (Jena) 9:108–112, 1974.
154. Lapin V. The pineal and neoplasia. Lancet 1:341, 1975.
155. Wrba H, Lapin V, Dostal V. The influence of pinealectomy and of pinealectomy combined with thymectomy on the oncogenesis caused by polyoma virus in rats. Oster Z Onkologie 2:37–39, 1975.
156. Dukor P, Salvin S B, Dietrich F M, Gelzer J, Hess R, Loustalot P. Effect of reserpine on immune reactions and tumor growth. Eur J Cancer 2:253–261, 1966.
157. Lapin V. Effects of reserpine on the incidence of 9,10-dimethyl-1,2-benzanthracene-induced tumors in pinealectomized and thymectomised rats. Oncology 35:132–135, 1978.
158. Welsch C W, Clemens J A, Meites J. Effects of hypothalamic and amygdaloid lesions and development and growth of carcinogen-induced mammary tumors in female rats. Cancer Res 29:1541–1549, 1969.
159. Lapin V, Ebels I. Effects of some low molecular weight sheep pineal fractions and melatonin on different tumors in rats and mice. Oncology 33:110–113, 1976.
160. Ebels I, Citharel A, Moszkowska A. Separation of pineal extracts by gelfiltration III. Sheep pineal factors acting either on the hypothalamus, or on the anterior hypophysis of mice and rats in *in vitro* experiments. J Neural Transm 36:281–302, 1975.
161. Aubert C, Janiaud P, Lecalvez J. Effect of pinealectomy and melatonin on mammary tumor growth in Sprague-Dawley rats under different conditions of lighting. J Neural Transm 47:121–130, 1980.
162. El-Domeiri A A, Das Gupta T K. The influence of pineal ablation and administration of melatonin on growth and spread of hamster melanoma. J Surg Oncol 8:197–205, 1976.
163. Quay W B, Gorray K C. Pineal effects on metabolism and glucose homeostasis: evidence for lines of humoral mediation of pineal influences on tumor growth. J Neural Transm 47:107–120, 1980.
164. Smythe GA, Lazarus L. Growth hormone regulation by melatonin and serotonin. Nature 244:230–231, 1973.
165. Pauly JE, Scheving LE. Circadian rhythms in blood glucose and the effect of different lighting schedules, hypophysectomy, adrenal medullectomy and starvation. Am J Anat 120:627–636, 1966.
166. Sothern RB, Nelson WL, Halberg F. A circadian rhythm in susceptibility of mice to the anti-tumor drug, adriamycin. *In* Proceedings XII International Conference, International Society for Chronobiology. Il Ponte, Milan, 1977, pp 433–437.

RICHARD RELKIN, M.D.

THE HUMAN PINEAL

CALCIFICATION

Short of total calcification, the calcification of the pineal that occurs with advancing age apparently has no effect on pineal function. Enzyme studies (1) of pineals from humans, aged 3–70 years, revealed the gland to retain the capacity to inactivate serotonin (5-hydroxytryptamine, 5-HT) and histamine and to synthesize melatonin. Other work (2) has also demonstrated that the human pineal remains functional through old age. Furthermore, absence of degeneration or loss of parenchymal cells has been observed in association with pineal calcification (3). Calcification has even been observed histologically in pineals of children dying in the first decade of life (4), and a fairly constant level of calcification has been observed beyond the age of 30 years (5). The latter study also revealed that pineals from females below the age of 60 years were significantly heavier than those of comparable males; this difference in gland weight was partly accounted for by an increased calcium content in female glands. Calcification apparently takes place in a ground substance that has been observed in both pinealocytes and interstitium.

From Easton Hospital, Easton, Pennsylvania 18042, and Hahnemann Medical College and Hospital, Philadelphia, Pennsylvania 19102.

This ground substance seems to be secreted soon after birth, as it has been identified in pineals of children less than 1 year of age (4). A theory, recently developed, proposed that a polypeptide hormone-carrier protein complex is released into the interstitium. The hormone then dissociates from the carrier protein by virtue of calcium ion exchange, the calcium then complexing with the protein (6). It was suggested that it is this latter complex which, in conjunction with exocytic debris, results in the formation of calcospherulites (also referred to as pineal acervuli, corpora arenacea, or pineal sand). Thus the degree of calcification in the pineal may actually be a reflection of past secretory activity rather than an indicator of degeneration (7).

One analysis of pineal calcifications reported the acervuli to have a granular substructure consisting of carbonate-containing hydroxyapatite, mineralogically similar to enamel (8). Other work (9–12) has reported a similar composition of pineal acervuli. One of these studies (9) also detected small amounts of magnesium and strontium, whereas another (10) revealed some detectable calcium sulfate. In one of these reports (12), the crystallinity of pineal sand was found to be higher than that of compact bone. As prior data had shown that the average size of pineal-sand hydroxyapatite was smaller than that in bone, it was concluded that the higher crystallinity of corpora arenacea is secondary to a lesser percentage of the submicrocrystalline fraction in their mineral.

Studying pineal calcification in skull roentgenograms in Nigeria, it was found that the incidence was less than that reported for other populations (13). In American blacks, the incidence of roentgenologically apparent pineal calcification has been reported to be approximately half that seen in American whites (14). In this study, the incidence of pineal calcification was slightly greater in American blacks as compared to indigenous African blacks. It was postulated that the low incidence of detectable pineal calcification in African blacks had a constitutional basis.

CHEMICAL CONSTITUENTS OTHER THAN INDOLEAMINES

In studying 144 human pineals obtained at autopsy, a significant correlation between pineal weight and calcium content was discovered in patients older than 60 years (15). On the average, calcium accounted for 1.9–7.4% of total pineal weight. Other findings were the presence of dopamine, epinephrine, and norepinephrine in most glands.

Since arginine vasotocin (AVT) apparently can be synthesized by the human pineal (16), an investigation (17) was performed to ascertain whether, like two other closely related nonapeptides, arginine vasopressin and oxytocin, AVT is also synthesized with a carrier protein, or neurophysin; the result was the finding of two neurophysins in the pineal. There was no readily available explanation for this phenomenon of two neurophysins for the one polypeptide neurohormone, AVT. It was suggested, however, that the situation may be analogous to that found in the pig posterior pituitary, where the presence of three neurophysins has been claimed (18), although only two neurohormones have been discovered there thus far.

As mentioned previously (see Chapter 6, Pineal, Vasotocin), melatonin has been reported to be the releasing hormone for AVT, causing its release into the cerebrospinal fluid (CSF) (19). Subsequently, it was found that the CSF of healthy males contained AVT when the CSF was withdrawn after their awakening from rapid-eye-movement (REM) sleep (20). No detectable AVT was found when the subjects awakened from non-REM sleep. These results were interpreted as evidence for REM-sleep-dependent release of AVT into the CSF of the human.

An enzyme having reninlike properties was recently described in human pineals obtained at necropsy (21).

Aside from those already mentioned, other constituents reported to be found in the pineal include histamine, inositol, taurine, pteridines, and iodinated compounds (22), as well as angiotensin I (23) and a peptide with melanotropic and lipotropic activities (24) (pro-opiocortin?). In addition, prolactin-releasing and prolactin-inhibiting activities have been identified in human pineal (25), as has a pineal antigonadotropic factor, which latter appears to be separate and distinct from melatonin (26).

EPILEPSY AND PARKINSON'S DISEASE

In addition to the finding that 200 mg of melatonin given intravenously could produce sedation in an adult male (27), subsequent investigation (28) focused on this hormone's effects in epileptic and Parkinsonian patients. Compared to normal subjects, epileptics and patients with Parkinsonism also manifested an increase in electroencephalographic alpha activity and synchronization, easily induced sleep, more frequent REM cycles during sleep, vivid dreams, unusual experiences in visual imagery, and feelings of elation. Melatonin was also found significantly to improve the manifestations of epilepsy and the Parkinsonian state.

INDOLEAMINES OTHER THAN MELATONIN

Five-methoxytryptophol (5-MTP) can be formed by the action of hydroxyindole-O-methyltransferase (HIOMT) on 5-hydroxytryptophol, the latter the result of monoamine oxidase acting on 5-hydroxytryptamine (serotonin, 5-HT); or 5-MTP can arise from the methylation of 5-HT to 5-methoxytryptamine (5-MeO-T), the latter then being deaminated to 5-MTP (29). In an investigation (30) of 5-MTP's effects in humans, it was found that this indoleamine was present in plasma throughout the 24 hours and that peaks of activity occurred during both light and dark phases. Plasma levels of 5-MTP also varied with the menstrual cycle, highest levels being found in the first 9 days of the cycle (all subjects having cycles of less than 30 days), with levels falling to a nadir in the last third of the cycle. Additionally, a fall in 5-MTP levels accompanied hypoglycemia, levels of 5-MTP recovering as blood glucose normalized.

In spite of these findings, the possibility was, nevertheless, presented that 5-MTP may represent an inactive metabolite.

Confirmation of some of the work just cited resulted from a study (31) in which 5-MTP levels were found to be lower in the final third of the menstrual cycle. Women taking oral contraceptives had low levels throughout the 28–30 days. It was suggested that the decrease in 5-MTP that occurred in the last third of the cycle may have been related to the higher levels of progesterone normally found at that time. The findings in women taking oral contraceptives would appear to support this postulate.

The indoleamines, 5-MeO-T and 5-methoxy-N, N-dimethyltryptamine (5-MeO-DMT) have now both been identified in the human pineal (32,33). Their significance will be discussed under Mental Illness.

LONGEVITY

Recently there has been the suggestion that the pineal may be involved in the determination of longevity (34,35). The basis of this hypothesis lies in the belief that longevity is regulated by a "biologic clock" (36), coupled with the implication that the pineal, with its ability to act as a transducer of environmental lighting, performs this function (37). In one study (38), it was observed that males and females under the age of 65 years who were afflicted with retrolental fibroplasia had better survival rates than other blind individuals. Unlike other causes of blindness, which are associated with systemic illness, only retrolental fibroplasia, corneal abnormalities, and myopia are not. However, survivorship in the latter two was not found to be enhanced. The reason for this may be that, compared to other causes of blindness, the blindness in retrolental fibroplasia is frequently total (i.e., no light perception), as well as the fact that such blindness almost invariably occurs within the first few weeks of life. Thus the pineal is chronically and maximally stimulated.

MELATONIN

Utilizing a bioassay, the daily rhythm of urinary melatonin was measured in healthy subjects of both sexes. Levels were found to be significantly higher between 23:00 and 07:00 hours than at other times (39). A confirmatory bioassay study (40) revealed urine levels of melatonin to be five to seven times greater during sleep, darkness, or recumbency (i.e., 23:00–07:00 hours) than during active, waking hours. Another investigation (41) determined that plasma levels of melatonin, measured by bioassay, were elevated during the dark (sleeping) phase of 14L:10D in both white and black men; nocturnal elevation of 5-hydroxyindole-acetic acid (5-HIAA) was also noted.

Using gas chromatography with electron capture detection, pineal melatonin concentration was observed to increase in the evening and through the night, decreasing in the morning and reaching a nadir about noon (42).

In all that follows, unless otherwise specified, measurement of melatonin has been by radioimmunoassay. Melatonin concentrations in the serum of children with leukemia in remission were found to be comparable to those in normal adults, whereas concentrations of melatonin in the CSF of these children were higher than those in respective serum samples (43). However, another investigation (44) revealed that in simultaneously obtained serum and CSF specimens from adult males and females, melatonin was lower in the CSF. Additional findings in both sexes were a circadian rhythm having peak values during the dark phase. In another study (45), the peak concentration of serum melatonin occurred at 02:00 hours with a nadir at 14:00 hours, these findings corresponding to those in the previous study. It was also demonstrated that serotonin-N-acetyltransferase (NAT) and HIOMT, both measured in pineals obtained at necropsy, displayed activity that was directly related to the time of death. Activity of each enzyme manifested a similar rhythm to that of serum melatonin.

After establishing the existence of similar diurnal rhythms of melatonin in healthy male subjects, with peak urinary and blood levels occurring during the period of darkness and sleep, the daily light-dark phases were shifted so that the dark phase occurred between 11:00–19:00 hours, instead of 23:00–07:00 hours. As a result of this shift, it took plasma and urinary melatonin rhythms 5–7 days to reentrain (46). The investigators also noted that there was a high degree of correlation between urinary melatonin levels and circulating melatonin levels.

Measurement of nocturnal plasma melatonin in healthy men yielded no correlation between the stages of sleep and melatonin concentrations. Neither was there any correlation between nocturnal melatonin levels and the levels of anterior pituitary hormones (47). It was concluded that nocturnal levels of melatonin are controlled differently from those of luteinizing hormone (LH), growth hormone (GH), and prolactin.

A comparison of the circadian variation of urinary melatonin in healthy American versus Japanese women revealed a circadian rhythm in both groups but lower levels in the Japanese subjects (48). Geographic as well as ethnic factors were among those implicated as causatively interacting to produce this difference.

Interest has recently focused on the intensity of light required to bring about changes in human pineal function. In one such study (49), using gas chromatography with negative chemical ionization mass spectrometry, it was found that bright artifical lighting (i.e., 2500 lux at eye level) suppressed nocturnal melatonin secretion in normal humans of both sexes. However, room light of a lesser intensity (500 lux at eye level) failed to suppress melatonin levels, although this latter lighting intensity has been shown to be sufficient to suppress melatonin secretion in other mammals (50). During the course of another investigation (51), it was observed that secretory episodes of melatonin persisted even in the presence of natural outdoor lighting, albeit these episodes were of a lesser magnitude than those observed during darkness. The rapid fall in melatonin levels that has been reported to follow the sudden exposure of other mammalian species to light, during darkness (52,53), was not observed in humans (54). This absence of an acute change in melatonin was postulated to be related to the influence of sleep-waking and prolonged-darkness alterations over an extended period of time.

It appears that not only does melatonin have a diurnal rhythm in man but it also has an annual rhythm characterized by January and July peaks (55).

In a study (56) of the effects of "jet lag" on melatonin in healthy males, a decrease in 24-hour sleep and daytime mean melatonin levels was found after a 7-hour westward time shift, during which the total daylight duration was 16 hours, instead of 10. A 7-hour eastward time shift, involving 33 hours of sleep deprivation, resulted in a total disruption of melatonin rhythm. On the day after completion of the westward trip, there was a shift in the acrophase, indicating partial adaptation. However, the amplitude of the acrophase diminished during the period of investigation (i.e., 10 weeks, October to January) pari passu with the decrease in duration of daylight. It was concluded that daylight may exert a major influence on the amplitude of the rhythm of melatonin.

Reasoning that, as the enterochromaffin cells of the gastrointestinal tract are the main site of synthesis of the melatonin-precursor, 5-HT, investigation (57,58) revealed evidence of active biosynthesis of melatonin in bioassay-tested extract of human appendiceal homogenates.

Evidence that melatonin may be involved in regulation of the human menstrual cycle was adduced from the finding of elevated levels of serum melatonin at the time of the menses, with a nadir at the time of ovulation (59). In this investigation, all women were healthy, having a mean age of 35 years and an average cycle length of 26 days. Although the possible participation of light was not mentioned in the preceding, a subsequent study (60) detailed a great deal of background material relating the degree of nocturnal moonlight to the time of ovulation and length of the menstrual cycle. Cited were the mean menstrual cycle length of 29 days as compared with the mean lunar month of 29.5 days. Considering the possibility that these figures may not be coincidental, 16 women, average age 29, with a history of menstrual irregularity and/or abnormally long cycles, were exposed to ordinary artificial lighting during sleep on the nights of cycle days 14–17. In 11 subjects exposed to light for more than one cycle, nine showed a decreased cycle length. The result was statistical evidence that the photic stimulation regularized the length of the menstrual cycle and, thus, presumably could influence the time of ovulation.

To ascertain whether the maximal human melatonin secretion that occurs with darkness is inhibitory to gonadotropin release, four pubertal boys were studied over a 24-hour period. Not only melatonin but LH as well were observed to increase during darkness and sleep (61). The data were interpreted to indicate that melatonin levels that occur during sleep are inadequate to prevent the spontaneous surges of LH seen in sleep during puberty (62). Further study (63) of the role of melatonin in human puberty revealed that, in young boys, there is an abrupt fall in blood melatonin levels (obtained between 11:00 and 13:00 hours) coincident with stage 2 (Tanner) of genital development.

MENTAL ILLNESS

The diurnal rhythm of melatonin in depressed patients has been found to be no different from that seen in healthy subjects (64).

Based on the observations that melanoctye-stimulating hormone (MSH), an antagonist of melatonin (65), can produce exaggerated responses to noxious stimuli in rats (66) and that MSH-inhibiting factor can act as an antidepressant (67), melatonin was administered either orally or intravenously to depressed patients (68); the result was an unexpected exacerbation of the patients' symptoms of dysphoria, as well as increased CSF levels of 5-HIAA. The latter contrasted with studies showing decreased CSF 5-HIAA following antidepressant drug administration (69). It was also noted that several of the most severely depressed patients developed psychotic symptoms during administration of melatonin. As pointed out in this study, melatonin synthesis has been reported to be increased by a number of psychotomimetic agents and stimulants, such as 5-MeO-DMT, bufotenin, mescaline, lysergic acid diethylamide, dimethoxyphenylethylamine (70), amphetamine (71), cocaine (72), and L-dopa (73); however, neuroleptics, such as fluphenazine and haloperidol, as well as the β-adrenergic blocker, propranolol, decrease such synthesis (74,75). As regards the foregoing, it is of interest that the psychotomimetic agent 5-MeO-DMT (76) has been identified in human pineal glands obtained at autopsy (31), as has its presumed precursor, 5-MeO-T (30), a psychotomimetic agent in its own right (77). Elevated levels of 5-MeO-T have been found in the CSF of schizophrenic patients (78), and 5-MeO-DMT as well as bufotenin have been identified in the urine of schizophrenics (79). Although the formation of 5-MeO-DMT apparently can occur via the action of either HIOMT or indoleethylamine-N-methyltransferase (INMT) on 5-HT, the intermediate compounds being 5-MeO-T and 5-hydroxydimethyltryptamine, respectively, one report (31) expressed the belief that the pathway utilizing HIOMT takes precedence in the pineal. However, in human and rabbit lung preparations, synthesis of 5-MeO-DMT has been found to proceed from 5-MeO-T through 5-methoxy-N-methyltryptamine (80); this latter metabolite has not yet been identified in the human pineal. Evidence tending to implicate INMT activity as being important in schizophrenics includes the demonstration that chlorpromazine, used in treating schizophrenia, inhibits rabbit lung INMT (81). Furthermore, as bovine pineal extract has been reported to have a salutory effect on some schizophrenics (82), an investigation (83) into the effect of bovine pineal extract on INMT revealed enzyme activity to be inhibited. Suggestion of HIOMT prominence in the apparently abnormal indoleamine metabolism in schizophrenia entails the findings that: (1) pyridoxal phosphate seems to be a powerful inhibitor of HIOMT in vitro (84), (2) psychotomimetics cause a decrease in rat brain pyridoxal phosphate (85), and (3) phenothiazines increase brain pyridoxal phosphate in vitro (85).

In a study (86) in humans of the effect of chlorpromazine on melatonin, it was found that the drug increased serum, but not CSF, melatonin levels. The low levels of serum melatonin in drug-free patients was adduced as evidence that HIOMT activity is either defective (87,88) or out of phase with its substrate (89) in schizophrenia. As chlorpromazine has already been mentioned as an indirect inhibitor of HIOMT, via its effects on pyridoxal phosphate, the results just presented would seem to be contradictory. Chlorpromazine would not be anticipated to decrease HIOMT activity on the one hand and increase melatonin levels on the other. The explanation could lie in the known ability of phenothiazines to inhibit melatonin degradation in the liver (90).

Other concepts, presented in a brief review (91) of suggested pathophysiology of schizophrenia, have included excess dopamine activity, overproduction of a normal endorphin or enkephalin or synthesis of an abnormal one, deficiency of prostaglandin synthesis or action, melatonin deficiency, zinc deficiency, wheat sensitivity, and hyperallergy. The hypothesis offered in this article is that the final common pathway involved in the causation of schizophrenia may be a failure of formation and action of prostaglandins of the 1 series.

Returning to the apparent efficacy of melatonin treatment for schizophrenia mentioned earlier, a study (92) of 10 young schizophrenics (average age 26 years) revealed that daily intramuscular injection of 1–2 ml of melatonin resulted in lower psychosis scores when compared to placebo-injected patients. All patients were continued on phenothiazine treatment throughout the experiment, the duration of which was never less than 3 weeks. Psychosis scores were based on responses of nurses to questions relating to hallucinations, delusions, paranoia, bizarre speech and/or behavior in the patients. Although this study is essentially in agreement with an earlier one (82), a later investigation (personal communication, quoted in reference 68) of two purportedly recovered schizophrenics revealed the production of a severe exacerbation in each following the administration of intravenous melatonin. This latter finding would tend to coincide with the production of psychotic symptoms in depressed patients (68) mentioned earlier.

MENTAL RETARDATION

The suggestion has been made that pineal hormones may be involved, via an inhibitory action, in the development of such states of mental retardation as found in mongols and morons (93).

MISCELLANEOUS

The effects of oral melatonin on skin color was studied in five adults; one with autoimmune Addison's disease, one with unrecognized adrenogenital syndrome, and three with idiopathic hyperpigmentation (94).

Prior experimentation had shown melatonin to be capable of causing skin blanching in tadpoles (95,96) and inhibition of MSH in weasels (97). Lightening of skin pigmentation was seen only in the subject with untreated adrenogenital syndrome. Explanation of these results is conjectural, with no clear-cut role for melatonin in human pigmentation having been established.

In comparing adrenal-cortex thickness versus pineal weights in autopsied patients dying of nonneoplastic disease, it was found that these two parameters varied inversely to a significant degree (98). It was concluded that an undefined mechanism is responsible for the apparent antagonism existing between the two glands (see Chapter 6 Adrenals).

It appears that the thyrotropin-releasing hormone (TRH) found in the pineal (99) (See Chapter 6 Pineal, Hypothalamic Peptides) may participate in the regulation of melatonin synthesis (100). This study was based on the previously demonstrated ability of norepinephrine and cyclic-adenosinemonophosphate (cyclic-AMP) to stimulate NAT (101), coupled with the postulate that the action of norepinephrine on NAT is mediated by cyclic-AMP (101). The result was the finding that TRH produced a significant inhibition of norepinephrine-induced cyclic-AMP formation.

NONPINEAL TUMORS

The background material for the effect of the pineal on malignancies has been detailed in Chapter 7 under the heading Tumor Growth.

It has been suggested that there may be a relationship in humans between the presence of malignancy and pineal weight, as heavier glands have been reported in patients over the age of 45 years who died of neoplasms (102). Other investigators, however, observed lighter weight pineals in patients who died of neoplasms than those found in patients who died from nonneoplastic causes (103). The heavier pineals found in the latter group were attributed to a greater mineral content. Children and adolescents who died of cancer were found to have multiple slitlike cystic cavities, gliosis, and large numbers of Rosenthal fibers in enlarged pineals (104).

A recent study (105) found no statistical difference between the weight of pineals in patients who died from malignancy versus pineal weight in those who expired from nonneoplastic disease. What was found in this investigation, however, was that patients who died from carcinoma of the breast and melanoma had heavier glands that those who died as a result of sarcoma. The one common hormonal association of these three types of malignancy appears to be with GH. GH levels in patients with melanomas or carcinoma of the breast have been reported to be low, whereas high GH levels have been found in patients with sarcomas (106). The reason for the inverse correlation of GH to pineal weight in these malignancies is uncertain.

In an attempt to link the pineal more firmly to the etiology of breast cancer, a hypothesis was advanced in which altered pineal function would lead to decreased melatonin secretion; the latter, in turn, would permit increased secretion of luteinizing-hormone-releasing factor, which would result in increased pituitary secretion of follicle-stimulating hormone (FSH) and LH. Increased ovarian secretion of estrogen and progesterone would follow and produce early and prolonged breast stimulation (107).

PINEAL TUMORS

Pinealomas and Teratomas

Examining a melanotic neuroectodermal tumor of the orbit and frontal region in a 6-month-old male, it was noted that the tumor, as with previously described neuroectodermal tumors, was characterized by melanin-containing epithelial cells, small undifferentiated cells, and a fibrovascular stroma. Since the human fetal pineal is characterized by the same histologic composition, it was hypothesized that the fetal pineal, believed to arise from neuroectoderm, may be a normally occurring precursor of melanotic neuroectodermal tumors of infancy (108).

A cytologic study (109) of 28 pinealomas revealed that the more undifferentiated tumors (i.e., pineoblastomas) histologically resembled medulloblastomas, whereas the lobular architecture of pineocytomas was similar to that of the mature pineal. Histologic features of pineoblastomas were also observed to merge with those of pineocytomas in some of the tumors. In addition, some pineocytomas differentiated toward astrocytes, some toward ganglion cells, and others represented a combination of the latter two; one pineoblastoma showed evidence of focal differentiation into retinoblastoma. Another case of pineoblastoma with retinoblastomatous differentiation was described, in which, in addition to widely divergent histologic changes, photoreceptor cells, typical of previously described "fleurettes" (110,111) were found (112). Such elements were also reported in the preceding study (109). Fleurettes appear to consist of clusters of cells possessing regular, round, hyperchromatic nuclei and elongated eosinophilic cytoplasmic processes. The distal portions of these processes frequently expand into a bulbous configuration. Many of these processes also group into bundles that perforate a membrane and then fan out from the fenestrated membrane; others coverge from the membrane. Electron microscopic examination of a pineoblastoma revealed characteristic granular bodies, whorls of smooth endoplasmic reticulum, and annulate lamellae (113). Some of these findings were thought to be reminiscent of the photoreceptor cells seen in the human fetal pineal.

Another study (114) of eight pineoblastomas and five pineocytomas resulted in the description of two clinicopathologic syndromes. The pineoblastomas clinically resembled the medulloblastoma-neuroblastoma group of tumors and were found mostly in young patients (average age 23 years); disease progression was rapid and, thus, the length of illness short (average, 21 months). These tumors were infiltrating and commonly spread via the CSF. Histologically, they also resembled the medulloblastoma-neuroblastoma tumor group, were characterized by a scarcity of cytoplasmic processes and Homer Wright rosettes, and contained giant cells. The latter provides some confirmation of the study (109) reported previously. The pineocytomas, in comparison, were tumors of older adults (average age 50 years) and evidenced slow progression with a long length of illness (average, 7 years). Their mode of progression entailed local expansion with compression of surrounding tissues. Histologically, they were characterized by abundant cytoplasmic processes, giant cells, and rosettes. Common variants included areas of neoplastic astrocytes and gangliocytes. These findings are also consonant with the previously described study (109).

In a series of 26 cases of pinealoma in children (only one case was labeled a pineoblastoma, the other 25 being categorized simply as pinealomas), pneumoencephalography, ventriculography, use of ventriculofiberoscopy millipore filter-cell culture of the CSF were all considered useful for diagnosis (115). Currently, metrizamide ventriculography should replace pneumoencephalography, and diagnosis can frequently be made with the use of computerized tomography (CT) alone.

A review (116), encompassing 53 years, of 34 patients with pineal tumors disclosed that most patients were male adolescents having increased intracranial pressure and Parinaud's syndrome (i.e., paralysis of upward and, sometimes, downward gaze, fixed pupils, and ocular divergence). Unexpectedly, hypothalamic symptoms were infrequent.

Two cases of pineocytoma were reported in which the initial presentation was that of a subarachnoid hemorrhage (117). Both tumors only became obvious later in the course of the disease. The first patient had three episodes of subarachnoid hemorrhage, the second, four. In another patient, presenting with the sudden onset of severe headache and brief unconsciousness, evidence of a subarachnoid hemorrhage was found (118). An encapsulated hematoma with surrounding clots were removed from the pineal region. Based on the operative findings and the histology of the hematoma capsule, it was concluded that bleeding had occurred into a pineal cyst, producing so-called pineal apoplexy.

An adolescent with a pineoblastoma has been described as presenting with what has been termed neurogenic, or essential, hypernatremia (119). This electolyte disturbance is characterized by sustained, but fluctuating, hypernatremia; failure of a fluid load to correct the elevated sodium concentration; normal glomerular filtration rate and blood urea nitrogen; absence of thirst or clinical dehydration; impaired antidiuretic hormone (ADH) response to osmotic stimuli, but normal ADH response to volume stimuli, and correction of hypernatremia with exogenous ADH. The electrolyte disturbance apparently is secondary to an elevated osmotic threshold for ADH release.

Of 32 cases of proven pineal tumor, radiologically demonstrable cacification was observed in 75% (120). When such calcification was studied by means of transmission electron microscopy, electron diffraction, and electron-induced x-ray fluorescence, it was found to be composed predominantly of amorphous calcium phosphate (121). This composition differs from that present in pineal calcospherulites, the latter being comprised mainly of crystalline hydroxyapatite (see the earlier section on Calcification).

Teratoma of the pineal has been reported to occur in two brothers, 2 years apart in age, at the respective ages of 13 and 17 years (122). This was the first reported familial occurrence of this type of tumor. Ill-defined intrauterine factors were implicated in the pathogenesis of these tumors.

Another rarity was reported in the case of a rapidly fatal rhabdomyosarcoma developing in a pineal teratoma of an adolescent (123).

Endodermal Sinus Tumors and Tumor Markers

Endodermal sinus tumors represent a selective overgrowth of yolk sac endoderm associated with extraembryonic mesoblast. These rare tumors are usually found in the gonads of young children (124–126). Other reported locations have been the mediastinum (127), the cervix and vagina (128), and the sacrococcygeal region (129). In the ninth report (130) of this tumor, it was found in the region of the pineal in a 12-year-old male. Histologic examination of the tumor revealed it to conform to similar, previously described tumors of the ovaries and testes (131). It was suggested that a disturbance in the region of the primitive streak could account for the exclusive midline location of this tumor in extragonadal sites.

In two other reports (132,133) of endodermal sinus tumors of the pineal in three adolescents, aged 14, 13, and 15 years, respectively, two of the patients were males. It was pointed out that the preponderance of this rare neoplasm is in young males, usually in their second decade, and that the diagnosis is usually established within 3 months of the onset of nonspecific symptoms of an intracranial mass. Most patients have died within 2 years of discovery, some with widespread intradural metastases (133).

Another instance, occurring in a 19-year-old female, provided the first electron microscopic study (134) of pineal endodermal sinus tumor. Tumor cells were seen to form glandlike structures lined by microvilli; tight junctions were observed between adjacent cells. Characteristic was a basement membranelike material in the intercellular spaces as well as within the endoplasmic reticulum of tumor cells. Also of note in this report was the finding of alphafetoprotein in the CSF, as measured by radioimmunoassay, and in the tumor, as measured by immunohistochemical techniques. Similarly, alphafetoprotein was detected in the CSF and serum of a 12-year-old female with this type of tumor (135). In this instance, the level of alphafetoprotein decreased after radiation treatment of the tumor, only to rise again prior to detectable tumor recurrence; the alphafetoprotein was, therefore, used as a tumor marker.

Because of the inaccessibility of the pineal, not only alphafetoprotein but other tumor markers as well have been sought. In the case of a 37-year-old male with a pineocytoma, tumor levels of HIOMT were five to seven times lower than normal, and serum melatonin levels were elevated fivefold during the day as compared to controls, but retained a circadian rhythmicity (136). However, this rhythmicity showed a reduced amplitude between the hours of 02:00 and 14:00 and an exaggerated amplitude between 14:00 and 24:00 hours; in addition to the daytime levels, during the remainder of the 24 hours the serum melatonin concentrations were also elevated when compared with controls. Because of the elevated daytime levels of melatonin, it was suggested that measurement of melatonin could be used as a pineal-tumor marker by obtaining midday serum samples. Despite several hypotheses, the low tumor HIOMT concentrations, in conjunction with elevated serum melatonin levels, were not satisfactorily taken into account. Two other male patients, aged 15 and 43 years, with pineal tumors were also evaluated for melatonin as a tumor marker; plasma melatonin, measured every 4 hours, was undetectable in both (137). The value of melatonin as a marker for pineal tumors was questioned. A 17-year-old male with a pineal neoplasm having elements of endodermal sinus tumor and choriocarcinoma was evaluated by measurement of human chorionic gonadotropin (HCG) and alphafetoprotein in the tumor, CSF, and blood; both markers were present in all three (138).

The presence of rosette formation was found in 81% of a single-cell suspension of large and small lymphoid-appearing cells from a pineal germinoma (139). The rosette-forming population was exclusively small mononuclear cells. Fifteen percent of the single-cell suspension bore surface kappa light chain immunoglobulin, and 18% bore lambda chains. Cells bearing these immunoglobulins were also small-cell in type. Thus T- and B-lymphocyte membrane markers were found in the small cells of this tumor. Also of note was the finding of plasma cells in the tumor. Similar studies performed on a pineoblastoma and a pineocytoma were negative for T- and B-cell markers.

Germinomas

Germinomas appear to be the commonest type of pineal neoplasm (140). Germ cells originate in the yolk sac endoderm and migrate widely throughout the embryo, including the head, before localizing in the gonadal ridges (141–144). By using ultrastructural, enzyme-histochemical, and fluorescence-histochemical methods of 43 cases of intracranial germinomas and 12 cases of pinealoma, a significant similarity between intracranial germinomas (usually termed pinealomas with a two-cell population), seminomas, and dysgerminomas was observed (145). True pinealomas were classified as either pineoblastomas or pineocytomas on the basis of architectural differences mentioned earlier (109).

In another study (146) or 15 cases of suprasellar germinomas—so-called ectopic pinealomas—histologic similarity to extracerebral germinomas, particularly testicular seminomas, was observed. No evidence of true pineal histology could be found in these cases.

Thus, according to one scheme of differentiation (126), germ cells of the yolk sac can differentiate into germinomas (encompassing the designation seminoma and dysgerminoma) or tumors of totipotential cells. The latter can differentiate into embryonal carcinomas, and thence to either teratomas, endodermal sinus tumors, or choriocarcinomas.

Unusual manifestations of pineal germinomas have included basal ganglia metastases, producing extrapyramidal dysfunction in a 12-year-old male (147); metastases to the posterior abdominal wall in a 17-year-old male, the metastases postulated to have occurred via direct extension through lumbar foramina from previously documented spinal metastases (148); and metastases to the lungs (149). This last report pointed out that primary intracranial tumors rarely metastasize outside the central nervous system in the absence of surgical manipulation (150).

PRECOCIOUS PUBERTY

The concomitant occurrence of pineal tumors and precocious puberty was first reported at the end of the last century (151,152). The association of these two conditions was confirmed in a study (153) performed some 55 years later. A review of such cases revealed that precocious puberty had been associated with nonparenchymatous pineal lesions, such as gliomas and teratomas, which were thought to be purely destructive, whereas depressed gonadal function had been associated with true pinealomas (154). The implications was that the pineal produced an antigonadotropic substance which could be secreted in excess from pinealomas, whereas this substance was rendered ineffectual by destructive lesions of the gland. However, recent reports (155–157) appear to have clarified this situation; ectopic secretion of HCG from pineal tumors has been incriminated as being primarily responsible for the associated precocious puberty, the biologic action of HCG being virtually equivalent to that of LH (158).

In the case of a 3-year-old male with precocious puberty, a choriocarcinoma of the pineal was demonstrated, immunohistochemically, to contain HCG, but not FSH or LH (155). In the discussion of this case, it was pointed out that Leydig cells are visible in the fetal testes after 8 months of gestation but disappear by the age of 3 years (159). When the child reaches approximately the age of 12 years, Leydig cells again appear in the testes and sexual development ensues as the result of increased gonadotropin secretion. Thus it was postulated that, in the case in point, the tumor must have been present in the pineal prior to birth, continuously secreting HCG, the Leydig cells then remaining in the testes from their first normal appearance until the age of 3 years, when the tumor was discovered. Dependence of Leydig cells on LH was demonstrated in this report by the immunohistochemical localization of endogenous LH, as well as exogenous HCG, in immature Leydig cells of an adult. Apparently, it is the immature Leydig cell that has the capacity to synthesize testosterone; mature Leydig cells have been described as not having this function (160). This concept was supported by the demonstration in this study (155) of endogenous LH localization in only a few mature Leydig cells.

Another report (156) described a 6-year, 9-month-old male who presented with polydipsia, lowered voice pitch, pubic hair, and penile enlargement without testicular enlargement. Serum HCG and its beta subunit, LH [which cross-reacts with HCG in most clinical assays (158)], and testosterone were elevated. The tumor contained HCG and beta-HCG activity.

High plasma HCG and testosterone levels were also demonstrated in the case of a $5^1/_2$-year-old male with a pineal tumor and precocious puberty (157). This patient's presentation was unusual, in that he also had enlarged testes. The testicular growth was hypothesized to be secondary to seminferous-tubule enlargement resulting from increased intratesticular testosterone production (161). The report stressed that, whereas pineal neoplasms occur in both sexes, sexual precocity has been virtually limited to males (153). It was suggested that this sex predominance could be explained if the sexual precocity produced by these tumors was incomplete, secondary to the secretion of HCG. Because ovarian follicular development depends on both FSH and LH (162), HCG, having essentially an LH-like action, would not be expected to cause female sexual precocity. This is substantiated by the literature; if one includes not only pineal neoplasms, but even so-called ectopic pinealomas, HCG-secreting tumors generally have not resulted in precocious puberty in afflicted females (163,164); one case of ectopic pinealoma with a two-cell population should be mentioned, however (165). In this case, a 5-year-old female presented with evidence of an intracranial mass and breast enlargement; a germinoma was located in the suprasellar region. Endocrine studies revealed a high plasma HCG and HCG beta subunit, a slightly elevated FSH, and nondetectable levels of estradiol. Additionally, tumor content of HCG was elevated, but FSH was not detectable. As breast tissue is so sensitive to estrogens (166)—even the minute amounts contained in cosmetics being capable of producing precocious breast enlargement—the undetectable estradiol here may simply have reflected the limit of assay sensitivity. Because the germinoma in this case was located in such a site as to be able to directly affect gonadotropin secretion, the relationship, if any, of the premature thelarche to the elevated tumor and serum levels of HCG remains speculative.

A syndrome comprising unusual facies, dental precocity and dysplasia, thickened nails, acanthosis nigricans, abdominal protuberance, insulin-resistant diabetes mellitus, hirsutism, and phallic enlargement was first described in three siblings more than 30 years ago (167). All three siblings died of their diabetes mellitus, autopsy revealing, among other things, pineal hyperplasia (168). This syndrome was subsequently considered to be a familial endrocrinopathy involving the pineal (169). More recently, two other siblings with this syndrome were described; one died, autopsy revealing pineal hyperplasia (170). Despite some intensive study of the mechanism of insulin resistance (171), apparently no investigation of the role of the pineal in this syndrome has been carried out.

Miscellaneous Tumors

In what was apparently the first such case to be reported, a cranio-pharyngioma of the pineal was an incidental autopsy finding in a 58-year-old female (172). As mentioned in this report, craniopharyngiomas are considered to be derived from Rathke pouch remnants, their location having been described in the hypothalamus, pituitary, nasopharynx (173), and third ventricle (174). It was postulated that multipotential pineal cells gave rise to the tumor in this unique location (172).

An embryonic carcinosarcoma of the pineal has been described in an 8-year-old male (175). Initially, the child has evidence of increased intracranial pressure and an early degree of genital development; no endocrine studies were performed.

A histologically classic primary glioblastoma multiforme (malignant astrocytoma) of the pineal was found at operation in a 68-year-old female who presented with Parinaud's syndrome, difficulty in walking, and dementia (176). The ability of pineal tumors to differentiate toward astrocytic cell lines has already been mentioned (109).

Several recent instances olf meningioma of the pineal region have been reported (177,178). Although such tumors are usually thought to arise from the junction of the falx and tentorium (179) or the velum interpositum (180), the suggestion has been made that the primary site of origin could be the connective tissue stroma of the pineal, which originates from the pia-arachnoid (181). This latter hypothesis was based on the finding of a total absence of identifiable pineal tissue at autopsy in three such cases (182). In the first report (177), there was also no identifiable pineal tissue in either of two patients.

Almost total replacement of the pineal by sarcoidosis was observed in a 13-year-old male who was determined to have obstructive hydrocephalus (183). No other evidence of organ involvement by sarcoidosis was detected at the time of admission or a year following operation. This appears to be the first record of such a case.

Treatment

There have been several different approaches to the treatment of pineal tumors. In one of these, the tumor would be localized by ventriculography, following which a ventriculoperitoneal or ventriculoatrial shunt would be created if there was significantly elevated intracranial pressure. Radiotherapy would then be given empirically and, subsequently, a repeat ventriculogram would be performed to determine whether there had been shrinkage of the tumor. Approximately 70% of pineal tumors are radiosensitive (184,185), and approximately 50% of patients receiving radiotherapy survive for 5–30 years (184,186,187). However, as this leaves approximately 30% of pineal tumors that are radioresistant, a direct surgical approach has been advocated (188–190). This philosophy is especially cogent when one realizes that, without a histologic diagnosis, it is not possible to predict the result of radiation therapy. As there are now microsurgical techniques for pineal tumor extirpation (191,192), it would appear that the empiric use of radiotherapy is no longer acceptable (193). Utilizing a standard procedure, such as the transcallosal Brunner-Dandy approach (194,195), the tumor could be biopsied and then partial or total removal accomplished, depending on the extent and type of tumor.

With the advent of CT scanning and stereotaxic biopsy (196,197), a new diagnostic approach has emerged (197). Tumor presence is looked for with a CT scan. If intracranial hypertension is marked, a shunt is created. Stereotaxic neuroradiology is then used to obtain superimposable roentgenograms of the cerebral vasculature, cisterns, and ventricles; at this time, a stereotaxic biopsy is obtained. Biopsied tissue is examined by smear preparations, frozen sections, and later by stained paraffin sections. The benefit of stereotaxic biopsy is that it frequently spares the patient having to undergo surgical exploration. Sequelae to stereotaxic biopsy have included transient meningismus, attributed to subarachnoid bleeding, and Parinaud's syndrome from peritumoral bleeding (197).

Once the type of tumor is established, and the extent of surgery defined, the problem arises as to what further therapy is required. Reports of results of radiation therapy are often difficult to evaluate, as pretreatment tissue diagnosis has frequently been lacking (198–204). The percentage of such cases in these series has varied from 45 to 100%. The diagnosis of pineal tumor, or pineal-region tumor, in those patients not having a tissue diagnosis was presumptively made by such findings as symptoms of increased intracranial pressure, Parinaud's syndrome, ataxia, cerebellar nystagmus, spasticity, and decreased hearing, as well as by the use of pneumoencephalography, ventriculography, and CT scanning.

In any event, there would appear to be a general consensus that pineal germinomas are radiosensitive and do well with this form of therapy (205,206). Conversely, pineal teratomas, teratoblastomas, teratocarcinomas, choriocarcinomas, and glial tumors are radioresistant (206), as are embryonal carcinomas (206,207), whereas in some instances, pineoblastomas and pineocytomas appear to have responded well to radiotherapy (208,209). However, others have found pineoblastomas to be insensitive to such treatment (206). Responses to radiation therapy can be followed by CT scanning and stereotaxic ventriculography (197). The latter provides radiographs that can be exactly superimposed on the initial stereotaxic studies, allowing assessment not only of change in tumor size but also of the patency of the aqueduct of Sylvius.

One of the unsettled problems in radiotherapy is whether to give prophylactic radiation to the entire craniospinal axis in cases of germinoma. The incidence of meningeal seeding can approach 60% with malignant pineal tumors, germinomas having the greatest tendency to seed (210). In one series (201), of the patients developing spinal cord metastases, none had received prophylactic spinal irradiation. Nevertheless, another review (211) found no evidence of spinal seeding in 19 patients seen over a 25-year span. It was recommended that CSF cytologic examination be performed following cranial radiation, as a screening procedure for meningeal seeding. However, another study (210) found tumor cells in the CSF in only 3 of 12 patients with proven meningeal metastases. Periodic myelography and/or body CT scanning, plus periodic CSF cytologic examination, have been suggested as alternatives to prophylactic spinal radiation (207). Reporting a probability of spinal metastases of less than 10% following adequate primary therapy, one review (202) did not recommend the routine use of prophylactic spinal radiation. A more definitive set of guidelines for germinomas, contained in a recent review (206) of 110 pineal tumors, suggested that, when the tumor is suspected by clinical evidence or CT scan to have extensively invaded the periventricular region, or the patient manifests meningismus or cranial nerve signs in addition to symptoms of pineal tumor, or when a direct operation has been performed prior to primary-tumor-area irradiation, prophylactic radiation of the entire spinal axis, as well as the whole brain, is in order. This report also suggested that a larger radiation field with a larger radiation dose for the primary lesion might prevent spinal metastases.

As regards decisions about surgery for various pineal tumors, it has been suggested that even stereotaxic biopsy prior to radiotherapy is unnecessary with germinomas, as diagnosis can be made by CSF cytology and CT scan (206). However, the value of such cytology has already been adversely commented on (210). Stereotaxic biopsy would appear to put the patient at the least risk, yet provide histologic confirmation of tumor type (197). For radioresistant tumors, the recommendation has been made that, prior to operation, radiation be delivered to the tumor site to reduce vascularity. At surgery, as much tumor as possible should be removed. Postoperatively, chemotherapy and radiotherapy should be used, followed by maintenance chemotherapy and immunotherapy (206). Postoperative radiation was also recommended by other investigators (207). In the latter instance, this modality was used whether or not complete surgical excision of the tumor had been accomplished.

Although tumors of the pineal that are of glial origin would appear, like glial tumors elsewhere in the CNS, to be unresponsive to chemotherapy (207), this is not the case with all pineal tumors. Thus it is not surprising that pineal germinomas, being histologically identical to testicular seminomas, have been reported to respond to such combination chemotherapy as bleomycin, cis-platinum, and vinblastine (207,212). Pulmonary metastases from a pineal germinoma have been reported to regress with the use of chlorambucil, dactinomycin, and methotrexate (213). Another study (214) noted a significant decrease in a histologically undiagnosed pineal-region tumor (presumed to be a germinoma) with the combination of bleomycin, daunorubicin, and vincristine. The ability of certain pineal tumors to respond to chemotherapy may be a function not only of the cell type involved but also of the absence of a blood-brain barrier in the pineal (215).

Not all reports regarding chemotherapy of pineal tumors have been encouraging, however; the use of bleomycin was unsuccessful in the case of an embryonal carcinoma of the pineal with spinal and extraneural metastases (216). As embryonal testicular carcinomas are highly sensitive to bleomycin plus cis-platinum and vinblastine (207), perhaps this combination would have yielded better results than bleomycin alone in the preceding case.

To keep this topic in perspective, it should be realized that pineal tumors have been found to comprise only 0.4–1% of all intracranial tumors in Europe and the United States (193,217–219). In Japan, however, for reasons that are not understood, these tumors represent 8–9% of all intracranial space-occupying lesions (220,221).

STRESS

Investigating the effects of stress, produced by pneumoencephalography, on blood melatonin levels in six patients, no significant elevation of melatonin levels was observed (222). The lower levels of melatonin at the conclusion of pneumoencephalography (i.e., 11:00 hours), along with a negative correlation with blood cortisol levels at that time, were postulated to be the result of a fall in melatonin due to diurnal variation, coincident with a rise in cortisol secondary to the stress of pneumoencephalography.

The relationship between stress and the pineal was studied in postmortem pineal glands from 20 men, aged 40–74 years, who apparently had died as a result of either bleeding or perforated peptic ulcers (223). Numerous glial plates, cavities, and acervuli were observed in the pineals. These morphologic alterations were interpreted as indicating pineal involution. If, as these findings would suggest, pineal function is, in fact, decreased in advanced peptic ulcer disease, the question arises as to whether this is cause or effect.

REFERENCES

1. Wurtman R J, Axelrod J, Barchas J D. Age and enzyme activity in the human pineal. J Clin Endocrinol Metab 24:299–301, 1964.
2. Tapp E, Huxley M. The histological appearance of the human pineal gland from puberty to old age. J Pathol 108:137–144, 1972.
3. Wurtman R J. The pineal gland. pp 117–132 in Endocrine Pathology. Williams & Wilkins, Baltimore, 1968.
4. Heidel G von. Die Haufigkeit des Vorkommens von Kalkkonkrementem im Corpus pineale des Kindes. Anat Anz 116:139–154, 1965.
5. Tapp E, Huxley M. The weight and degree of calcification of the pineal gland. J Pathol 105:31–39, 1971.
6. Lukaszyk A, Reiter R J. Histophysiological evidence for the secretion of polypeptides by the pineal gland. Am J Anat 143:451–464, 1975.
7. Tapp E. The histology and pathology of the human pineal gland. Prog Brain Res 52:481–499, 1979.
8. Mabie C P, Wallace B M. Optical physical and chemical properties of pineal gland calcifications. Cell Tissue Res 16:59–71, 1974.

9. Krstić R. A combined scanning and transmission electron microscopic study and electron probe microanalysis of human pineal acervuli. Cell Tissue Res 174:129–137, 1976.

10. Michotte Y, Lowenthal A, Knaepen L, Collard M, Massart D L. A morphological and chemical study of calcification of the pineal gland. J Neurol 215:209–219, 1977.

11. Krstić R, Golaz J. Ultrastructural and x-ray microprobe comparison of gerbil and human pineal acervuli. Experientia. 33:507–508, 1977.

12. Ostrowski K, Dziedzic-Goclawska A, Michalik J, Stachowicz W. Calcif Tissue Int 30:179–182, 1980.

13. Daramola G F, Olowu A O. Physiological and radiological implications of a low incidence of pineal calcification in Nigeria. Neuroendocrinology 9:41–57, 1972.

14. Adelove A, Felson B. Incidence of normal pineal gland calcification in skull roentgenograms of black and white Americans. Am J Roentgenol Radium Ther Nucl Med 122:503–506, 1974.

15. Hinterberger H, Pickering J. Catecholamine, indolealkylamine and calcium levels of human pineal glands in various clinical conditions. Pathology 8:221–229, 1976.

16. Pavel S, Dorcescu M, Petrescu-Holban R, Ghinea E. Biosynthesis of a vasotocinlike peptide in cell cultures from pineal glands of human fetuses. Science 181:1252–1253, 1973.

17. Reinharz A C, Vallotton M B. Presence of two neurophysins in the human pineal gland. Endocrinology 100:994–1001, 1977.

18. Uttenthal L O, Hope D B. The isolation of three neurophysins from porcine posterior pituitary lobes. Biochem J 116:899–909, 1970.

19. Pavel S, Goldstein R. Further evidence that melatonin represents the releasing hormone for pineal vasotocin. J Endocrinol 82:1–6, 1979.

20. Pavel S, Goldstein R, Popoviciu L, Corfariu O, Földes A, Farkas E. Pineal vasotocin: REM sleep dependent release into cerebrospinal fluid of man. Waking Sleeping 3:347–352, 1979.

21. Hăulică I, Ianovici I, Rosca V, Ionescu G. Presence of isorenin in human pineal gland. Rev Roum Med Endocrinol 17:277–279, 1979.

22. Lerner A B. Hormones in the pineal other than melatonin. J Neural Transm (Suppl) 13:131–133, 1978.

23. Coculescu M, Oprescu M, Zagrean L. Angiotensin I-like immunoreactive substance in pineal gland of normal and Brattleboro rats with hereditary diabetes insipidus. Rev Roum Morphol Embryol Physiol 14:47–51, 1977.

24. Rudman D, Del Rio A E, Hollins B M, Houser D H, Keeling M E, Sutin J, Scott J W, Sears R A, Rosenberg M Z. Melantropic-lipolytic peptides in various regions of bovine, simian and human brains and in simian and human cerebrospinal fluid. Endocrinology 92:372–379, 1973.

25. Blask D E, Vaughan M K, Reiter R J, Johnson L Y, Vaughan G M. Prolactin-releasing and release-inhibiting factor activities in the bovine, rat and human pineal gland: in vitro and in vivo studies. Endocrinology 99:152–162, 1976.

26. Matthews M J, Benson B, Rodin A E. Antigonadotropic activity in a melatonin-free extract of human pineal glands. Life Sci 10:1375–1379, 1971.

27. Lerner A B, Case J D. Melatonin. Fed Proc 19:590–592, 1960.

28. Anton-Tay F, Diaz J L, Fernandez-Guardiola A. On the effect of melatonin upon human brain: its possible therapeutic implications. In The Pineal Gland, ed G E W Wolstenholme, J Knight. Churchill Livingstone, Edinburgh, 1971, pp 363–364.

29. Otani T, Creaven P J, Farrell G, McIsaac W M. Studies on the biosynthesis of 5-methoxytryptophol in the pineal. Biochim Biophys Acta 184:184–190, 1969.

30. Mullen P E, Leone R M, Hooper J, Smith I, Silman R E, Finnie M, Carter S, Linsell C. Pineal 5-methoxytryptophol in man. Psychoneuroendocrinology 2:117–126, 1979.

31. Hooper R J L, Silman R E, Leone R M, Finnie M D A, Carter S J, Grudzinskas J G, Gordon Y B, Holland D T, Chard T, Mullen P E, Smith I. Changes in the concentration

of 5-methoxytryptophol in the circulation at different phases of the human menstrual cycle. J Endocrinol 82:269–274, 1979.

32. Bosin T R, Beck O. 5-methoxytryptamine in the human pineal gland: identification and quantitation by mass fragmentography. J Neurochem 32:1853–1855, 1979.

33. Guchhait R B. Biogenesis of 5-methoxy-N, N-dimethyltryptamine in human pineal gland. J Neurochem 26:187–190, 1976.

34. Lehrer S. Possible pineal-suprachiasmatic clock regulation of development and life span. Arch Ophthalmol 97:359, 1979.

35. Lehrer S. Pineal effect on longevity. J Chronic Dis 32:411–412, 1979.

36. Denckla W D. A time to die. Life Sci 16:31–44, 1975.

37. Binkley S. Pineal gland biorhythms: N-acetyltransferase in chickens and rats. Fed Proc 35:2347–2352, 1976.

38. Rogot E, Goldberg I D, Goldstein H. Survivorship and causes of death among the blind. J Chronic Dis 19:179–197, 1966.

39. Lynch H J, Wurtman R J, Moskowitz M A, Archer M C, Ho M H. Daily rhythm in human urinary melatonin. Science 187:169–171, 1975.

40. Lynch H J, Ozaki Y, Shakal D, Wurtman R J. Melatonin excretion of man and rats: effect of time of day, sleep, pinealectomy and food consumption. Int J Biometeorol 19:267–279, 1975.

41. Vaughan G M, Pelham R W, Pang S F, Loughlin L L, Wilson K M, Sandock K L, Vaughan M K, Koslow S H, Reiter R J. Nocturnal elevation of plasma melatonin and urinary 5-hydroxyindoleacetic acid in young men: attempts at modification by brief changes in environmental lighting and sleep and by autonomic drugs. J Clin Endocrinol Metab 42:752–764, 1976.

42. Greiner A C, Chan S C. Melatonin content of the human pineal gland. Science 199:83–84, 1978.

43. Smith J A, Mee T J X, Barnes N D, Thorburn R J, Barnes J L C. Melatonin in serum and cerebrospinal fluid. Lancet 2:425, 1976.

44. Arendt J, Wetterberg L, Heyden T, Sizonenko P C, Paunier L. Radioimmunoassay of melatonin: human serum and cerebrospinal fluid. Horm Res 8:65–75, 1977.

45. Smith J A, Padwick D, Mee T J X, Minneman K P, Bird E D. Synchronous nyctohemeral rhythms in human blood melatonin and in human post-mortem pineal enzyme. Clin Endocrinol 6:219–225, 1977.

46. Lynch H J, Jimerson D C, Ozaki Y, Post R M, Bunney W E Jr, Wurtman R J. Entrainment of rhythmic melatonin secretion in man to a 12-hour phase shift in the light/dark cycle. Life Sci 23:1557–1564, 1978.

47. Vaughan G M, Allen J P, Tullis W, Siler-Khodr T M, de la Pena A, Sackman J W. Overnight plasma profiles of melatonin and certain adenohypophyseal hormones in men. J Clin Endocrinol Metab 47:566–571, 1978.

48. Wetterberg L, Halberg F, Tarquini B, Cagnoni M, Haus E, Griffith K, Kawasaki T, Wallach L A, Ueno M, Uezo K, Matsuoka M, Kuzel M, Halberg E, Omae T. Circadian variation in urinary melatonin in clinically healthy women in Japan and the United States of America. Experientia 35:416–419, 1979.

49. Lewy A J, Wehr T A, Goodwin F K. Light suppresses melatonin secretion in humans. Science 210:1267–1269, 1980.

50. Minneman K P, Lynch H, Wurtman R J. Relationship between environmental light intensity and retina-mediated suppression of rat pineal serotonin-N-acetyltransferase. Life Sci 15:1791–1796, 1974.

51. Weinberg U, D'Eletto R D, Weitzman E D, Erlich S, Hollander C S. Circulating melatonin in man: episodic secretion throughout the light-dark cycle. J Clin Endocrinol Metab 48:114–118, 1979.

52. Illnerova H, Backström M, Sääf J, Wetterberg L, Vangbo B. Melatonin in rat pineal gland and serum; rapid parallel decline after light exposure at night. Neurosci Lett 9:189–193, 1978.

53. Rollag M D, Morgan R J, Niswender G D. Route of melatonin secretion in sheep. Endocrinology 102:1–8, 1978.

54. Vaughan G M, Bell R, de la Pena A. Nocturnal plasma melatonin in humans: episodic pattern and influence of light. Neurosci Lett 14:81–84, 1979.

55. Arendt J, Wirz-Justice A, Bradtke J. Annual rhythm of serum melatonin in man. Neurosci Lett 7:327–330, 1977.

56. Fèvre-Montange M, Van Cauter E, Refetoff S, Désir D, Tourniaire J, Copinschi G. Effects of "jet lag" on hormonal patterns. II. Adaptation of melatonin circadian periodicity. J Clin Endocrinol Metab 52:642–649, 1981.

57. Raikhlin N T, Kvetnoy I M, Tolkachev V N. Melatonin may be synthesised in enterochromaffin cells. Nature 255:344–345, 1975.

58. Raikhlin N T, Kvetnoy I M. Melatonin and enterochromaffine cells. Acta Histochem (Jena) 55:19–24, 1976.

59. Wetterberg L, Arendt J, Paunier L, Sizonenko P C, van Donselaar W, Heyden T. Human serum melatonin changes during the menstrual cycle. J Clin Endocrinol Metab 42:185–188, 1976.

60. Dewan E M, Menkin M F, Rock J. Effect of photic stimulation on the human menstrual cycle. Photochem Photobiol 27:581–585, 1978.

61. Fevre M, Segel T, Marks J F, Boyar R M. LH and melatonin secretion patterns in pubertal boys. J Clin Endocrinol Metab 47:1383–1386, 1978.

62. Boyar R M, Perlow M, Hellman L, Kapen S, Weitzman E. Twenty-four hour pattern of luteinizing hormone secretion in normal men with sleep stage recording. J Clin Endocrinol Metab 35:73–81, 1972.

63. Silman R E, Leone R M, Hooper R J L. Melatonin, the pineal gland and human puberty. Nature 282:301–303, 1979.

64. Jimerson D C, Lynch H J, Post R M, Wurtman R J, Bunney W E Jr. Urinary melatonin rhythms during sleep deprivation in depressed patients and normals. Life Sci 20:1501–1508, 1977.

65. Kastin A J, Viosca S, Nair R M G, Schally A V, Miller M C. Interactions between pineal hypothalamus and pituitary involving melatonin, MSH release-inhibiting factor and MSH. Endocrinology 91:1323–1328, 1972.

66. Kastin A J, Miller M C, Ferrel L, Schally A V. General activity in intact and hypophysectomized rats after administration of MSH, melatonin, and Pro-Leu-Gly-NH₂. Physiol Behav 10:399–401, 1973.

67. Ehrensing R H, Kastin A J. Melanocyte-stimulating hormone-release-inhibitory hormone as an antidepressant. Arch Gen Psychiatry 30:63–65, 1974.

68. Carmen J S, Post R M, Buswell R, Goodwin F K. Negative effects of melatonin on depression. Am J Psychiatry 133:1181–1186, 1976.

69. Post R M, Goodwin F K. Effects of amitriptyline and imipramine on amine metabolites in CSF of depressed patients. Arch Gen Psychiatry 30:234–239, 1974.

70. Hartley R, Smith J A. The activation of pineal hydroxyindole-O-methyltransferase by psychotomimetic drugs. J Pharm Pharmacol 25:751–752, 1973.

71. Backström M, Wetterberg L. Increased N-acetyl serotonin and melatonin formation induced by d-amphetamine in rat pineal gland organ culture via β-adrenergic receptor mechanism. Acta Physiol Scand 87:113–120, 1973.

72. Holtz R W, Deguchi T, Axelrod J. Stimulation of serotonin N-acetyltransferase in pineal organ culture by drugs. J Neurochem 22:205–209, 1974.

73. Lynch H J, Wang P, Wurtman R J. Increase in rat pineal melatonin content following L-dopa administration. Life Sci 12:145–151, 1973.

74. Hartley R, Padwick D, Smith J A. The inhibition of pineal hydroxyindole-O-methyltransferase by haloperidol and fluphenazine. J Pharm Pharmacol 24 (Suppl):100–103, 1972.

75. Deguchi T, Axelrod J. Induction and superinduction of serotonin N-acetyltransferase by adrenergic drugs and denervation in the rat pineal. Proc Natl Acad Sci USA 69:2208–2211, 1972.

76. Holmstedt B, Lindgren J E. Chemical constituents and pharmacology of South American snuffs. In Ethnopharmacologic Search for Psychoactive Drugs, ed D H Efron. US Public Health Service, Washington, 1967, pp 339–373.

77. De Montigny C, Aghajanian G K. Preferential action of 5-methoxytryptamine and 5-methyoxydimethyltryptamine on presynaptic serotonin receptors: a comparative iontophoretic study with LSD and serotonin. Neuropharmacology 16:811–818, 1977.

78. Koslow S H. The biochemical and biobehavioral profile of 5-methoxytryptamine. In Trace Amines and the Brain, ed E Usdin, M Sandler. Dekker, New York, 1976, pp 103–130.

79. Narasimhachari N, Baumann P, Pak H S, Carpenter W T, Zocchi A F, Hokanson L, Fujimori M, Himwich H E. Gas chromatographic-mass spectrometric identification of urinary bufotenin and dimethyltryptamine in drug-free chronic schizophrenic patients. Biol Psychiatry 8:203–305, 1974.

80. Mandel L R, Walker R W. Biosynthesis of 5-methoxy-N,N-dimethyltryptamine in vitro. Life Sci 15:1457–1463, 1974.

81. Narasimhachari N, Lin R L. A possible mechanism for the antischizophrenic action of chlorpromazine: inhibition of the formation of dimethyltryptamine by chlorpromazine metabolites. Res Commun Chem Pathol Pharmacol 8:341–351, 1974.

82. Altschule M D. Some effects of aqueous extracts of acetone-dried beef-pineal substance in chronic schizophrenia. N Engl J Med 257:919–922, 1957.

83. Narasimhachari N, Lin R L, Himwich H E. Inhibitor of indoleethylamide N-methyltransferase in pineal extract. Res Commun Chem Pathol Pharmacol 9:375–378, 1974.

84. Nir I, Hirschmann N, Sulman F G. Inhibition of pineal HIOMT by pyridoxal-5'-phosphate. Biochem Pharmacol 25:581–583, 1976.

85. Gey K F, Georgi H. Effect of neurotropic agents on total pyridoxal phosphate and on the activity of the decarboxylase of aromatic amino acids as well as of other pyridoxal phosphate-dependent enzymes in rat brain. J Neurochem 23:725–738, 1974.

86. Smith J A, Barnes J L, Mee T J. The effect of neuroleptic drugs on serum and cerebrospinal fluid melatonin concentrations in psychiatric subjects. J Pharm Pharmacol 31:246–248, 1979.

87. McIsaac W M, Khairallah P A, Page I H. 10-methoxyharmalan, a potent serotonin antagonist which affects conditioned behavior. Science 134:674–675, 1961.

88. Greiner A C. Schizophrenia and the pineal gland. Can Psychiatr Assoc J 15:433–447, 1970.

89. Hartley R, Smith J A. Formation in vitro of N-acetyl-3, 4-dimethoxyphenethylamine by pineal hydroxyindole-O-methyltransferase. Biochem Pharmacol 22:2425–2428, 1973.

90. Wurtman R J, Axelrod J, Anton-Tay F. Inhibition of the metabolism of H^3-melatonin by phenothiazines. J Pharmacol Exp Ther 161:367–372, 1968.

91. Horrobin D F. Schizophrenia: reconciliation of the dopamine, prostaglandin, and opioid concepts and the role of the pineal. Lancet 1:529–531, 1979.

92. Bigelow L B. Some effects of aqueous pineal extract administration on schizophrenia symptoms. In Frontiers of Pineal Physiology, ed M D Altschule. MIT Press, Cambridge, Mass., and London, 1975, pp 225–263.

93. Reiss M. Inhibitory substances in body fluids of morons and mongols. Their possible significance in mental retardation. International Copenhagen Congress of the Scientific Study of Mental Retardation, 1964, pp 808–811.

94. Nordlund J J, Lerner A B. The effects of oral melatonin on skin color and on the release of pituitary hormones. J Clin Endocrinol Metab 45:768–774, 1977.

95. McCord C P, Allen F P. Evidences associating pineal gland function with alterations in pigmentation. J Exp Zool 23:207–224, 1917.

96. Lerner A B, Case J D, Takahashi Y, Lee T H, Mori W. Isolation of melatonin, the pineal gland factor that lightens melanocytes. J Am Chem Soc 80:2587, 1958.

97. Rust C C, Meyer R K. Hair color, molt, and testis size in male, short-tailed weasels treated with melatonin. Science 165:921–922, 1969.

98. Hasegawa A, Mori W. Morphometry of the human pineal gland: relationship to the adrenal cortex. Acta Pathol Jap 30:407–410, 1980.

99. White W F, Hedlund M T, Weber G F, Rippel R H, Johnson E S, Wilber J F. The pineal gland: a supplemental source of hypothalamic-releasing hormones. Endocrinology 94:1422–1426, 1974.

100. Tsang D, Lal S, Finlayson M H. Effect of TRH on cyclic AMP formation in human pineal gland homogenates. Brain Res 188:278–281, 1980.

101. Axelrod J. The pineal gland: a neurochemical transducer. Science 184:1341–1348, 1974.

102. Rodin A E, Overall J. Statistical relationships of weight of the human pineal to age and malignancy. Cancer 20:1203–1214, 1967.

103. Tapp E, Blumfield M. The weight of the pineal gland in malignancy. Br J Cancer 24:67–70, 1970.

104. Hajdu S I, Porro R S, Lieberman P H, Foote F W Jr. Degeneration of the pineal gland of patients with cancer. Cancer 29:706–709, 1972.

105. Tapp E. The human pineal gland in malignancy. J Neural Transm 48:119–129, 1980.

106. Starr K W. Growth and new growth, environmental carcinogens in the process of human ontogeny. Prog Clin Cancer 4:1–29, 1970.

107. Cohen M, Lippman M, Chabner B. Role of pineal gland in aetiology and treatment of breast cancer. Lancet 2:814–816, 1978.

108. Dooling E C, Chi J G, Gilles F H. Melanotic neuroectodermal tumor of infancy. Cancer 39:1535–1541, 1977.

109. Herrick M K, Rubinstein L J. The cytological differentiating potential of pineal parenchymal neoplasms (true pinealomas). Brain 102:289–320, 1979.

110. Tso M O M, Fine B S, Zimmerman L E, Vogel M H. Photoreceptor elements in retinoblastoma. Arch Ophthalmol 82:57–59, 1969.

111. Tso M O M, Zimmerman L E, Fine B S. The nature of retinoblastoma. I. Photoreceptor differentiation: a clinical and histopathologic study. Am J Ophthalmol 69:339–349, 1970.

112. Stefanko S Z, Manschot W A. Pinealoblastoma with retinoblastomatous differentiation. Brain 102:321–332, 1979.

113. Kline K T, Damjanov I, Katz S M, Schmidek H. Pineoblastoma: an electron microscopic study. Cancer 44:1692–1699, 1979.

114. Borit A, Blackwood W, Mair W G P. The separation of pineocytoma from pineoblastoma. Cancer 45:1408–1418, 1980.

115. Sano K. Pinealoma in children. Childs Brain 2:67–72, 1976.

116. Donat J F, Okazaki H, Gomez M R, Reagen T J, Baker H L Jr, Laws E R Jr. Pineal tumors. Arch Neurol 35:736–740, 1978.

117. Steinbok P, Dolman C L, Kaan K. Pineocytomas presenting as subarachnoid hemorrhage. J Neurosurg 47:776–780, 1977.

118. Higashi K, Katayama S, Orita T. Pineal apoplexy. J Neurol Neurosurg Psychiatry 42:1050–1053, 1979.

119. Khomami-Asadi F, Norman M E, Parks J S, Schwartz M W. Hypernatremia associated with pineal tumor. J Pediatr 90:605–606, 1977.

120. Lin S R, Crane M D, Lin Z S, Bilaniuk L, Plassche W M Jr, Marshall L, Spataro R F. Characteristics of calcification in tumors of the pineal gland. Radiology 126:721–726, 1978.

121. Møller M, Gjerris F, Hansen H J, Johnson E. Calcification in a pineal tumour studied by transmission electron microscopy, electron diffraction and x-ray microanalysis. Acta Neurol Scand 59:178–187, 1979.

122. Wakai S, Segawa H, Kitahara S, Asano T, Sano K, Ogihara R, Tomita S. Teratoma in the pineal region in two brothers. J Neurosurg 53:239–243, 1980.

123. Preissig S H, Smith M T, Huntington H W. Rhabdomyosarcoma arising in a pineal teratoma. Cancer 44:281–284, 1979.

124. Teilum G. Endodermal sinus tumors of the ovary and testis. Comparative morphogenesis of the so-called mesonephroma ovarii (Schiller) and extraembryonic (yolk sac-allantoic) structures of the rat's placenta. Cancer 12:1092–1105, 1959.

125. Huntington R W Jr, Morgenstern N L, Sargent J A, Giem R N, Richards A, Hanford K C. Germinal tumors exhibiting the endodermal sinus pattern of Teilum in young children. Cancer 16:34–47, 1963.

126. Teilum G. Classification of endodermal sinus tumor (mesoblastoma vitellinum) and so-called "embryonal carcinoma" of the ovary. Acta Pathol Microbiol Scand 64:407–429, 1965.

127. Teilmann I, Kassis H, Pietra G. Primary germ cell tumor of the anterior mediastinum with features of endodermal sinus tumor (mesoblastoma vitellinum). Acta Pathol Microbiol Scand 70:267–278, 1967.

128. Allyn D C, Silverberg S G, Salzberg Z M. Endodermal sinus tumor of the vagina. Report of a case with 7-year survival and literature review of so-called "mesonephromas." Cancer 27:1231–1238, 1971.

129. Thiele J, Castro S, Lee K D. Extragonadal endodermal sinus tumor (yolk sac tumor) of the pelvis. Cancer 27:391–396, 1971.

130. Prioleau G, Wilson C B. Endodermal sinus tumor of the pineal region. Cancer 38:2489–2493, 1976.

131. Teilum G. Special Tumors of Ovary and Testis, and Related Extragonadal Lesions. Lippincott, Philadelphia, 1971.

132. Ho K L, Rassekh Z S. Endodermal sinus tumor of the pineal region. Cancer 44:1081–1086, 1979.

133. Tavcar D, Robboy S J, Chapman P. Endodermal sinus tumor of the pineal region. Cancer 45:2646–2651, 1980.

134. Stachura I, Mendelow H. Endodermal sinus tumor originating in the region of the pineal gland. Cancer 45:2131–2137, 1980.

135. Arita N, Bitoh S, Ushio Y, Hayakawa T, Hasegawa H, Fujiwara M, Ozaki K, Par-Ken L, Mori T. Primary pineal endodermal sinus tumor with elevated serum and CSF alphafetoprotein levels. J Neurosurg 53:244–248, 1980.

136. Barber S G, Smith J A, Hughes R C. Melatonin as a tumour marker in a patient with pineal tumour. Br Med J 29:328, 1978.

137. Kennaway D J, McCulloch G, Matthews C D, Seamark R F. Plasma melatonin, luteinizing hormone, follicle-stimulating hormone, prolactin, and corticoids in two patients with pinealoma. J Clin Endocrinol Metab 49:144–145, 1979.

138. Haase J, Nielsen K. Value of tumor markers in the treatment of endodermal sinus tumors and choriocarcinomas in the pineal region. Neurosurgery 5:485–488, 1979.

139. Neuwelt E A, Smith R G. Presence of lymphocyte membrane surface markers on "small cells" in a pineal germinoma. Ann Neurol 6:133–136, 1979.

140. So S C, Ho J. Multiple primary germinomas (ectopic pinealoma) of the brain. Neurochirurgia (Stuttg) 23:147–150, 1980.

141. Askanazy M. Die Teratome nach ihrem Bau, ihrem Ban, ihrem Verlauf, ihrer Genese und in Vergleich zum experimentellen Teratoid. Verh Dtsch Ges Pathol 1:39–82, 1907.

142. Witschi E. Migration of the germ cells of human embryos from the yolk sac to the primitive gonadal folds. Contrib Embryol Carnegie Inst No. 209, 67–80, 1948.

143. Mintz B, Russell E S. Gene-induced embryological modifications of primordial germ cells in the mouse. J Exp Zool 134:207–237, 1957.

144. Mintz B. Formation and early development of germ cells. In Symposium on the Germ Cells and Earliest Stages of Development. Fondazione A. Baselli, Instituto Lombardo, Milan, 1961.

145. Koide O, Watanabe Y, Sato K. A pathological study of intracranial germinoma and pinealoma in Japan. Cancer 45:2119–2130, 1980.

146. Izquierdo J M, Rougerie J, Lapras C, Sanz F. The so-called ectopic pinealomas. Childs Brain 5:505–512, 1979.

147. Lins M M, McDonnell D E, Aschenbrener C A, Cancilla P A. Extrapyramidal disorder with pineal germinoma. J Neurosurg 48:108–116, 1978.

148. Rubery E D, Wheeler T K. Metastases outside the central nervous system from a presumed pineal germinoma. J Neurosurg 53:562–565, 1980.

149. Gindhart T D, Tsukahara Y C. Cytologic diagnosis of pineal germinoma in cerebrospinal fluid and sputum. Acta Cytol (Baltimore) 23:341–346, 1979.

150. Spriggs A I. Malignant cells in cerebrospinal fluid. J Clin Pathol 7:122–130, 1954.

151. Heubner O. Tumor der glandula pinealis. Dtsch Med Wochenschr 24:214–215, 1898.

152. Ogle C. A case of pineal tumour. Trans Pathol Soc Lond 1:4, 1899.

153. Kitay J I. Pineal lesions and precocious puberty: review. J Clin Endocrinol Metab 14:622–625, 1954.

154. Relkin R. Pineal effects on the reproductive system. In The Pineal. Eden Press, Montreal and Lancaster, England, 1976, pp 34–45.

155. Kurisaka M, Moriyasu N, Kitajima K. Immunohistochemical studies of brain tumors associated with precocious puberty: a preliminary report of correlation between tumor secreting hormone and Leydig cells in precocious puberty. Neurol Med Chir (Tokyo) 19:675–682, 1979.

156. Rosenberg D. Puberté précoce par tumeur pinéale sécrétant des gonadotrophines chorioniques. Ann Pediatr (Paris) 27:179–184, 1980.

157. Sklar C A, Conte F S, Kaplan S L, Grumbach M M. Human chorionic gonadotropin-secreting pineal tumor: relation to pathogenesis and sex limitation of sexual precocity. J Clin Endocrinol Metab 53:656–660, 1981.

158. Vaitukaitis J L. Ectopic hormonal syndromes. In Reproductive Endocrinology, ed S S C Yen, R B Jaffe. Saunders, Philadelphia, 1978, pp 388–397.

159. Gorski R A, Wagner J W. Gonadal activity and sexual differentiation of the hypothalamus. Endocrinology 76:226–239, 1965.

160. Zahor von Z, Raboch J. Ein Beitrag zum Problem der Hodenbiopsie bei Kryptorchismus unter besonderer Berucksichtigung des Optimalalters für die Orchidopexie. Schweiz Med Wochenschr 86:311–314, 1956.

161. Paulsen C A, Espeland D H, Michals E L. Effects of HCG, HMG, HLH and HGH administration on testicular function. In The Human Testis. Serono Foundation Symposium, ed E Rosenberg, C A Paulsen. Plenum, New York and London, 1970, pp 547–562.

162. Ross G T, Schreiber J R. The ovary. In Reproductive Endocrinology, ed S S C Yen, R B Jaffe. Saunders, Philadelphia, 1978, pp. 63–79.

163. Mori K, Iwayama K, Fujita Y. Malignant suprasellar teratoma in a girl with elevated serum gonadotropin. Case report and some considerations for development of precocious puberty. No Shinkei Geka 2:243–248, 1974.

164. Case records of the Massachusetts General Hospital (Case 38–1975). N Engl J Med 293:653–660, 1975.

165. Kubo O, Yamasaki N, Kamijo Y, Amano K, Kitamura K, Demura R. Human chorionic gonadotropin produced by ectopic pinealoma in a girl with precocious puberty. J Neurosurg 47:101–105, 1977.

166. Wilkins L, Bizzard R M, Migeon C J. Adolescent sexual development and its varia-
     tions. *In* The Diagnosis and Treatment of Endocrine Disorders in Childhood and
     Adolescence, 3 ed. Charles C Thomas, Springfield, Ill., 1965, pp 195–221.
167. Mendenhall E N. Tumor of the pineal body with high insulin resistance. J Indiana
     State Med Assoc 43:32–36, 1950.
168. Rabson S M, Mendenhall E N. Familial hypertrophy of pineal body, hyperplasia of
     adrenal cortex, and diabetes mellitus. Am J Clin Pathol 26:283–290, 1956.
169. Schimke R N. Familial tumor endocrinopathies. Birth Defects 7:55–65, 1971.
170. West R J, Lloyd K, Turner W M L. Familial insulin resistant diabetes, multiple somatic
     anomalies, and pineal hyperplasia. Arch Dis Child 50:703–708, 1975.
171. West R J, Leonard J V. Familial insulin resistance with pineal hyperplasia: metabolic
     studies and effect of hypophysectomy. Arch Dis Child 55:619–621, 1980.
172. Solarski A, Panke E S, Panke T W. Craniopharyngioma in the pineal gland. Arch
     Pathol Lab Med 102:490–491, 1971.
173. Prasad U, Kwi N K. Nasopharyngeal craniopharyngioma. J Laryngol Otol 89:445–452,
     1975.
174. Cashion E L, Young J M. Intraventricular cranipharyngioma: report of two cases. J
     Neurosurg 34:84–87, 1971.
175. Vuia O. Embryonic carcinosarcoma (mixed tumor) of the pineal gland. Neurochirurgia
     (Stuttg) 23:47–54, 1980.
176. Kalyanaraman U P. Primary glioblastoma of the pineal gland. Arch Neurol 36:717–718,
     1979.
177. Rozario R, Adelman L, Prager R J, Stein B M. Meningiomas of the pineal region and
     third ventricle. Neurosurgery 5:489–495, 1979.
178. Nakayama K, Miyasaka Y, Ohwada T, Yada K. Meningioma in the pineal region.
     Neurol Med Chir (Tokyo) 20:265–271, 1980.
179. Ameli N O, Armin K, Saleh H. Incisural meningiomas of the falco-tentorial junction:
     a report of two cases. J Neurosurg 24:1027–1030, 1966.
180. Sachs E Jr, Avman N, Fisher R G. Meningiomas of pineal region and posterior part
     of 3d ventricle. J Neurosurg 19:325–331, 1962.
181. Araki C, Kyoto M D. Meningioma in the pineal region. Report of 2 cases removed
     by operation. Nippon Geka Hokan 14:1181–1192, 1937.
182. Zeitlin H. Tumors in the region of the pineal body: a clinicopathologic report of three
     cases. Arch Neurol Psychiatry 34:567–586, 1935.
183. Schaefer M, Lapras C, Thomalske G, Grau H, Schober R. Sarcoidosis of the pineal
     gland. J Neurosurg 47:630–632, 1977.
184. De Girolami U, Schmidek H. Clinicopathological study of 53 tumors of the pineal
     region. J Neurosurg 39:455–462, 1973.
185. Smith R A, Estridge M N. Pineal tumors. *In* Handbook of Clinical Neurology, vol
     17, Tumors of the Brain and Skull, part II, ed P J Vinken, B R Bruyn. Elsevier North-
     Holland, Amsterdam, 1974, pp 648–665.
186. Cummins F M, Taveras J M, Schlesinger E B. Treatment of gliomas of the third
     ventricle and pinealomas: with special reference to the value of radiotherapy. Neu-
     rology 10:1031–1036, 1960.
187. Smith R A. Pineal tumors. Univ Mich Med Bull 27:33–43, 1961.
188. Poppen J L, Marino R Jr. Pinealomas and tumors of the posterior portion of the third
     ventricle. J Neurosurg 28:357–364, 1968.
189. Stein B M. The infratentorial supracerebellar approach to pineal lesions. J Neurosurg
     35:197–202, 1971.
190. Jamieson K G. Excision of pineal tumors. J Neurosurg 35:550–553, 1971.
191. Yamamoto I, Kageyama N. Microsurgical anatomy of the pineal region. J Neurosurg
     53:205–221, 1980.

192. Quest D O, Kleriga E. Microsurgical anatomy of the pineal region. Neurosurgery 6:385–390, 1980.

193. Obrador S, Soto M, Gutierrez-Diaz J A. Surgical management of tumours of the pineal region. Acta Neurochir (Wien) 34:159–171, 1976.

194. Brunner C. Cited by Rorschach H. Zur Pathologie und operabilität der Tumoren der Zirbeldrüse. Beitr Klin Chir 83:451–474, 1913.

195. Dandy W E. An operation for the removal of pineal tumors. Surg Gynecol Obstet 33:113–119, 1921.

196. Pecker J, Scarabin J M, Brucher J M, Vallee B. Apport des techniques stéréotaxiques au diagnostic et au traitement des tumeurs de la région pinéale. Rev Neurol (Paris) 134:287–294, 1978.

197. Pecker J, Scarabin J M, Vallee B, Brucher J M. Treatment in tumours of the pineal region: value of stereotaxic biopsy. Surg Neurol 12:341–348, 1979.

198. Smith N J, El-Mahdi A M, Constable W C. Results of irradiation of tumors in the region of the pineal body. Acta Radiol Therapy Phys Biol 15:17–22, 1975.

199. Onoyama Y, Ono K, Nakajima T, Hiraoka M, Abe M. Radiation therapy of pineal tumors. Radiology 130:757–760, 1979.

200. Jenkin R D T, Simpson W J K, Keen C W. Pineal and suprasellar germinomas. Results of radiation treatment. J Neurosurg 48:99–107, 1978.

201. Wara W M, Jenkin R D T, Evans A, Ertel I, Hittle R, Ortega J, Wilson C B, Hammond D. Tumors of the pineal and suprasellar region: childrens cancer study group treatment results 1960–1975. Cancer 43:698–701, 1979.

202. Salazar O M, Castro-Vita H, Bakos R S, Feldstein M L, Keller B, Rubin P. Radiation therapy for tumors of the pineal region. Int J Radiat Oncol Biol Phys 5:491–499, 1979.

203. Mincer F, Meltzer J, Botstein C. Pinealoma. A report of twelve irradiated cases. Cancer 37:2713–2718, 1976.

204. Takaki S, Hikita T, Ishii C, Nakayama K, Aiba H. Serial computed tomographic studies of pineal region tumor treated by irradiation. Kurume Med J 26: 163–173, 1979.

205. Ishii R, Honda H, Tanaka R, Ishikawa N, Ueki S. Abnormality of blood vessels in 2 cases of two cell pattern pinealoma and effects of the radiotherapy. Jap J Clin Radiol 19:219–220, 1974.

206. Ueki K, Tanaka R. Treatments and prognoses of pineal tumors—experience of 110 cases. Neurol Med Chir (Tokyo) 20:1–26, 1980.

207. Neuwelt E A, Glasberg M, Frenkel E, Clark W K. Malignant pineal region tumors. J Neurosurg 51:597–607, 1979.

208. Sano K. Diagnosis and treatment of tumours in the pineal region. Acta Neurochir (Wien) 34:153–157, 1976.

209. Turpin G, Metzger J, Bataini J, de Gennes J L. Ann Endocrinol (Paris) 40:371–384, 1979.

210. Sung D I, Harisiadis L, Chang C H. Midline pineal tumors and suprasellar germinomas: highly curable by irradiation. Radiology 128:745–751, 1978.

211. Wara W M, Fellows C F, Sheline G E, Wilson C B, Townsend J J. Radiation therapy for pineal tumors and suprasellar germinomas. Radiology 124:221–223, 1977.

212. Einhorn L H. Combination chemotherapy of disseminated testicular carcinoma with cis-diammine-dichloroplatinum, vinblastine, and bleomycin (PVB): an update (Abstract). In Proceedings of the American Society of Clinical Oncology, Washington, DC, April, 1978, p 306.

213. Borden S IV, Weber A L, Toch R, Wang C C. Pineal germinoma. Long-term survival despite hematogenous metastases. Am J Dis Child 126:214–216, 1973.

214. de Tribolet N, Barrelet L. Successful chemotherapy of pinealoma. Lancet 2:1228–1229, 1977.

215. Rapoport S I. Sites and function of the blood-brain barrier. *In* Blood Brain Barrier in Physiology and Medicine. Raven Press, New York, 1976, pp 43–86.

216. Sakata K, Yamada H, Sakai N, Hosono Y, Kawasako T, Sasaoka I. Extraneural metastasis of pineal tumor. Surg Neurol 3:49–54, 1975.

217. Cushing H. Pinealomas. *In* Intracranial Tumors: Notes Upon a Series of Two Thousand Verified Cases With Surgical Mortality Pertaining Thereto. Charles C Thomas, Springfield, Ill., 1932, pp 62–65.

218. Grant F C. A study of the results of surgical treatment in 2,326 consecutive patients with brain tumor. J Neurosurg 13:479–488, 1956.

INDEX

Sciatic nerve, 259
Sea lion, pineal size, 6
Seals, pineal size, 6
Seasonal reproduction, 7, 39–40, 158–160
Seizures, following pinealectomy, 230
Seminal vesicles, 163, 227
Seminoma, 285
Serotonin (5-hydroxytryptamine, 5-HT),
    11, 15, 26–30, 45, 51–52, 85–87, 175,
    176, 180, 184, 210, 230, 237, 251,
    273
Serotonin-N-acetyltransferase (NAT), 4,
    82, 102, 114, 182, 217, 228, 254, 258,
    277
Seven-day cycle. *See* Circadian rhythm
Sheep
    hypothalamic peptides in, 230
    innervation, 19
    secretory activity, 26, 142
Sleep, pineal effects on (cats), 253
Sloth, pineal size, 6
Smooth endoplasmic reticulum, 30, 47,
    57, 282
Social isolation, 250
Somatomedin, 263
Somatostatin, 32, 203–205, 230
Spectrophotofluorometric assay, 134–135
Sperm production, 153, 179
Spinal cord, 251
Squirrel monkey, innervation, 15f, 21
Stress, 227–228, 291
    melatonin effect on (rats), 250
Subarachnoid hemorrhage, 283
Subcommissural organ, 20, 203
Subsurface cistern, 47
Superior cervical ganglia, 183, 185
Superior cervical ganglionectomy, 11, 37,
    56, 79, 85, 185
Superior salivary nucleus, 16
Supportive cell. *See* Glial cell
Suprachiasmatic nucleus (SCN), 96–97,
    98, 116, 142
Suprapineal recess, 5
Sympathetic innervation, 36–37, 89,
    96–97, 115, 130
Sympathetic nerve fibers, 11–15, 26, 37
Synaptic ribbons. *See* Vesicle-crowned
    rodlet

T
Tadpole culturing program, 133
Tanycytes, 236
Taurine, 213, 275
Tau (τ) (the period of the free-running
    endogenous circadian pacemaker),
    98–101, 104, 106

Tay-Sachs disease, 252, 253
Telencephalon, 230
Temperate zone, effects on pineal gland,
    6, 10, 40–41
Temperature information, integrated by
    pineal gland, 6, 62
Teratoblastoma, 289
Teratocarcinoma, 289
Teratoma, 282–284, 289
Testes, 154, 157–158, 162–163, 166, 231,
    260
Testosterone, 156, 182–183, 215, 250, 260,
    286, 287
Thelarche, 287
Thermoregulation, 260–2
Third ventricle, 2, 35, 61–62, 142, 231,
    251–252, 288
Threonylseryllysine (TSL), 211–213
Thymus, 257, 259, 262
Thyroid, 236–238
Thyrotropin (TSH), 237–238
Thyrotropin releasing hormone (TRH),
    168, 204–205, 217, 230, 238,
    281
Thyroxine (T₄), 236–238
Triiodothyronine (T₃), 238
Tritiated melatonin, 135
Tropical zone
    effects on pineal gland, 7–8, 10, 40,
    58
    mammals in, 6
Tryptamine, 259
Tryptophan, 26, 28, 31, 51, 52–3, 85, 238,
    251
Tryptophan-5-hydroxylase, 27–28, 51–52,
    79, 251
Tumor growth, 262–265
Turtle, vesicle-crowned rodlets in, 57
Tyrosine, 79, 229
Tyrosine hydroxylase, 79

U
Ubiquinone, 226
Unilateral ovariectomy, 212
Uterus, 163
Uveitis, allergic, 254

V
Vacuolar system, 49–51, 59–60
Vacuoles containing flocculent material,
    25, 35, 41, 42, 45, 47, 48
Vasoactive intestinal polypeptide (VIP),
    21–22, 235